Advanced Yoga Practices

—

Easy Lessons for Ecstatic Living

The Original Internet Lessons with Additions by the Author

Yogani

Cover image of radiating *OM* symbol drawn by the author.

AYP Publishing

For ordering information go to:

www.advancedyogapractices.com
or
www.geocities.com/advancedyogapractices

Library of Congress Control Number: 2004195185

Published simultaneously in:

Nashville, Tennessee, U.S.A.
and
London, England, U.K.

This title is also available as an eBook – ISBN: 0-9764655-2-3 (for Adobe Reader)

ISBN: 0-9764655-0-7 (Paperback)

If you are interested in other writings by the author, or would like to submit questions or comments on any of the lessons in this book, please visit the Advanced Yoga Practices (AYP) Internet sites at:

AYP Web Site:
www.advancedyogapractices.com

Alternate AYP Web Site:
www.geocities.com/advancedyogapractices

Main Lessons Forum:
http://groups.yahoo.com/group/advancedyogapractices

Tantra Lessons Forum:
http://groups.yahoo.com/group/advancedyogapractices_tantra

This is dedicated to you who seek the truth within…

Introduction

The theory of yoga is simple. It states that there is an outer reality and an inner one, and that the human nervous system is the doorway between them. To engage in the practices of yoga is to promote the opening of that doorway. The fascinating thing about this is that when we do yoga practices such as meditation, breathing techniques (pranayama) and bodily maneuvers (asanas, mudras and bandhas) in a coordinated way on a regular basis, something happens. We can observe changes inside us. As these inner changes occur, our experience of everyday living is changed in positive ways. So yoga is about much more than theory. It is about practice. It is about cause and effect. Over time, the quality of our life can be dramatically transformed by doing yoga practices. We become filled with lasting inner peace and happiness. We come to know that the possibility of achieving "enlightenment" is real – the ultimate destination of every human being. That is what happens as the doorway of our nervous system gradually opens and there is less and less division between our outer and inner realities. In the end, they merge to become one glorious reality of unending joy, and then we know that we are home. This is the journey recorded by saints and sages in every culture throughout history. It is the journey we can all take by choosing to engage in daily yoga practices.

What is the essence of effective yoga practice? Are there ways to optimize our practices to maximize our progress? This is the perennial question. It is a question that calls for a scientific investigative approach. As we survey the landscape, we find that the field of yoga often appears complex, confusing and mysterious. In every direction we turn, something seems to be missing. The purpose of this book is to try and clear some of that up, fill in the gaps, simplify things, and help make the application of yoga practices a more practical and self-directed endeavor than it has been in the past. As part of this, we will be exploring beyond the limits of what has been publicly available about yoga practices. We will look at the so-called "esoteric" practices, along with those that are well known, and combine them into an optimized routine that anyone can follow every day. We will be integrating together the best methods from the ancient traditions of mantra yoga, kriya yoga, hatha yoga, kundalini yoga, tantra yoga, bhakti yoga and others. If these terms are not familiar to you, don't be concerned. It is the nuts and bolts of practice that really matter, and that is what you will find in this book – in plain English. We will not be dwelling on the many yoga traditions and philosophies – only touching on them enough to clarify what is going on during and after our daily practices. The yoga methods in this book act directly through heart, mind, body, breath and sexuality. So you can be sure we will be dealing with your personal experiences in yoga, rather than abstract philosophical concepts.

These lessons can be used as a stand-alone teaching, or to supplement any other path. This is a non-sectarian resource that is open to everyone, and makes a claim on no one. If you are looking for a hands-on instruction manual covering all levels of yoga practice, from the beginning to the most advanced, you have come to the right place. Because so many powerful methods of practice are discussed in these lessons, everyone is strongly encouraged to go at their own safe pace. Much attention in the lessons is devoted to developing skills in "self-pacing," with the aim of assisting every practitioner to become self-sufficient in applying yoga practices for achieving maximum progress while maintaining good safety. Each is responsible for their own progress, and for the means applied.

Most of what is in these lessons was first written on the Internet. The author, an American, is a long time spiritual scientist who, over a lifetime, has developed an integrated system of yoga practices which has proven to be highly effective and easily incorporated into the modern lifestyle. It is a flexible, scientific approach, rather than a rigid, arbitrary one. Wanting to leave something useful behind, he started posting lessons in an open online forum in 2003. Before long, thousands of yoga enthusiasts from all over the world joined the forum, with hundreds submitting comments and questions via email. Numerous correspondences resulted between the author and readers, and many of the questions and answers (Q&As) were posted in the forum, becoming an integral part of the lessons. Because the questions in the Q&As come from yoga practitioners in many countries around the globe, you will see variations in writing style. The original writing is edited only minimally to preserve the energy and spirit of the interactions. Because the lessons originated in an online forum/group, they contain terms such as "members," "group," and so on. You will also notice that the numbering of the lessons is a little unusual. That is explained on a separate page.

This book is a preservation of the original online lessons of Advanced Yoga Practices, with significant additions by the author. The additions can be found at the end of many of the lessons, and are indicated by asterisks (*) in the table of contents and lesson titles. A summary of the additions is provided after the table of contents.

The online Internet lessons include an extensive "links section" with over 100 yoga-related web sites. Because this is a dynamic list, subject to ongoing revision, it has not been included in this book. Instead, the links section can easily be accessed by going to the Advanced Yoga Practices web site provided at beginning of the book. The "AYP links section" is referred to in several lessons to provide supplementary information, as necessary.

We owe our everlasting gratitude to all of the great spiritual masters and teachers who have researched, exemplified and generously shared the knowledge of spiritual practices with humanity for thousands of years. It is on their shoulders that we stand today as we reach for the heights of ecstatic bliss and outpouring divine love – our destiny as human beings. We also owe our heartfelt thanks to the many yoga practitioners around the world who have stepped forward and contributed to the development of these lessons through their sincere sharing of experiences and questions. Because of them, these lessons are far more comprehensive than would have been possible otherwise. Finally, without the wonder of instant worldwide communications through the Internet, this in-depth exploration of the methods of human spiritual transformation could not have happened. A much deserved thank you goes to all those who provide the technology that has enabled this book to become a reality.

It is hoped you will find the Advanced Yoga Practices lessons to be a useful resource as you travel along your chosen spiritual path. Practice wisely, and enjoy!

The guru is in you.

Table of Contents

Note: An asterisk (*) indicates that a lesson includes additional material at the end, beyond what is in the original online lessons. A summary of the additions follows the Table of Contents.

The Tantra Lessons

Additional Resources

Summary of Additions and Illustrations

The following list provides a summary of the additions that have been included at the end of the designated lessons. These are also indicated by asterisks (*) in the table of contents and in the lesson titles. **If you are already familiar with the AYP online lessons, this page identifies what has been added in the book.**

Lesson 13 – Clarifications on mantra, language and meaning.
Lesson 29 – Discussion on alcoholism, addiction and yoga.
Lesson 41 – Discussion on nadi shodana (alternate nostril breathing) and spinal breathing.
Lesson 44 – Additional discussion on visualization of spinal nerve during spinal breathing.
Lesson 47 – Descriptions for the seven major chakras.
Lesson 71 – An "Asana Starter Kit," including instructions and illustrations for postures.
Lesson 80 – Instructions for a routine of aerobic and muscle toning exercises in support of yoga.
Lesson 91 – Discussion on risks of external kumbhaka (retaining the breath outside).
Lesson 108 – Introduction to kechari stage 5, and illustrations of kechari stages 1-5.
Lesson 114 – Additional discussion on kechari stages 1 and 2.
Lesson 135 – Discussion on hand mudra (jnana or chin mudra).
Lesson 140 – Discussion on chin pump and automatic movements.
Lesson 173 – Discussion on spinal bastrika and the sequencing of pranayamas.
Lesson 182 – Explaining spinal breathing and meditation to a skeptic.
Lesson 188 – The third enhancement to the mantra.
Lesson 200 – Additional follow-up with a sensitive meditator.
Lesson 204 – Summary of sequence and times for a complete yoga routine.
Lesson 229 – Instructions for brahmari ("bee sound") pranayama with spinal breathing.
Lesson 230 – On allowing crown experiences to evolve safely and naturally with practices.
Lesson T13 – On higher frequency of urination during kundalini awakening.
Lesson T25 – Existing lesson on Sri Vidya is expanded, and a Sri Yantra diagram is included.
Lesson T28 – Additional discussion on advanced siddhasana.
Lesson T30 – Additional discussion on vajroli mudra.
Lesson T32 – Instructions for amaroli practice.
Lesson T34 – Discussion on the kechari "secret spot" from female and male points of view.

The following lessons have clarifying notes added at the end – 12, 30, 33, 39, 55, 56, 85, 132, 160, 166 and 235.

A Glossary of Sanskrit Terms is included in the Additional Resources at the back of the book.

Illustrations:

Lesson 33 – Cross-legged Sitting with Back Support
Lesson 71 – Asanas (postures) for the "Asana Starter Kit"
Lesson 108 – Kechari Mudra Stages 1-5
Lesson T25 – Sri Yantra

About Those Unused Lesson Numbers

You will notice in the table of contents, and throughout this book, that certain lesson numbers are unused. There are two reasons for this. A mysterious numerology is not one of them.

First, in the original online forum, the format was not designed for editing of already posted messages. A posting needing correction could be deleted and then re-posted after editing, leaving an unused number in the overall series. Because some editing did occur using this method, especially in the early lessons, there are some unused numbers in the lesson sequence, and they are marked "not used" in the table of contents.

The second reason for unused lesson numbers occurs only in this book. These were online postings pertaining to administrative matters relating only to the Internet lessons, and having no bearing on the actual content of the Advanced Yoga Practices lessons. They have been left out of this book, and those numbers are marked "omitted" in the table of contents.

The question arises, "Why didn't you just renumber the lessons from scratch in this book, starting with the number "1," and go straight through without skipping any numbers? The reason this has not been done is because it is important to maintain consistency in numbering between the several versions of the lessons. So, lesson #13 on meditation will be lesson #13 no matter which source of the lessons you are looking at. This is true of the actual content in the lessons also. The content is nearly the same in all venues, except that this book includes "fine-tuning" of the original lessons, plus substantial new instructional material added to many of the lessons (see list on previous page), going well beyond what is available in the online lessons.

The numbering of the lessons is the same in this book as it is on the Advanced Yoga Practices web site, in the online forums, and also in the several translations of the lessons to other languages that are underway. So, while the lesson numbering looks a bit unusual, it is practical. The lesson numbers will always be the same, no matter where you happen to be reading them.

When all of the unused and omitted lesson numbers are subtracted from the total, there are 242 lessons in all in this volume.

If you go to the AYP web site or online forums, you will find that the lessons are continuing there. This book goes to #235 in the main lessons, and to #35 in the tantra lessons. So anything you see beyond that on the Internet is new material. Feel free to partake, both here and there!

The guru is in you.

Disclaimer

"Each is responsible for his or her own spiritual progress, and for the methods applied. What you do with the information in these lessons is your call."

This is what is posted in the introduction to the online Advanced Yoga Practices lessons. It applies to this book also. There is no one who can be responsible for the conduct of your yoga practices but you. All efforts have been made to render an accurate presentation and effective integration of the ancient methods of yoga. Additionally, safety measures (the methods of "self-pacing") are discussed throughout the lessons for the purpose of facilitating good progress while maintaining stability. However, none of the methods in this book are guaranteed. You engage in these practices at your own risk.

The remarkable capabilities for higher functioning inherent in every human being are the touchstone for all the lessons in this book. The lessons are therefore experience-based. The practices discussed herein are intended to be applied in a flexible manner according to observed causes and effects, and managed responsibly by each individual practitioner.

These lessons do not represent the teachings of any other organization, school, or person, and should not be construed as such. They are the author's best effort to integrate yogic knowledge from a variety of ancient traditions in a scientific manner. To that end, certain traditions and teachers of yoga are sometimes mentioned in the lessons to add perspective. While it is common for modern teachings to claim a connection to one tradition or another, these lessons claim no such connection. The lessons are an integrated approach to yoga, and must stand on their own merit. It is you, the reader, who will decide their value by how they resonate in both theory and practice.

The Main Lessons

Lesson 10 – Why This Discussion?
(This is the first lesson)

Everyone knows they are special, that there is something more than this birth, life and death. It resonates somewhere deep inside all of us. We spend our lifetime trying to reach beyond what we are to be more in one way or another. Sometimes we make a mess of it. Sometimes we make progress. But too often we drift along hoping someone will open a door for us. If only they would, we'd run right through. Or would we?

This is the first crucial step, wanting to run through to that something more in us. Being willing to do it. Craving it. Being desperate for it. I am here because I have been one of those for many years, and I know there must be others. I want to throw out some methods, some methods that work. Tools, you know. They are for your consideration. The rest is up to you.

We will talk about philosophy, but not too much. Mostly we will talk about yoga practices, how they work, what they do, and how to do them. And how they can blend together and leverage each other like magic. That is why you will be hearing the phrase "integrated practice" a lot here. It is not a new idea. The *Yoga Sutras* of Patanjali lay out an eight-limbed path of practice. Most traditions lean toward one limb or another. It is natural enough. How many balls can anyone keep in the air? But if you want to really make progress in this life, you must multi-channel your efforts in the direction you want to go. It is like that in all things. Spiritual practice is no different.

We will be talking about many inward ways here – the ways into the divine you. How to really open things up. Are you ready for that? Do you long for it? Not everyone does. But everyone will sooner or later. In fact, a little practice fans the fire of divine longing. Just a little bit of practice opens the door enough so the divine desire wells up. Then we are on fire and want more practice and more powerful ways in. It is a kind of addiction – a divine addiction. I confess to being an addict for this spiritual practice game. It is an ecstatic spiral that pulls us out of our limited earth perception. Everything will look different, first just a little, and, later on, a lot different. So if you do not want to become divinely inspired or divinely addicted, better stay away – because the best means are here. If you set your heart and mind to it, you can do it. Honest. And then nothing will ever be the same. You will laugh and laugh when you see how it really is.

This discussion is for wise souls, those who are ready to do what it takes for as long as it takes. Were the sages of old less committed than this? Of course not. We marvel at their remarkable stories in the scriptures. It is just the same now. You will get out of your practices what you put in. It has always been like that.

Why bother with all this? To be honest, it is the greatest high we can have. The pleasure is beyond anything on earth. Really. The essence of divine experience is unending devastating bliss and an unshakable silent peace. It seems contradictory, doesn't it? That's how it is. But don't take my word for it. Try some of these methods and see for yourself. It's all waiting in you. Take a few baby steps, and soon you can be opening by leaps and bounds. That is assuming you are ready, and choose each day to go for more. Remember, it is the one thing we can take with us when we move on from this life.

Some of the practices we will be discussing include:

■ Cultivating permanent inner silence through deep meditation.

- Opening the subtle nerves through pranayama (breath control).

- Stimulating divine energy through advanced physical postures and maneuvers.

- Cultivating divine desire and conduct.

- Cultivating sexual energy to a new purpose.

- Cultivating silent inner awareness outward in powerful ways.

Some of these practices will seem familiar. Others will seem radical. Combined together in particular ways, they comprise a powerful system of yoga. These means are too useful to be reserved for the few. They belong to the many. So indulge yourself. If you long for the knowledge of human spiritual transformation, you are worthy, and you have come to the right place.

The guru is in you.

Lesson 11 – What is Yoga? What is Religion?

Yoga. Religion. These two words conjure up so many images, don't they? Not all of them clear. Not all of them good. Let's not get into the foibles of humanity right now. Let's stick to the basics. For spiritual practice is best seen in terms of the basics, and often is clouded by the cultural coloring of these two simple words.

Yoga means, "to join." Religion means, "to bind back together." Hmmm ... similar meanings. But to join or bind back together what? Ah ... this is the essence of it. We are, or seem to be, two things that are to be put back together. On the one hand we are in the world of space and time, a world we perceive through our senses. On the other hand we are observers of the world, something behind it all, within it all. We are conscious. Aware. We are both subject (observer) and object (observed). And these two things are separate. But must they be? Are they really? Yoga and religion say, "No." So the putting together process starts there. No matter what else you may have heard, that is what yoga and religion are really about.

But why the separation in the first place? If the two are really one, why are there two? Think about yourself for a minute. Who are you? Most of us point to our body and say, "This is me." We all sense something more, but the best we can do is observe our body and say, "This is me. This is my body. My name is Joe Schmo. I can think and feel, and that is part of me too."

If you were to say to someone, "I am something behind all this that you see, and behind all this that I think and feel. I am consciousness," might it seem a bit strange? Why strange? Because we are identified with our perceptions of our body/minds and this world. It is a habit, a deep biologically and neurologically ingrained habit. Not only that. Because we habitually imprint our sense of self on our body/mind, we see our physical surroundings as separate from ourselves. So the world becomes a stranger to itself. Through our process of identified perception the one has become many.

Yoga and religion are about clearing up the identification of awareness that has led to the one becoming many. Not that the world will go away. It is only to be seen for what it really is, a flow of the one, the real you. Then it becomes a much friendlier place. That's the whole point, to find happiness in our lives in the world. Even as the whole thing keeps lurching forward through the shadows of apparent separateness, we don't have to go on seeing it that way. This is the promise of yoga and religion. This is the promise of spiritual practices. It's a good promise. It is up to us to fulfill the promise of yoga and religion, using the best means we can find.

The joining is not just about an intellectual understanding of the situation, though that can't hurt. It is about changing our deepest functioning, biologically and neurologically. Then does our experience change. From that, our thoughts, feelings and actions change, becoming full of love and purpose. We could all use more of that. The identification gradually dissolves, and something stupendous comes up from within us. Yoga is not just an intellectual process. It is physical, as anyone who has taken a yoga class knows. Yoga practices operate on many levels – physical, mental, emotional, neurological – and in galaxies of inner ecstatic energy!

The process of joining begins with making direct contact with our inner self, our consciousness. Once we have established a foothold in consciousness, we can proceed from there with many other things. Becoming aware of our deepest consciousness on a regular basis is peaceful and pleasant and can bring immediate relief to a hectic, busy life. It is accomplished with meditation. A very particular kind of meditation called deep meditation. This is the first advanced yoga practice we will learn on our road to union, on the way to binding ourselves back together. It is a good first step that brings a big return for a small daily effort.

"Daily effort?" you say. This is what we will talk about next. For without a commitment to a daily effort, you will be wasting your time here, and anywhere else.

The guru is in you.

Lesson 12 – The Essential Ingredient – Desire

It is common knowledge that if we want to be successful at something, at anything, we must desire it continuously, and be willing to act to fulfill that desire every day. Think of the most successful people you know. Isn't this what they have in common? If we look at their lives, we see that they have worked long and hard to achieve excellence in their chosen field. Behind that, an insatiable desire to succeed in their efforts kept them driving forward, overcoming obstacles, working for years toward their objective. It is like that in yoga, which is working toward divine union.

Jesus said, "Blessed are those who hunger and thirst after righteousness, for they shall be filled." He also said, "Seek and you will find. Knock and the door will open to you."

This is the magic formula – desire toward a goal, which spawns action toward that goal. Continuous desire is the fuel. Daily action is the fire. The word "continuous" is important, as is the word "goal." Without these two operative functions, desires are scattered, actions are unfocused, and not much happens. With them, anything is achievable.

If we cultivate our desire to become continuously focused on a particular goal, such as the achievement of divine union, we are cultivating a special kind of desire. It is called "devotion." Devotion is the continuous flow of desire toward an object or goal. We are all familiar with the concept of devotion. It is how we explain the success of great achievers: "Oh, she is so devoted to her work." Or of great mystics: "Oh, she is so devoted to God." It is no coincidence that devotion and greatness are found in the same place. The first invariably leads to the second. The second cannot happen without the first.

Whatever your concept of enlightenment may be, whatever tradition or creed you hail from, whatever inspires you in the direction of spiritual unfoldment, cultivate that. It is the engine of practice. It is what enables us to sustain daily spiritual practice for as long as it takes. As we practice, our divine experience grows, and, with that, devotion grows. Increased devotion intensifies our commitment to practice, and more dedicated practice yields more divine experience which in turn increases devotion further. This is how it progresses – devotion yielding practice ... yielding divine experience ... yielding more devotion ... and so on. Devotion sustained at a fever pitch by every means possible is the spiritual aspirant's best friend. It is not always an easy life being constantly consumed by spiritual "hunger and thirst," but it puts us on the royal road to enlightenment. Intense devotion to transforming our lives through yoga practices assures that what must be done will be done.

Speaking of what must be done, now let's talk about the next step – developing the habit of cultivating our eternal silent depths on a daily basis. Let's talk about meditation.

The guru is in you.

Note: This lesson points out the importance of desire in the overall process of yoga. In later lessons the role of desire is discussed further as "bhakti," which means, "love of Truth" or "love of God." This is much more than an emotional indulgence. Bhakti is one of the most powerful of all spiritual practices. Emotional energy has a huge influence on the process of human spiritual transformation, and on the course of all our endeavors in yoga. So, the principles and practical methods of bhakti are returned to again and again in the lessons.

Lesson 13* – Meditation – Awakening the Silent Seed

Your mind has a natural ability to be quiet. When it becomes quiet, you are in touch with your genius. Albert Einstein said the ideas that led him to the theory of relativity came during moments of quiet reflection. Mozart heard sonatas and symphonies resonating through the silent reaches of his mind. All he had to do was write them down. We know that Isaac Newton came up with laws of motion and gravity while relaxing under an apple tree. Whether he actually got hit in the head by that apple or not, no one knows, but there is no doubt that his quiet mind yielded a treasure of knowledge. We could cite more examples, but you get the point. Silent mind has great creativity. But this is not all. Silent mind is peaceful, blissful and healthy, and radiates these qualities out through the person to the surroundings. People who know how to cultivate quiet mind not only are in touch with their inner creativity; they also radiate a youthfulness and optimism that effects everyone nearby. They have "good vibrations."

Earlier we spoke of consciousness (awareness – the observer), and the objective world (the observed). The essential nature of our consciousness is blissful silence. It is what is behind the mind, what is experienced when the mind becomes still. It is an infinite storehouse of the qualities just mentioned – the realm of what we know as God, always right here within us. This is why it is proclaimed in the *Psalms*, "Be still and know I am God." To access the divine all we have to do is know how to be still.

Meditation is the process of systematically allowing the mind to become still for specific periods of time each day. In doing this daily over weeks, months and years, quietness, consciousness, gradually becomes more evident when the mind is active while we are not meditating, and worldly life is enriched. Through meditation, the relationship between consciousness and the world gradually changes. This is a process of yoga, the joining. It is the first step. Once blissful silence is coming on in daily experience, many other things can be done to enhance and expand it. But first we have to establish a base in consciousness, awaken the silent inner seed of who we are, so to speak.

It was mentioned that your mind has a natural ability to become quiet. In the deep meditation method we will practice here, we will harness that natural ability. In fact, all of the practices which will be taught here (and there are quite a few), we will be harnessing your natural abilities. The idea is to show you how to utilize the gifts you have already. We will just be adding special levers here and there to activate your natural abilities. The rest will be up to you. If you apply what you learn, and keep at it, one day you will know that you are a perpetual bliss machine, capable of experience far beyond the imaginings of the mind. Oh yes, you really are. Meditation is the first step.

Thoughts are coming up in the mind from the minute we wake up in the morning until the minute we fall asleep at night, and then more are coming during dreaming. Yet we say the mind has a natural ability to be quiet. How?

We will use a thought to do it. Not just any thought. A special thought called a "mantra." We will use a particular method of thinking this mantra that allows the mind to do what it can easily do if given the opportunity, settle down.

Actually, any thought can be used to meditate, as been amply demonstrated by researchers over the past thirty years. But we'd like to use a particular thought, one that has certain vibratory qualities, one that produces a certain effect in the nervous system. It is also one we can enhance as our practice advances, but more about that later. The mantra we will begin with here is:

... I AM ...

We will not be focusing on the meaning of *I AM* during meditation. No doubt it has sacred meaning in the Judeo/Christian tradition in particular, and also bears similarity to the sacred sounds of other traditions. It is the sound we are interested in, not the meaning. It is the sound we will be using, within. We are after the profound vibratory quality of the sound when it is used effectively deep inside the mind and nervous system. Perhaps these profound effects inside the human being are the reason why *I AM* has been revered for centuries. What we will be doing is focusing on the correct utilization of the mantra in the practice of meditation. Then we will have the best results.

Here is how we will use it:

Find a quiet, comfortable place where you can sit, preferably with back support. We want to remove unnecessary distractions. Just sit and relax somewhere where you can close your eyes for twenty minutes without interruptions.

Once you have gotten comfortable, slowly close your eyes. You will notice thoughts, streams of thoughts. That is fine. Just observe them without minding them. After about a minute, gently introduce the thought ... *I AM* ... and begin to repeat it easily and effortlessly in your mind. If your mind wanders off into other thoughts, you will eventually realize this has happened. Don't be concerned about it. It is natural. When you realize you are not repeating the mantra, gently go back to it. This is all you have to do. Easily repeat the mantra silently inside. When you realize you are not thinking it, then easily come back to it. The goal is not to stay on it. The goal is to follow the simple procedure of thinking the mantra, losing it, and coming back to it when you find you have lost it. Do not resist if the mantra tends to become less distinct. Thinking the mantra does not have to be with clear pronunciation. *I AM* can be experienced at many levels in your mind and nervous system. When you come back to it, come back to a level that is comfortable, not straining for either a clear or fuzzy pronunciation.

Do this procedure for twenty minutes, and then, with your eyes closed, take a few minutes to rest before you get up.

This practice is to be done twice each day, before you start your day and before you begin your evening activities. It is best done before meals, as digestion can interfere with the process of meditation. Make a commitment to yourself to do it for a few months. Give it some time to work. You will be amazed at the results, and then you will want to keep going forward to more and more.

That's enough for now.

In the following lessons, we will go into more detail about the process and consequences of meditation. After that we will begin to work with another natural ability we each have, our ability to use the breath to move silence in us with endless ecstasy.

The guru is in you.

Addition – Following the online publication of this lesson, inquires were received from time to time about the English meaning of the *I AM* mantra in relation to the process of meditation, and whether those with other languages should translate the meaning of "I AM" to their own language and use that as the mantra. As it says in the lesson, meditation is not on the meaning of *I AM*. It is on the sound. The effectiveness of the sound in the depths of the mind is related to the characteristics of the human nervous system, not to any particular meaning (or lack of meaning) that may be assigned to the sound in language. For example, the sound of *I AM* is equally well represented using the spelling *AYAM*, which has the same pronunciation, but no known meaning in English. It may have a meaning in some other language, but it does not matter, because we are not concerned with meaning in using the mantra in the easy process of meditation. If per-chance the spelling of *I AM* distracts you in some way, then assign another spelling that enables you to use the sound for meditation unencumbered by meaning. Or forget spelling altogether! This matter is further discussed in lessons #115, #117 and #188. You don't have to go and read those lessons now. Better to continue step by step through the lessons from here. Just be aware that it is the sound of the mantra we are using inside during meditation, not the meaning, just like it says in this lesson.

Lesson 14 – Not Much Happening in Meditation

Q: Thank you for the meditation instructions. It doesn't seem to be working for me though. I repeat the mantra and nothing much happens. I just wander off into everyday thoughts and come back to the mantra when I remember to, like you said, over and over again for the twenty minutes. It is pretty boring. Am I just not suited for this?

A: Our nervous systems are wired for the experience of blissful silence. Indeed, we are created for this. No human being is an exception. However, every nervous system contains obstructions which are to be released and flushed out – lifetimes of accumulated impurities that block our natural state from manifesting in the world, blocking us from inward seeing. The practices of yoga are concerned with the removal of these obstructions. Yoga is a cleaning process. It is the cleaning that brings union between our inner and outer nature. During meditation, we know the process is working when we lose the mantra and later find ourselves in some other thoughts. During the meditation procedure, these other thoughts are a symptom that something has been released. Recognizing that, we go back to the mantra and continue the process. It is important to be easy with the mantra, not hanging on to a clear mental pronunciation, not hanging on to an unclear mental pronunciation, no hanging on at all, just easily being with it. If we develop this habit if easiness, the mind will settle into its silence naturally. It is a natural process of our mind we are facilitating.

Until now, all of our conscious thoughts have been for going outward into manifestation in the mind, and into the world. The mantra, *I AM*, is for going inward into de-manifestation, taking us to the source of our thoughts, the source of us, pure consciousness, unbounded awareness. But it isn't always experienced in such glorious terms. Often it is just losing the mantra, having some pleasant unaccounted for time of no mantra and no thoughts, then becoming aware of thoughts again, and then going back to the mantra. The cleansing process goes on. This is perfect meditation. This is the habit we want to cultivate in meditation every day, for it will lead us to the infinite. The experiences will be there as the cleansing process continues. But the experiences, or lack of them, are not the measure of the correctness of the meditation procedure. The procedure is very specific, and we may or may not feel inner expansion on any given day. You see?

In a way, it is like digging for treasure. Good digging is moving earth in a very particular way that efficiently takes us down to where the box full of gold sits waiting for us. The digging itself may not seem to resemble a box full of gold. Nevertheless, it is the digging that leads to the gold. The good news with meditation is that we will glimpse the gold often during the digging process, and also while we are not digging during our regular daily activities. Our experience of the gold accumulates gradually over time as we practice meditation daily. Then, one day, we realize that we are the gold. We kept at it for a long time and everything has changed. From day one we begin to see the world differently, for through the inner cleansing process we are becoming that which underlies the world. From the very beginning we have been that. With yoga we clean the window of our nervous system and develop a clear perception that this is the truth. This is who we are. The mystery of life is being uncovered. We are that which underlies everything. We are eternal bliss!

So stick with it. Continuously fan the fire of your desire to know the truth within you. This will keep you going. Along the way, you will get positive feedback from within yourself. Keep following the procedure of meditation twice-daily for twenty minutes. As your experiences go deeper you will not want to stop facilitating this natural ability you have to go within, because it is your own self you are uncovering. You will be self-propelled.

In time, we will add advanced yoga practices that will greatly increase the power of meditation. If a sturdy garden hose is not getting all the dirt, we have the option to hook the hose up to a pressure washer.

The guru is in you.

Lesson 15 – Restlessness in Meditation

Q: Since beginning, I felt some nice peacefulness and calmness for a few days. Then I started getting restless during meditation and irritable during the day. What's going on?

A: While cleansing the nervous system with meditation seems a simple enough process, it is quite delicate. The procedure we use is simple – easily thinking the mantra, letting it refine naturally, losing the mantra, later realizing we are off it, then easily going back to it without attempting to hold it clearly or unclearly ... and so on for twenty minutes twice each day. But do not be deceived by the simplicity. Do not take it lightly. This is an advanced and powerful practice. We are facilitating lifetimes of obstructions to be released naturally from deep within us. These are stresses and strains embedded in our nervous system that restrict our vision of the truth in and around us. Some restrictions we were born with. Others we have added in this life. It all is being released bit by bit during meditation. It is a huge undertaking, with profound results.

If the purification process is a little out of balance, some discomfort can happen – Restlessness. Irritability. Unpleasant physical sensations. Fidgeting. Unpleasant thoughts. Things like that. Fortunately, there are ways to balance the process of meditation if there is some discomfort. The first thing to do is take plenty of time coming out of meditation. Remember that during meditation a process of inner cleansing is going on. You might not feel like much is happening, but if you jump up from meditation without resting first, you could feel irritable for some time afterwards – maybe even all day. Don't take it out on your loved ones, friends and coworkers. See it for what it is – an imbalance in your practice. Always take at least a few minutes of doing nothing with eyes closed (relaxing, not thinking the mantra) at the end of meditation. This allows stresses and strains being released from the nervous system during meditation to dissipate harmlessly. Then, when you get up, you will feel light and refreshed. If you don't, you are probably not resting long enough. So rest at the end as long as necessary to enable a smooth transition from meditation to activity. You may even wish to lie down for a while at the end of meditation. Everyone is different. Find what is the best for you coming out of meditation.

Some people respond very quickly to meditation. A little bit may go a long way. This is a good thing. If you are one of these, you are blessed, but you must be careful to balance your routine so you won't be uncomfortable due to a high rate of inner cleansing going on. If lying down and resting for a while after twenty minutes of meditation does not settle things down, then it may be necessary to shorten the time of meditation to fifteen minutes. If it is still uncomfortable, try ten minutes. Find your balance. And always take your time coming out.

Sometimes physical discomfort can happen during meditation. This is usually a symptom of the release of obstructions in the nervous system. If it interferes with the easy process of meditation, then pause with the mantra and allow the attention to be drawn to the physical discomfort. Just be with it for a while. Usually, this will dissolve the discomfort naturally. Once it does, go back to the mantra and continue your meditation until your time is up. Count the time you spent with your attention on the physical discomfort as part of your meditation time. If the sensation does not dissolve, lie down for while, until the sensation subsides. It is a good thing. A big obstruction is going. Let it go easily, naturally. The same procedure applies if you are overcome with a barrage of overbearing thoughts, which may or may not be accompanied by physical sensations. If you can't easily go back to the mantra, just be with the thoughts until they dissipate enough so you can easily pick up the mantra again. Remember, meditation is not a fight with physical or mental activity we may have. These are all symptoms of the release of obstructions from deep in the nervous system. We just let them go. Our job is to follow the easy procedure of thinking the mantra and allowing the process of inner cleansing to happen. This is not a war on the level of the conscious mind. You can never win it that way. We are working from the inside, within and beyond the subconscious mind. In order to do this we must allow the natural ability of the mind to take us in. So learn to think the mantra easily, and let it go in.

Meditation is the most effective means of operating deep inside the subconscious mind and cleaning it out. With meditation we easily go beyond the subconscious mind to our underlying consciousness, the source of all that is true and evolutionary. It is our consciousness that removes the inner obstructions, if we give it the opportunity through meditation. Over time, as the obstructions are removed, we find more and more peaceful silence in our daily lives. This is the dawning of enlightenment, our natural state. So keep cleaning the window of your nervous system every day.

The guru is in you.

Lesson 16 – Bliss in Meditation

Q: I have been filled with bliss since beginning meditation. I sit and think *I AM* a few times and I am gone into a tingly silence inside. I disappeared for ten minutes yesterday before I realized it. I thought *I AM*, and was gone in bliss again. I have such feelings of gratitude. My background is devout Catholic and it has been difficult for me to relate to the Eastern traditions, though I have sensed there is much value there. This seems a wonderful approach – a bridge. I feel closer to Christ. Is it for real?

A: As our experience grows, stabilizes on a higher plane, and then keeps growing with practice, never ceasing to expand, then we have the answer to the question: Is it for real? The answer is in you. This is the truth of spiritual life – as we practice and open from within, the experience becomes self-validating. There is nowhere else you have to go to find it, to prove it to yourself. Once we know, our life becomes a joyous never-ending journey of self-discovery. Under these conditions, human life gradually morphs into a kaleidoscope of bliss.

Jesus said, "Seek first the kingdom of God within, and all will be added to you."

Bliss is our birthright, our true nature. It is time for us to step forward and claim it by awakening the natural abilities we were born with.

It is a long journey for most of us. It took a long time for us to become blocked so completely from our true nature. It stands to reason that it will take a while for us to open back up, even with the best of tools. At times we will experience a clear view of the bliss bubbling up in us. Other times we will feel blocked, or like we are getting reamed from the inside as we continue our daily meditations. The process will unfold in many ways. In time, bliss will predominate, and we will see the world as we have not before. Bliss will be seen bubbling up everywhere, constantly. A dirty pipe can't stay dirty forever if we are flushing it through with the pure water of consciousness every day.

So, while the bliss you feel is a treasure, and certainly for real, keep in mind that there will be cycles of experience as your meditation proceeds. Sometimes you will feel like you did when you wrote of your bliss. Other times you may not feel so blissful as deep cleansing is going on. There may even be periods where you feel like you are stuck on a plateau of experience. Just keep meditating every day, no matter what. In the long run, what matters is your daily practice. Whatever the experience may be, if our practice is correct and consistent, we will have the results in the end.

You will experience many emotions in connection with your journey: wonderment, awe, gratitude, impatience, boredom, anger, frustration, pain ... whatever the feelings are, use these to redouble your commitment to practice. If you can transmute your feelings, whatever they may be, into an unceasing desire to do your daily practice, then you cannot fail. For then you are devoted. Those who are steadily devoted always succeed, sooner or later. Your desire will always be the essential ingredient. Cultivate it well.

The guru is in you.

Lesson 17 – Was I Asleep in Meditation?

Q: I think I fell asleep during meditation, though I don't think I lost consciousness. It seemed I was awake, but I had no sense of time or anything. Then I realized my head was on my chest and looked at my watch. Thirty minutes had gone by. I felt pretty groggy. I felt pretty unsteady and it didn't feel right to just get up, so I lay down for a while. Then I was okay. Was I asleep?

A: No sensory experience, no mantra, no thoughts, but still conscious inside – were you asleep? Probably not. Meditation sometimes produces a sleep-like state, like you described, but the physiological parameters are different. The metabolism goes much lower than in sleep. Heart rate and breathing are much slower than in sleep, nearly stopped. The body and mind come to a state of complete silence, while still awake inside. The level of rest in the body and mind in meditation is deeper than sleep. It is a different kind of rest that removes impurities; obstructions to consciousness that sleep cannot reach. However, meditation is not a replacement for sleep, which has its own dynamics in the daily rejuvenation cycle.

People who have been meditating for years may have less need for sleep due to the accumulated purity in their nervous systems. It is not that meditation replaces sleep. It is that the body and mind gradually have become purified over time and the body needs less purification during its daily sleep cycle. It is the purity resulting from long-term meditation and other advanced yoga practices that generally reduces the need for sleep. In time, consciousness remains present twenty-four hours a day. Then, daily activities, dreaming and deep sleep are all playing like a movie on the screen of our silent, blissful awareness. In this state we are never asleep anymore. This is the kind of freedom and happiness we all are capable of achieving naturally – our unalienable birthright.

You did just right by lying down at the end of your session until you were able to get up feeling clear and smooth. This is another circumstance where extra rest after meditation is needed. Much cleansing went on during the meditation. Many different kinds of experiences can happen during meditation, ranging from the sublime to the ridiculous. It is all part of the same process of easily thinking the mantra and letting it settle in. Then the purification happens. We let it happen. Then, when we become aware, we return to the mantra and let the mind dive again. This process, done twice-daily for twenty minutes, will gradually transform your life to bliss.

Remember to count any experiences while off the mantra as part of your meditation time. It is okay that you became aware of the time again after thirty minutes. It was a natural event in your meditation. Whenever anything like that happens and you go past your allotted time, be sure to go through the appropriate rest period to finish the session. If you keep your meditation balanced with the right amount of rest at the end, you will always get up feeling refreshed and ready for activity.

The guru is in you.

Lesson 18 – Finding the Time for Meditation

Q: Meditation is very relaxing and I want to keep it up, but doing it twice a day will be hard for me. I travel a lot and have a wife and kids who I love to spend time with when I'm home. Time for meditation is short. What is your advice?

A: We who have families, responsibilities, busy lives, have an advantage when it comes to utilizing meditation, assuming we are able to make the time to do it. This is because the evolution of enlightenment depends on regular interaction between consciousness and worldly living. How can the true nature of the world be known if we are not in it, stabilizing the blissful silence we experience in meditation in our daily activities?

The trick is to make the time to do our two meditations each day so the benefits will be there. This "making the time" is a test of our desire, our devotion to the possibilities in us. It is a test that we all face every day – to do the things we want to do that require some discipline. Honestly, it is not a matter of how much time we have or do not have. It is a matter of deciding what is important to us, and doing what is necessary.

No one can tell you what is most important to you. Only you can know. It is entirely in your hands, always your choice. But you have an inner voice, you know. Something inside calls you to experience more, always to more. The seed wants to grow into a strong tree with beautiful, fragrant flowers blooming out all over. It must. We are all called by that evolutionary current inside us. Whatever else may be going on in our lives, the current will be there. It is not just for us, it is for everyone, and we do everyone a great service by deciding to cultivate it, first by favoring the rise of the desire, and then with practices that naturally bring out the peace and bliss residing within us.

Given that a choice is made to pursue meditation, it boils down to practical considerations. How to make the time? It is pretty mundane really. How do we find time to brush our teeth, bathe, eat right, wash the dishes, pay the bills and take out the trash? These are things we do because we know they must be done. We do them because we know that if we do not, life becomes a mess, a shambles, and we feel rotten. We could get along without doing any of these things for a while, but eventually it would catch up with us. People who have been regularly practicing meditation for some time develop a similar attitude about it. They know it has to be taken care of, or the desired result will not be there, and life will not be all it can be. They come to the same conclusion about meditation that they have about brushing teeth, bathing and taking out the trash. So they just make meditation a habit.

What about circumstances arising that make doing normal meditation seem impossible? You are on an airplane at 5:00 PM with an hour to go to get home. It's a no-brainer. Meditate on the plane. What about the noise, the banking of the plane, the turbulence? None of it matters. In meditation, you treat it all the same as other diversions from the mantra. Easily come back to the mantra when you realize you are off into thoughts, noise, movements of the body or surroundings, or whatever. It is not difficult to meditate in planes, trains, automobiles (not while driving!), waiting rooms, just about anywhere you are not required to be interacting with others for a while. Of course, at home in your regular meditation spot is best. But when in a pinch at the appointed time, if there is the opportunity, take it.

If it is impossible to meditate at the regular time, consider doing it at another time during the day, earlier or later. Don't make a habit of meditating right before bed though. It is better than not meditating at all, but it is much better to go into activity after meditation. The purification process and integration of consciousness in the nervous system is best accomplished during activity rather than in sleep. In fact, meditating right before bed might keep you awake for a while. Try it sometime and see what happens.

Suppose you get home from work and find that you have to go out to dinner with friends in half an hour. This is meditation time, and normally you would leave more time before having to go out. But this time it didn't work out. What do you do? Sit and meditate for five minutes, ten minutes, or fifteen minutes – whatever you can swing. Take the time you have to meditate and use it as best you can, allowing time to rest adequately after meditation and still make your date. There are a hundred ways to squeeze in a meditation, if you really want to. Don't make squeezing it in a daily habit though. If you plan ahead you will be on the mark with your practice most of the time. When something goes haywire, you can still take a few dives into your pure bliss consciousness. It aids in the continued cultivation of your meditation habit, and gives you an infusion of peace and bliss. Every little bit of meditation is a big step forward.

Your success will be in the wanting, and in doing the best you can to act on that every day. If you do, it will certainly enhance your full and active life. It is one of the best things you can do for your family. In the long run it will work an invisible magic in all of their lives, and the outer results will be very evident.

The guru is in you.

Lesson 19 – What Tradition to follow?

Q: I have been practicing yoga and meditation (a different kind) for five years, and I'm not sure how to proceed. Your meditation is very good. I experienced that right away. I'm not even supposed to be here, as the tradition I follow forbids learning outside practices. What shall I do?

A: As mentioned in the introduction, these lessons do not promote a particular sectarian view. Neither are they opposed to traditions that may adhere to the teachings of a specific individual or lineage of teachers. Everything has its purpose. It is up to each individual to weigh the pros and cons of the various approaches and carefully choose a course that promises to bring the best results. Everyone is different. At the same time, everyone has the same potential, for we are all spun from the same divine thread – pure silent bliss consciousness. If we are in touch with that on a daily basis, and keep on cultivating it with increasingly more powerful means, we cannot miss.

If your path is serving you well, stay with it. If you are finding fulfillment over time, you are in the right place. However, if your tradition is mostly serving you well, yet seems to be lacking in some way, find the courage and flexibility to try and fill in what is missing. In the end, it is you who will unfold bliss consciousness by your own efforts through devotion and application of the most comprehensive practices you can find. This point of view may fly in the face of traditions that insist we cannot achieve salvation by any other means but theirs. Maybe so, but that approach also shuts the door on further inquiry and scientific investigation into the practices of human spiritual transformation. The methods of Western science can offer much in this regard – highly integrated and collaborative approaches for discovering and applying knowledge. The success of Western science in many fields has been astounding. It is time for these methods of knowledge development to be applied in the arena of spiritual knowledge.

This discussion is the result of an open inquiry into many advanced yoga practices over a long period of time. The fruit of this journey has been an integrated system of practices. If there is something here that helps enhance your progress, it is good. If, at the same time, it creates friction with your current tradition, you will have to sort that out yourself. Ultimately, the answer is in you. Follow your heart. The potential conflict is not a bad thing. It will test your resolve and help lead you to the truth.

The venerable spiritual traditions are of great value. However, times are changing, and today we are seeing the emergence of more open approaches to examining and applying spiritual knowledge that are well suited for wise spiritual practitioners. Ultimately, this will have profound effects on all of humanity. Change is in the air, and it is a good thing.

The guru is in you.

Lesson 20 – Enlightenment without God?

Q: I am an atheist. A friend told me about this group. Frankly, I find the religious overtones annoying. But I was curious and tried the meditation, and have been pleasantly surprised. I would like to continue because it calms my nerves, and I remain curious as to what I might learn about myself. But I am still an atheist! Is there such a thing as enlightenment without God?

A: There is enlightenment both with and without God. This is because human beings are inherently enlightenable, transformable to a higher state of evolution, regardless of the belief system utilized. We could say that all of existence is headed in that direction, from the rocks up through all the kingdoms of living things. Everything is moving forward. Humanity is no exception. We humans have an added ability to consciously accelerate the process, to choose a fast track, which is what advanced yoga practices are about. We can turbo-charge the evolutionary process.

There has always been a mystique about human spiritual evolution. It is a practical mystique, a mystique with a purpose. The conception of God by humanity has been a necessary relationship structure. It has enabled humanity to surrender to its higher destiny, and approach it enthusiastically. At it's best, this is what belief in God is – belief in humanity's highest destiny, emerging from within us, and ultimately experienced all around us. Belief in God helps people to personally participate in the most exciting part of the human journey – the enlightenment process.

Is it necessary to believe in God for this unfoldment to occur? No. But it is necessary to believe in something in order to move in the direction of enlightenment.

If we are sitting in a café in New York, and I tell you there is a wonderful place called California three thousand miles away and that you should go see it, why would you go? Suppose you didn't believe me, didn't believe such a place existed at all. How could you find the motivation to go? It would be hard. Having never been west of the Mississippi River, you might believe that everyone who has gone past the Mississippi fell off the edge of the earth. This is, in fact, how Europeans felt about the Atlantic Ocean until people like Columbus and Magellan proved that there was a new world on the other side, and more.

To be motivated to do something about moving forward, we have to believe in the possibility of the destination. For many, the journey toward salvation is fueled by a belief in God. But it doesn't have to be about God. It can also be about truth, and believing that there is a final truth about us, in us, and that we can live it, become it. It can also be a belief in a personal process of transformation, and our own experience of it as we practice meditation and other yoga methods. Experiencing the journey naturally unfolding through practices can be more than enough to believe in, once the process has gotten underway and our experiences of deep silence and bliss light the fire of our desire to go for more and more. Whether we are selling out to our own rising experience of peace and bliss, or to the idea of pursuing the ultimate truth of life, or to a relationship with God, the result will be the same – an unwavering devotion to becoming one with "That" which is true.

Jesus said, "You will know the truth, and the truth will set you free." No mention of God there.

The word "God" does not exist in Buddhism or Taoism. Each has found its own intellectual and emotional motivation for approaching the infinite within. In all approaches it is the same thing that is sought, that great inner truth which lies deep within our heart, mind and senses – that which we can merge with by direct means, which, in turn, brightly illuminates our heart, mind and senses. This is the joining. By any name or belief structure, the outcome will be the same, so long as the aspirant has found the motivation to apply the methods of transformation on a daily basis.

So, it does not matter exactly how you have come to believe in a place called, "California." You may even call it by some other name. If you believe enough to keep putting one foot in front of the other, you will eventually be dipping your toes into the Pacific Ocean. If you don't believe it is there, you aren't likely to put forth the effort to get there. It's that simple.

Think of enlightenment in whatever way that inspires you the most, and use that inspiration to meditate every day.

Be tolerant of your brothers and sisters who cherish beliefs that are different from yours. We will each develop our own unique passion for the journey, and we are all headed home.

The guru is in you.

Lesson 21 – Objects of Meditation

Q: What is the difference between meditation on a mantra, chakras, a religious icon, a candle, etc?

A: Meditation is the bridge between attention on an object and the great beyond we know as bliss consciousness without thoughts or external sensory experience. The goal is to make that journey repeatedly, like clockwork, on a daily basis.

The technique we use is simple, yet delicate, relying on the natural ability of our mind to become quiet. Other forms of meditation may not be so simple and natural, and may involve focusing on intellectual meanings or on multiple objects. This can bog down passage of the attention to the expanded realm of bliss consciousness residing within us. This is not to say other forms of meditation will not work. But in our approach, simplicity and efficiency are at the forefront. This is an advanced method of meditation anyone can do. We will discuss meditation on other objects from the point of view of the method we are using here.

What is the difference between meditating with our technique using a mantra, versus using chakras (energy centers in the body), a religious icon or other physical objects? Again, it is a matter of simplicity and efficiency. The goal is to bring the attention beyond the thinking process, and, in doing so, take the attention beyond outer sensory experience.

The mind is the neurological process in us that links consciousness with the outer world. It is a very intimate connection. Our attention, engaged in the dynamics of the mind, is always an inch away from experiencing the divine bliss of pure consciousness. When the mind is allowed to come to rest, we are there.

So we begin with the mind, the most intimate connection to bliss consciousness we have. We begin inside, so we can quickly and easily go deeply inside. If we were to begin with a physical location in the body or a physical object, we could still go deep. No question about it. But it is a longer journey, a more complicated journey. The further outside we are when we start, the more physical, intellectual and emotional baggage we have to shed on the way in. This is also why we do not verbally utter the mantra during meditation, or give our attention to meanings while meditating. It is an inner process right from the start. By beginning meditation with a thought, using the specific procedure, we bypass external obstacles in the nervous system that can bind our attention. Ultimately we dissolve them naturally from the inside going out, rather than trying to dissolve them from the outside going in, which is not easy.

We begin with a thought, not focusing on any meaning, just picking up the repetition of the thought of the mantra's sound easily, on the edge of letting go. We let the mantra go its own way naturally to less and less – this is the simplest and most efficient way to dive into the infinite sea of bliss consciousness within us. Having done so repeatedly, we come back out after twenty minutes soaked with peace and bliss, achieving much purification during the process.

In time, the distance between consciousness and outside experiences evaporates as the obstructions become less and less. There was really no distance at all! Then it becomes natural to experience many shades of bliss consciousness while gazing upon chakras, religious icons, our loved ones, beautiful landscapes, scriptures, or even a book on theoretical physics. When bliss consciousness has arisen, everything is seen in terms of that. But this is not the procedure of meditation. This is enjoying the fruit of meditation – living life with an increasing appreciation of its many gifts. The rise of this appreciation inspires us all the more to carry on with our practice.

The guru is in you.

Lesson 22 – Vibratory Quality of Mantra

Q: You mentioned the "profound vibratory quality" of the sound *I AM*. What does this mean? If I choose to meditate on any sound I like, will it work just as well?

A: Certain sounds resonate in our nervous system. Deep in the silence of the mind they have a vibratory footprint that awakens our nervous system in particular ways. *I AM* is such a sound. As you continue to practice, you will see that your nervous system is being awakened in a particular way. It will be self-evident. You will say, "Ah Ha!" because it will be obvious. When we learn advanced pranayama (breathing) methods, we gradually begin to see and feel the mantra unfolding the subtle nerves. So many flavors of bliss. That is when the profound vibratory quality of the sound becomes obvious.

So there is a method to the mantra. It is not just any sound. Still, you can meditate using any sound you like. If you use the sound, "banana," you will be able to take it to very silent levels of mind. But there is no guarantee you will not end up with bananas growing out of your ears. Only kidding...

As you become advanced, you will know exactly what the mantra is doing as it vibrates through your subtle nerves, spreading out inside your vast ecstatic regions. As you become familiar with your cosmic realms, options for using certain kinds of sounds, and also thoughts with meaning, will become apparent. But we must take it one step at a time. Today the mantra, tomorrow the cosmos. It all belongs to you. It is all you.

The guru is in you.

Lesson 23 – Watching the Clock in Meditation

Q: I keep peeking at the clock while I am meditating, afraid I will go over my time. How do I break this distracting habit?

A: You have a biological clock that is quite accurate. Give it the opportunity to work. It only needs to be spot checked with a clock occasionally. As you get settled in the habit of regular meditations, keeping the time will become second nature. So, trust yourself. It's okay if you go over your time a bit inadvertently. Better that than being distracted. First let go of the habit of watching the clock. Don't mind the time at all. Be easy about it. Your body knows pretty much when twenty minutes are up. After a few weeks of daily practice you will open your eyes for the first time during a meditation and the clock will show that twenty minutes have gone by. You will be amazed how easy it is. Then timekeeping will continue automatically with no effort at all.

The guru is in you.

Lesson 24 – Does Meditation Cure Sickness?

Q: If I am sick, will meditation help me get better?

A: It can, but it is a far better prevention than a cure. As the nervous system becomes more balanced over time from a regular routine of daily meditation, the body's immune system functions much more efficiently, and there is far less chance of falling sick. Other advanced yoga practices we will be discussing here will further enhance the body's resistance to illness. Balance and purity of body and mind are known to be among the best defenses against disease. Meditation and other methods of yoga are important contributors. You could say that good health is a coincident benefit of long-term meditation practice, a foundation upon which we are building a much greater thing – enlightenment.

In our Western culture, we tend to think in terms of fighting disease when it has come upon us after months and years of unhealthy living, rather than cultivating a state of balance within ourselves in advance that will practically nullify the occurrence of disease. No doubt, achieving good prevention through balanced, healthy living is the best course of action. But if we get sick, meditation can help us there too. If you are bedridden, meditate as much as is comfortable, alternating with sleep periods. Be very relaxed about it, leaning back on a pile of pillows. Meditation will help the healing process. But do not expect it to be a magic bullet that will instantly correct a situation that has finally tipped toward sickness after a period of unbalanced living. Instead, think of working your way back into good daily habits, including meditation, which will lead to long term balance. Then sickness will be much less of a factor in life.

Of course, sooner or later, these bodies of ours will disintegrate and die. The longer we have cultivated pure bliss consciousness within, the less overwhelming and confusing will the transition be. This is the greatest cure of all.

The guru is in you.

Lesson 25 – Effect of Meditation on High Stress Situations

Q: I am going through a difficult divorce. Will meditation help me get through it?

A: Yes it will, but keep in mind that meditation is not a Band-Aid designed to deal with only the crisis at hand. It is a long-term practice that has many benefits. One of these is the development of an increasing tolerance for high stress situations. So, meditation will help in your current situation, but will also, over time of regular practice, make you permanently more resilient in high stress situations in general.

Why is this so? It is an interesting and observable phenomenon relating to the gradual rise of pure bliss consciousness in the nervous system. As we meditate, we find, over time, that there is more "silence" in us. It is not that we become silent in our outer life. We will probably seem much the same to others – perhaps a bit calmer. But inside we are more still, not moving around randomly in our thoughts, feelings and inner physical reactions as much as before. Less jangled, you know. This experience of inner silence continues to grow as we continue to meditate every day for weeks, months and years. As this is occurring, we notice that daily upheavals in life do not throw us off as much. Things that used to upset us don't as much. We become steady inside. If there is a sudden event, like a bang, that used to make us jump before, we may not even move now. We will experience it from someplace inside that is not affected. It goes right through, leaving little trace of tension. Does this mean we become cold and unfeeling? Not at all. We still feel, actually become more compassionate, but we are not swept away by emotions as we were before.

This is the essential thing about not being undone by stressful situations: this inner silence, this inner immovability.

From a spiritual perspective, it is well described by Jesus when he says, "The wise man built his house upon a rock. And the rain descended, and the floods came, and the winds blew, and beat upon the house, and it fell not: for it was founded upon a rock."

If you build your house upon the rock of your inner silence, nothing will be able to knock you off center. This is why meditation is one of the best stress therapies known. As with preserving good health, meditation is best for cultivating the nervous system in advance, stabilizing balance and inner silence before the storms of life rear up.

Besides these practical, everyday-living benefits, inner silence also is the foundation for the rise of divine ecstasy in the nervous system, and refining our perception of the world around us in a celestial way. The rise of silence in the nervous system is the first stage of the enlightenment process.

The guru is in you.

Lesson 27 – Location of Mantra in Meditation

Q: Am I supposed to think the mantra in particular locations in the body? Sometimes it gravitates to physical locations in me.

A: No, we do not deliberately physically locate the mantra. This is a delicate question because the mantra has a vibratory quality that awakens the nervous system in particular ways, as previously discussed on the question about the vibratory quality of the mantra. So it might be experienced in some place or another, as you said. But we do not favor that. We continue with the simple procedure for using the mantra, always.

The nervous system in its most subtle realms is like a tuning fork – rather, like a multitude of tuning forks, with just a few tuning forks harmonizing the vibrations of all the others. The mantra resonates with these few leading tuning forks. Later on, we will enhance the mantra to broaden the influence of this tuning fork effect. The result will be broader and deeper immovable inner silence, also experienced as pure bliss consciousness coming up in us. If you find the mantra occurring in particular locations, that is okay. We don't resist that. Nor do we encourage it. Just as we let the mantra settle down naturally to quieter and quieter levels, so too do we let it occur in the body wherever it is naturally. If it doesn't occur in any particular place, that is okay too. It is not about physical locations. The mantra naturally resonates according to the complex purification process going on inside us while we are meditating. All we have to do is follow the simple procedure of thinking the mantra easily, and picking it back up easily when we realize we have been off it.

Another reason this question you ask about location of the mantra is a delicate one is because soon we will be discussing pranayama, and taking up an advanced breathing practice before each meditation session. This will involve moving the attention in a particular way through the physical body in concert with the breath. We will be using two practices in succession – pranayama and meditation, each quite different in its procedure. They will complement each other tremendously, as you will see. This will be the beginning of the all-important integration of advanced yoga practices. Each part will be done independently. Yet, with these two methods taken in succession, an integration will begin to occur in us. The whole will be greater than the sum of the parts. Instead of using one natural pathway to the divine in us (the mind), we will be using two (adding the breath). Together, these will transform the nervous system at a more rapid rate, and the greater purification and corresponding experiences will reflect this. This process of integration of practices will be gradually expanded to more fully embrace all of the natural pathways leading inward through us, and coax pure bliss consciousness out through us in increasingly dynamic ways. This integration of practices is a delicate process, much like playing a musical instrument. We must be able to do one thing at one time and do another different thing at another time. With some practices, we will be doing several different things at the same time. It is all part of a natural unfoldment in us, and the practices themselves will become natural in due course, and automatic. The results experientially cannot be done justice with the written word, except perhaps in poetry. You have to go there and see what it is for yourself. It is the real "final frontier." It is the glorious cosmos, and you are the doorway.

The guru is in you.

Lesson 28 – Will I become a Milquetoast from Meditation?

Q: My employees tell me I am less crabby. I'm not sure this is a good thing. Will I become a milquetoast from meditation?

A: It's not likely. You will become much stronger from meditation, which means becoming who you are at the most fundamental level. At the same time, you will engage in tense and harmful behavior less and less. You will be less crabby and be more calmly resolute about the things that matter to you. People have noticed something already. This is a good thing. You will be in a much better position to motivate your employees because you will act more from a level of inner strength, instead of from a level of anger and tension.

Of course, there is the belief that tension is necessary to motivate people, especially in business. "Fear is the greatest motivator," they say. Fear is a motivator. But it is only useful if it spurs people to attain a greater realization of inner truth, which includes growing beyond the reach of fear. If fear does not motivate us to find the truth, then is just a grind, an endless wheel of misery. Nobody really wants to be on that wheel, not even those who are turning it, rolling it over others. Until now, there may not have seemed to be any other alternative. But there is, and things can change. Go within daily with meditation and you will get off the wheel, and help others to get off it as well. You will find that business, and all of life, is much more fulfilling as crabbiness fades. Crabbiness fades as pure bliss consciousness rises. There are no limits to what you can accomplish then.

The guru is in you.

Lesson 29* – Alcohol, Tobacco and Drugs

Q: I enjoy having a drink when I get home from work. That doesn't seem to work so well before meditation, and it doesn't feel so good after meditation either. Are drinking and meditation incompatible?

A: Meditation is about cultivating purity deep in the nervous system. Many positive results in life come up from this. It stands to reason that taking in substances that retard purification of the nervous system will not be helpful to the meditation process.

This is not a moral lesson. It is common sense. Most importantly, it is experiential. If something makes us feel bad, we will eventually stop doing it. Maybe before beginning meditation a drink or two gave us some relief from the tensions of life. It dulled our perception, or altered it in some way to give us a temporary feeling of wellbeing. After beginning meditation, the experience changes. The peace, happiness and clarity we discover coming from within are quite different from the temporary chemical states we have previously engaged in. There is no comparison between the two, and we begin to have a different perspective. The transitory pleasure of drinking loses it luster in comparison to the permanent joyful results of meditation.

Again, this is not a moral lesson. It is not a "Thou shalt not." It is your choice, always. If your choice is to go for more in life, to take up the path of meditation and other advanced yoga practices, it will be a no-brainer. The rising experience of pure bliss consciousness will change your attitude about alcohol. Give regular practice of meditation a fair chance, and the things that are not good for you will tend to drop off naturally over time. Besides alcohol, people find the same thing happens with recreational drugs, tobacco and even caffeine. There are no rules – just the rise of pure bliss consciousness, our true nature. All we have to do is meditate twice a day, and listen to what our inner silence is telling us. We will know what to do.

Prescription drugs are a different story. Stay with your doctor's instructions on those. If you think a prescription drug you are taking is interfering with meditation, talk to your doctor. See if there is some way to accommodate both your medical need and your meditation need.

The guru is in you.

Addition – And another question on alcohol and tobacco:

Q: I am a heavy drinker and smoker, and want to stop both. I have tried meditating per your instructions, but don't experience anything, and my desire to drink and smoke has not been affected. About all I am getting out of meditation is a headache during and after, so I am losing faith. Can meditation help me?

A: Drinking and smoking put obstacles in the nervous system that limit the ability of pure bliss consciousness to be expressed. If the drinking and smoking are light to moderate, then meditation may be enough to clear things out, and then those behaviors will become less attractive as the inner cleansing process overcomes the obstructions, with more natural bliss is coming up from within.

On the other hand, if the drinking and smoking are very heavy, meditation may not be enough to overcome the obstructions.

Think of your nervous system as a dirty window. The methods of yoga are for cleaning the window so the light of your divine consciousness can shine through. Meditation is a very refined tool for this, and is capable of making the window very clean. However, if the dirt is very thick on the window, with more being thrown on every day, then meditation may not be able to keep up. So, if we want the window to get clean, we will be wise to reduce the amount of dirt we are throwing on it. In other words, in approaching yoga practices, some change in our habits may be necessary to help facilitate forward progress. It is common sense, yes?

If addiction to alcohol, tobacco, or other substances exists, we will be wise to deal with that through additional methods that are designed specifically for overcoming those habits. The 12-step program pioneered by *Alcoholics Anonymous*, and now used in many behavior modification support programs, is an excellent approach for overcoming self-destructive habits. At its core is the principle of giving our life to a higher purpose, and that is certainly consistent with yoga. This higher purpose is our own divine destiny. With a 12-step program, we are systematically shifting our identification of self from the narrowness of destructive behavior to our divine destiny. This is worth doing, and is an excellent way to prepare for yoga practices if drinking, smoking or other limiting habits are blocking the way. Check the AYP links section on the web site for more information on "Twelve-Step Programs."

As for the headaches, they are proof that meditation is doing something, though this is not the ideal symptom. If the inner obstructions are heavy and/or we are forcing the mantra, there can be a headache like that. If there is a headache in meditation, we just easily back off the mantra and be with the sensation without trying to do anything with it. After a few minutes we can gently come back to the mantra again. If there is still pain and it is too uncomfortable, then we should take the rest of our meditation time lying down, letting the mind be relaxed without the mantra.

Always remember to take plenty of time coming out of meditation – at least a few minutes. 5-10 minutes lying down is good if there has been discomfort in meditation. Coming out of meditation too fast can cause a headache or irritability in activity, because we have not allowed the cycle of purification to complete itself. So, easy in meditation and good rest coming out is the formula. If that does not eliminate the headaches, then consider shortening the time of meditation until a balance has been found. And, by all means, consider taking additional steps to deal with the heavy drinking and smoking. Then your meditation will be able to carry the purification process forward more quickly and enjoyably.

As the window of your nervous system becomes clean, your divine light will be shining through more and more every day. That's how it works.

Lesson 30 – Diet and Meditation

Q: If I become a vegetarian, will meditation be better?

A: Only if you are naturally inclined that way. Forced diets are not usually the best diets, because they introduce stress and self-judgement. The first chance it gets, the body rushes back to the old diet. This is why regimented diet programs rarely work over the long run. It has to come from within.

If you meditate regularly, you will find that, in time, you will be drawn to a lighter, more nutritious diet. Your preferences will change naturally. Go with that. The body knows what it needs to sustain the process of purification fostered by meditation. As pure bliss consciousness rises, the eating habits will change accordingly.

"Light and nutritious" is about all the diet description you will see here in these lessons. "Light" to aid in easy cleansing of the nervous system through advanced yoga practices, and "nutritious" to help keep the body in good health. Too light is not usually nutritious, and too nutritious is not usually light. Balance is the key, and regular meditation will naturally lead us in that direction. A preoccupation with diet is not an aid to meditation. So take it easy and meditate twice each day. If you do that, the diet will take care of itself.

The guru is in you.

Note: Later in the lessons (see #69), diet is also discussed from the point of view of helping stabilize inner energy imbalances.

Lesson 31 – Enjoying the Great Outdoors

Q: We went to the mountains last weekend and I meditated outdoors overlooking a huge valley. It was beautiful, and my meditation was wonderful. I was blissfully intermingled with the soft mountain air. Is there a benefit in meditating outdoors in beautiful places?

A: There is great benefit in being outdoors in beautiful places, but not necessarily in meditating there. To be able to appreciate the profound beauty of nature is the greatest joy in life. For what greater purpose could we be here than to enjoy the infinite sea of harmony in and all around us? Regular meditation gradually cultivates our inherent ability to appreciate the beauty in life.

But remember what we are doing in meditation. We are easily picking up the mantra and letting it go however it will. Then we are picking it back up again when we realize we have been off it. This procedure we do for twenty minutes twice a day. We do not meditate for a particular experience while we are doing it. The purification process has its own way to go. We cannot direct it or predict it. We do the easy procedure of meditation and let it happen.

So, doing the meditation procedure is not about sitting on a mountaintop or in any particular place, except to take advantage of the best place we have available at meditation time where we will have the least distraction. Jesus said, "Go into your closet to pray." This is the idea. Meditation is an inner process, so we withdraw to do it.

If we are on an airplane, in a waiting room, or some other busy place, we may not have a choice, so we make the best of it and meditate there. As discussed previously, it can easily be done. However, we do not go sit outdoors on a mountaintop for the purpose of meditating. It's much better to be in the cabin where it is quiet and subdued. Then we can meditate, go inward, with the least stimulation of the outer senses. Later on we can go out and appreciate the grand display of the valley below, having soaked ourselves with the perception-illuminating qualities of pure bliss consciousness. Close your eyes then, if you wish, and be one with the glory of nature all around you. Enjoy!

Meditation is a preparation for enriching the experience of everything else. It is a retreat from the outer world to pure bliss consciousness within so we can come back and know the outer world in a much more refined way. If we try and blend our meditation practice with experiencing the outer world at the same time, the results will not be optimal. First we go in. Then we come back out. Our meditation is not about trying to be in and out at the same time. That state of being both in and out at the same time comes naturally with regular daily meditation. Being in and out at the same time is not the practice of meditation. It is the fruit of meditation.

Do be inspired by the beauty of nature. Know that you can experience nature in increasingly refined ways as a result of daily practice of meditation. Use your inspiration to redouble your commitment to daily practice. Then, in time, you will know nature in a way that will permanently melt you in bliss. Then your natural state will be to be completely in and completely out at the same time. You will become the great outdoors. This is the fruit of true yoga and true religion. This is enlightenment.

The guru is in you.

Lesson 33 – A New Way to Sit in Meditation

Q: In a yoga class I went to, the instructor said one should always sit vertically without back support on a floor mat or pillow when meditating. I have been trying this and getting pretty sore in the process. Is this necessary for successful meditation?

A: In a word, no. Meditation works just fine while sitting on a soft surface with back support. An easy chair is good. Being on a bed with a couple of pillows behind us is better, for reasons that will become clear shortly. Don't meditate in a reclined position, as this can result in sleep rather than meditation. The idea is to be sitting upright comfortably. We don't want unnecessary discomfort in the body competing with the simple procedure of meditation. If it is natural for you to sit on a hard surface without back support for twenty minutes or more, this is okay for meditation. But few will be able to do this, and it is not necessary. Less comfort is synonymous with unnecessary distraction in meditation. So keep it comfortable.

Having said all that, here comes a curve ball. Once you are steady in your daily meditation routine and feel you are ready for the next step in your yoga practice, it is a good idea to put your legs in a crossed position while you are meditating. This is where the bed comes in handy. If you can get one leg in so the sole of your foot is against the inside of your thigh with your heel near your crotch, this is good. The other leg can come in with its sole resting under the shin of the first leg. It doesn't matter which leg goes inside first to the thigh. It is your choice. Over time, you can develop the ability to switch legs, so that either one can be the inside leg during meditation. Comfort will be the determining factor on which leg to use on the inside.

If you are new at this, it may seem difficult. For most it will take some doing, but we will not be approaching it in an extreme way. We will take a very gentle, gradual approach. There are important long-term reasons why we are tackling this now, so give it the necessary consideration, as long as it does not jeopardize your regular meditation routine.

Making first attempts, you may find that you are not able to get your inside foot to your thigh. You may find your knees sticking up in the air, not wanting to lie flat on the bed. Go as far as you comfortably can, and use pillows to prop up your knees if necessary, so you can be as comfortable as possible while meditating. Don't torture yourself, or your meditation, by forcing yourself into an uncomfortable position. What we want is to gently coax our legs into a cross-legged position over a period of time. It might happen immediately for some. For others it might take weeks or months of gentle coaxing. It is the direction we gradually want to go in. Rome was not built in a day.

As you become familiar with the physics of your legs, you will find that your knees will more easily come down and lie comfortably on the bed when the soles of your feet are turned up a bit. The toes of the inside foot can then tuck under the thigh with the heel remaining near the crotch, and the toes of the outside foot can then tuck under the shin. A bed is very good for this, as the soles of the feet can easily turn up while the tops of the feet sink into the mattress a bit. Having turned the soles of the feet up, if the knees still have not come down, feel free to use pillows to fill in the void under them. But if you are turning the soles up, the knees should come down, just as though you are heading toward kneeling on the bed with your knees spread wide apart. Use back support while meditating and developing this new way of sitting in meditation. You will find that you can get comfortable in this position after a gentle coaxing period of several weeks or months. If your legs get uncomfortable during meditation it is okay to extend one or both of them out on the bed as needed and continue meditating. Or you can switch the inside leg from one to the other from time to time, and continue that way. Do whatever it takes to keep comfortable during meditation, while gently favoring the cross-legged way of sitting at the same time. Back support is recommended for all but the most hearty. The hands can be folded in the lap or placed on the thighs, knees, or wherever they are most comfortable. In time, sitting cross-legged will become second nature, and you will be able to meditate easily and not even notice how you are sitting.

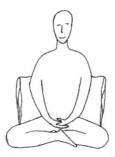

Cross-legged sitting with back support

If there is a disability or other limiting factor you can't overcome, and sitting cross-legged is not going to be possible for you, it is okay. You can still meditate and derive all the benefits. Nothing is lost. As we take on new advanced yoga practices down the road, there are ways we can get around the lack of crossed legs. Crossed legs are preferable, but not mandatory.

Obviously, when we find ourselves in situations where we will be meditating in planes, offices, waiting rooms, etc., we just sit normally on our chair without any special position for the legs. But when we are meditating at home, we always favor (with comfort) the cross-legged way of sitting just described. It is an important preparation that will form the foundation for a dramatic stage of our spiritual transformation as we add additional advanced yoga practices.

The guru is in you.

Note: This lesson is preparation for an important practice called "siddhasana," which will be introduced further on.

Lesson 34 – Meditation and World Problems

Q: Certainly there must be more important things to think about than *I AM*. What about the pressing problems of the world: terrorism and war, poverty, hunger? I don't get it. Are you sure meditation isn't an escape from reality?

A: Keep in mind that meditation is not about thinking *I AM* in a haphazard way. As has been discussed in detail, it is a precise procedure that brings us to the deepest level of peace and bliss in us, and brings these qualities out into our daily activity. Meditation is not an escape from reality. Rather, it is a preparation for it. You could even say that meditation is a revealer of reality, because what we consider to be reality is almost entirely a product of our perception. Specifically, do we see the glass as half full, or half empty?

If we see the glass as half full, there is hope. There is boundless energy to do good, even in the most daunting of circumstances. We see ways for things to get better, and we work toward that. When we see the glass as half empty, there is little hope, little energy to work for something better. There is misery, and we become a drag on everyone around us. We become part of the problem, rather than part of the solution. So, if you find that meditation is a source of peace, inner happiness, optimism and strength in your life, then this is a formula for bettering your surroundings, and the world.

The results of meditation are infectious. When we meditate, others are affected not only by our inspired actions, but also by the invisible radiation of pure bliss consciousness emanating from us. We can induce peace and optimism in others by opening ourselves to the infinite within.

Jesus said, "You are the light of the world."

If millions of people engaged in meditation each day, the world would be illuminated. We can each do our part by bringing out the divine light within us. It is not an escape. It is a responsibility. To become more is not only about us. It is about everyone on the earth.

So meditate every day, and wholeheartedly go do the work you feel in your heart is most important. May your glass overflow for the benefit of the world.

The guru is in you.

Lesson 35 – Enlightenment Milestones

Q: What is the ultimate destination of meditation, how will experiences evolve along the way, and how long will it take to complete the journey?

A: The ultimate destination is enlightenment. What is enlightenment? A state of balanced union between our two natures: pure bliss consciousness, and our sensory involvement on this physical earth. That is the definition of yoga, and the destination of all religion.

The evolution of experiences is a complex and personal journey, but has a certain pattern to it. There are three identifiable stages:

First comes the rise of silence from regular meditation. It is also experienced as an increasingly steady state of peace, happiness and bliss. Most of all it is experienced as an inner stability that is not shaken by any outer experience. Inner silence is the foundation for further experiences that are facilitated by additional advanced yoga practices that awaken the silence of pure bliss consciousness to a dynamic state in our nervous system.

Second comes the rise of ecstatic experience in the body and surroundings. It comes from an awakening of the life force in the body and a gradual refinement of sensory perception. Through pranayama (breath control) and other means, meditation is enhanced so that the senses are opened in an inward direction, enabling us to perceive the ecstatic energies coursing within and around us. You could say that silence moves within us, and this creates a new and captivating kind of experience. During this stage, appreciation for the divine flow of life is naturally heightened, leading to increased desire to enter and merge with the deepening sensory experience. One surrenders to the process as it advances, and this accelerates it. The second stage is like falling into an endless abyss of ecstasy. We function in the world with increasing joy as our attention becomes absorbed in the ever-present living beauty moving beneath the surface of all things. For us, the boundaries are dissolving.

Third, as our attention comes to reside naturally in the omnipresent, undulating blissful silence in all things, we become that ever-present harmony. We find our own self to be the essence of all things. This is the experience of unity, union, enlightenment. The world does not disappear. It becomes transparent. Boundaries become like veils, thinly covering the essence of life, which we have come to know as an expression of our own nature. Can we still act in the world? Yes, but our motives are different than before when we could only see ourselves as separate. We now act in the interest of a broader self. In doing so, we may seem to become selfless. The truth is that we always are acting for our own self-interest. But our self has become universal, so our interest is for the whole of humanity, and for the whole of life.

From the beginning of advanced yoga practices (and perhaps even before), we may experience shades of any of these three stages, depending on the dynamics of our unique purification process. We may experience elements of all three stages at the same time. Over time, we come to recognize the telltale experiences as mileposts on the way to enlightenment. There will be many more sub-mileposts discussed as we get into additional advanced yoga practices. The mileposts are useful to keep us going, to keep us inspired and regular in our daily practices. The mileposts are not so useful for proclaiming, "Today I am here along the road to enlightenment." Indeed, we may well be, but it will only be significant when we have gone past there and our experience has become permanent and unnoticed. When the experience becomes natural and normal it becomes real. It is life as we are meant to live it. The mileposts will be dissolved in the journey. Enlightenment, ultimately, is not so much about the mileposts. It is about enjoying becoming that which we always were.

If you made that trip to California we were talking about earlier, would you spend your time marveling about how you got there? Probably not. Much better to enjoy the beauty of California in the present moment. However, it is useful to review the particulars of the long journey for the benefit of others. After all, everyone emanates from the same divine consciousness as we do, so we are naturally concerned that all should have a safe and speedy journey.

Jesus said, "Do unto others as you would have them do unto you." The truth is that all others are you. So this is not only good moral advice, it is good practical advice. Experientially, we come to know that others are our own self as our inner doors are opened to the divine realms within.

How long does the journey take? It depends mainly on us – on our past actions that have produced the obstructions lodged deep in our nervous system, and on what we do from now on. We can't change the past. But we can do much in the present that will shape our future. No one else can make the choice but us. If we take up advanced yoga practices with sincere devotion, there will be a new direction in our life. Once we have committed ourselves unswervingly to the path, it is only a matter of time. Then we see it is not even so much about the final destination. It is about experiencing increasing joy in the present each day, each month and each year. This is a path of bliss, a path of pleasure, as we naturally unfold from within. Get on it and begin to enjoy the ride today. You will get to the end, bye and bye.

The guru is in you.

Lesson 36 – Meditation and the Fifth Dimension

Q: When I meditate, I feel like I am gone someplace else. It is very pleasant, and it is gradually changing my view of life. Where am I when I meditate? What is being added to me?

A: When we meditate we are allowing the mind to naturally bring our awareness out of the familiar realm of time and space to the realm of unadulterated bliss consciousness. Consciousness is neither time nor space. We could say it is the infinite dimension underlying the world we perceive with our physical senses. Besides having no boundaries, it is eternally "now." Consciousness is another dimension beyond time and space – we could call it the fifth dimension. With meditation, we are gradually marrying the fifth dimension of consciousness with the four dimensions of time and space, so all five dimensions come to coexist together. Our nervous system is gradually cultured to give us the experience of all five dimensions simultaneously.

This has profound implications in our everyday life. Before meditating, everything we did was in time and space. All our action, our problem solving, was limited to the four dimensions. The options we saw before us were always time and space limited. With meditation, we are bringing in an additional dimension, consciousness. It makes a big difference. Now we see situations in ways we could not see before. We are able to influence the course of life in ways we could not before.

Imagine you are trying to solve a puzzle lying on a table. You are looking at it in two dimensions, on the flat surface of the table. Try as you may, the pieces won't fit together. Then a friend walks into the room and says, "Try this." She picks up two edges of the puzzle and curls them together above the table, and they fit together perfectly. By moving into the third dimension, the space above the table, the puzzle has been solved easily. Life is like that. Dealing with it only in time and space, four dimensions, it is often an unsolvable puzzle. We go round and round, never quite getting the pieces to fit together. When we begin to meditate, we are adding a new dimension, a new perspective. Then the pieces start to fit together, and it all begins to make sense.

The guru is in you.

Lesson 37 – Group Meditations

Q: If I can find others who do this practice, can we meditate together in a group? I have heard there are benefits in this.

A: Group meditations are a good thing. Any gathering that is for the purpose of studying and encouraging paths of spiritual unfoldment can be good for you. If you can commune with others of like interest on a regular basis, there will be significant benefits, particularly in inspiring you to press forward with your daily practice. No doubt you will inspire others to practice as well.

It is good to do a group meditation of ten minutes or so at the beginning or end of a gathering. You may structure your own discussion group, or you may be a guest at someone else's. Regardless, you will find that group meditations have their own quality. They can be deep and pervasive as individual quieting minds mingle and reinforce each other. It is a noticeable effect, and radiates outward to the surroundings. It is good if members of the group are doing the same practice, but not mandatory, as long as all can operate quietly within the same time period. Group meditations are good for individual meditators, and uplifting for the world.

Some people go for "guided meditations." You will not find this style of group meditation to be compatible with using the mantra, because your practice is for going inward quickly and efficiently. As your meditation becomes habit, you will be gone within as soon as you close your eyes, and a talking meditation guide will be counter-productive for you. The same goes for meditations using music, chanting, drumming, etc. These all have their purpose and benefits, but are not compatible with taking the mantra inward quickly toward pure bliss consciousness. This is not to say you cannot participate in guided meditations, chanting, or whatever. But it will be a distinctly different procedure from your daily meditation using the mantra. You will find the connections that are appropriate for you with the many groups that are available. Or maybe you will start your own group geared to this open approach to advanced yoga practices. Whatever works for you.

Jesus said, "For where two or three are gathered in my name, there I am in the midst of them." This quote is not given from a sectarian point of view. It describes a well-known principle. When people gather for a spiritual purpose, consciousness is stimulated and rises. This rising can be experienced as deepening silence and pervading bliss consciousness. This experience occurs in every faith, in every gathering for a high spiritual ideal, in every gathering for truth. The group experience of pervading silent bliss consciousness is maximized during group meditations where multiple minds are systematically brought to quietness.

Group meditations are not a substitute for your regular twice-daily meditations. Your individual practice is your primary practice, and should always be. This keeps your spiritual destiny in your hands, in your daily practice, regardless of other circumstances. Groups come and go. Group meditations can be a wonderful boost, but they will come and go too. Don't rely on them as core practice. Think of them as bonuses. Life is always changing on the outside. Be sure that your daily practice is ingrained as an inside aspect of your life, not subject to being waylaid by outer events. We have talked about the various strategies for sustaining daily meditation practice in non-routine situations. Keeping your regularity in practice is very important as you travel along the byways of life. Whatever you ultimately choose your daily practice to be, this should be sacred. It is your primary pathway inward. You can count on it, because you are committed to doing it every day without fail. Everything else is passing scenery, inspiring at times, and not so inspiring at other times. Lean toward the inspiring, let it light the fire of your desire for progress, and let your daily practice continue to do the work of ongoing inner purification. We will be adding additional practices for you to consider. You will build your own daily routine. A daily routine is the key. It is the surest path to enlightenment.

Explore groups and engage in the ongoing discussion of spiritual transformation. You have entered a new realm of citizenry – spiritual citizenry. Bring your inner silence to each gathering and to each group meditation. And always remember you are building your house daily upon the rock of pure bliss consciousness.

The guru is in you.

Lesson 38 – What is Your Time Line?

We have a bit of a dilemma. It has to do with time. We are now ready to move the discussion on into the next area of advanced yoga practices. The question is, are you ready?

"Yes," you say, "I want to read about it."

The dilemma is not so much in the reading. It is in the application of the knowledge, how to go about that.

The lessons being written here are the result of decades of experience in yoga. It will take six months or so to fully describe for you how to do the most important advanced yoga practices, and what their effects will be. Once the writing is complete, you will be able to read it all in just a few days. Obviously, it would not be advisable for you to begin all of these advanced yoga practices in the time it would take you to read about them. It would not be possible. Each stage of practice requires a substantial period of acclimation before the next stage can be successfully entered. If one tries to run before they have become reasonably adept at walking, there is a strong likelihood they will fall flat on their face. This is also true in taking on advanced yoga practices. A gradual build-up is not a luxury – it is a necessity.

So, that is the dilemma. Having received all this powerful information on the front end, how will you build up your practices in an appropriate manner over time? It boils down to finding what your unique time line will be, your pace, and being methodical about building up, being careful not to take on too much at once. Everyone is different and has a different capacity for taking on new practices. You will have to find your own pace, your own time line that is progressive for you, yet stable.

The challenge used to be in finding the knowledge. Here, the challenge is in applying it as expeditiously as you are inspired to without overdoing it and falling off the wagon, so to speak.

In the old days, it was said that it was better to receive powerful spiritual techniques lifetimes late, rather than a minute too soon. Practices were doled out sparingly over long periods of time on an individualized basis. This hardly fits with the face-paced, mass-market information age we now live in, where, in many fields, new applications of knowledge supercede the old every few years.

There is a need to speed up the transmission and integration of the knowledge of advanced yoga practices. It needs to be simplified and codified in ways that will bring it into the mainstream of this scientific age. It has to be turned over to the people, and the people must decide how it will be applied for practical benefit for present and future generations. It must happen, or the methods of transmitting this knowledge will remain in the dark ages, and few will benefit. The world can no longer afford to be without effective and freely available methods for unfolding the inner nature of humanity.

There are those who say, "Do not throw pearls before swine." Two thousand years ago this may have been good advice for those who had spiritual knowledge. If they were too open in its dissemination, it was likely they would be attacked by an angry, superstitious mob, and executed soon after. Consequently, spiritual practices have been kept secret, even as the scientific age has blossomed all around us. Times have changed, but the methods of sharing spiritual knowledge have remained largely frozen in the past.

Today, we need a more open approach. We stand at an important juncture in history. Can we continue to sit by and regard the human race as a mob, as swine, undeserving of the knowledge that will transform it? No. Humanity is more than that, and deserves to have the means to experience its true nature. It is time for change.

We stand on the edge of a massive shift in human awareness. Its consequences exceed the realization centuries ago that the earth is round and not flat, and that the sun is the center of the solar system and not the earth. The realization occurring in the present is that the interior of the human being is the center of divine experience, of God, and of Truth. It is not somewhere else. External experiences, whether they appear divine or not, are but mirrors of the internal experience of the human being. Every human being is a window, a portal, from this world to the infinite, and from the infinite to this world.

These lessons give you the most important tools of human transformation, the means to open the portal in you. The decision-making on what practices to do is in your hands. It is no different than applying any form of knowledge. We are all familiar with learning to apply powerful technologies prudently and beneficially – automobiles, household machinery, modern medicine, electricity, the unlimited information of the Internet... We can use these things effectively within a reasonable learning period. This is an instruction manual on advanced yoga practices. Wise practitioners will know what to do with it. Others will let it go by, and it will incubate for a while, which is part of the awakening process also.

The knowledge is here. It is suggested you take it in. But don't act on it all at once. Take it one step at a time. Become comfortable in a practice before you add on the next one. The more we evolve in our practice to a comfortable routine, the easier it will be to take on something new. It takes time.

We have already added cross-legged sitting to our meditation routine. Have you been making good progress with that? We are about to embark on a new leg of the journey – pranayama. Pranayama will evolve into a complex practice with far-reaching effects. We will build it up with simple, logical steps. Even so, if you are uneven in your meditation practice, and trying to get in cross-legged position at the same time, taking on pranayama will be too much for now. Way too much. So wait until the meditation and crossed legs are stable. You may be one who skips the crossed legs altogether. That's okay. Still, be sure your meditation is comfortable and in a steady routine before taking on pranayama.

This message of taking it gradually will be repeated over and over again as we, in very few pages, step though eons of powerful spiritual knowledge designed for opening your inner doors.

The dilemma of timing will be resolved if you respect the power and delicacy of this knowledge, and apply it responsibly in your life. It is recommended you err on the side of sticking with regular, stable practice. Always consider carefully before you add a new practice. If you overdo and feel instability, back off to your last stable platform of practice. There you can regroup and take your time while considering the best way to move ahead.

Meditation is the core practice. With it alone you will go far. Everything else is designed to enhance the process of meditation, to enhance the flow of pure bliss consciousness through the body and in the surroundings. If it is only meditation you are interested in, it will be enough. If you are interested in more, there will be plenty for you here.

The guru is in you.

Note: Further along in the lessons, the application of this concept of each person finding their own time line is given a name – "self-pacing." It turns out to be one of the most important teachings in the lessons, returned to again and again – a practice in itself, as important as any of the powerful yogic techniques discussed. As you will see in the Q&As, self-pacing becomes one of the biggest challenges for many on this path of yoga. It lies at the heart of each one of us finding a relationship with our spiritual condition and working systematically to unfold the divine within. There is no question that developing skill in self-pacing is the key to achieving self-sufficiency in yoga. With that, we know exactly what to do in practices each day, and then the features of enlightenment can be clearly seen emerging in us.

Lesson 39 – Pranayama – Cultivating the Soil of the Nervous System

It is common knowledge that when a friend is upset, really upset, it is good to tell him to breathe, to take slow, deep breaths in and out for a while. This invariably has a calming effect on the nervous system, mind and emotions.

Why? Because it loosens the nerves. Tension constricts our nerves, and this restricts the flow of consciousness through us. Breathing slowly and deeply loosens our nerves, facilitating the flow of consciousness through us, and this has the desired relaxing effect.

To say that consciousness flows through us is a bit of an over-simplification. While, in truth, all is the flow of consciousness, it is more descriptive to say that the "life force" flows through us. What is the life force? It is the first manifestation of consciousness in matter. It is called, "prana," which means, "first unit." In the string theory of modern physics, the miniscule, subatomic energy strings thought to be the building blocks of everything in the universe might well be analogous to prana. In any case, we know that influencing prana (the life force) in the human body has significant effects on our nervous system, and our experience.

Meditation is a way of influencing prana with the mind taking the lead. The human mind arises from a flow of energy through the nerves of the brain. In meditation, we systematically allow that energy (prana) to become still, which brings us to the underlying cause of that energy. We experience it as pure silent bliss consciousness. In meditation, the attention is easily brought beyond the mind, and beyond prana. It is an extraordinary natural ability we have.

Besides meditation, there are other ways to influence prana to facilitate the purification of the nervous system for joining of our inner and outer nature. As mentioned, managing the breath can have a noticeable effect on our experience. By restraining the breath in certain ways we can produce certain predictable effects. This is the science of "pranayama," which means, "restraint of prana." In terms of what we do externally, it is called breath control. But there is more to pranayama than physical control of the breath. Other actions are brought to bear that deepen and broaden the effects of the breath. The mind is involved, and so is the body in ways other than by controlling the breath. Taken together, these actions loosen and cultivate the nervous system in ways that greatly enhance the effects of our core practice of meditation.

Think of the nervous system as the soil, and of pure bliss consciousness as the seed. We have been awakening the silent seed through regular daily meditation. Now we will be cultivating the soil of our nervous system so the seed of pure bliss consciousness will grow to be dynamic and strong in us.

How does the breath affect the flow of prana in the body? There is an electromagnetic relationship in the body between the breath, the mind, the flow of prana, and every aspect of our biological functioning. All of these are connected. This is why, when we meditate, the breath is automatically subdued and the whole metabolism slows down. During pranayama, when we consciously slow down the breath and mentally take it along a particular pathway, we influence the flow of prana in that pathway. It is a kind of induction. It is like inducing an electrical current in a wire with a magnet. So, using the breath in coordination with the mind, we are able to engage in selective purification of a particular channel in our nervous system that plays a leading role in the rise of enlightenment. This channel is the tiny thread-like nerve that runs up inside the spine and through the brain. It is called the "sushumna." Purifying and opening this nerve is where pranayama and additional advanced yoga practices will be focused.

We will begin with a breathing technique to be done right before each meditation session. As we become comfortable with it we will add on new elements, step by step, that will greatly increase the power of our practice.

The guru is in you.

Lesson 41* – Spinal Breathing Pranayama

We will now begin an advanced pranayama practice called spinal breathing. It has several components to it, and is done right before our daily meditation sessions. The procedure of meditation will not change in any way. First we do our pranayama. Then we do our meditation.

Sit comfortably with back support, and close your eyes just as you do when you meditate. Now, keeping your mouth closed, breathe in and out slowly and deeply through your nose, but not to the extreme. Be relaxed and easy about it, breathing as slowly and deeply as possible without discomfort. There is no need to be heroic. Work your muscles so each breath begins in your belly and fills you up through your chest to the top of your collarbones, and then comes back down slowly. Next, with each rising inhalation of the breath, allow your attention to travel upward inside a tiny thread, or tube, you visualize beginning at your perineum, continuing up through the center of your spine, and up through the stem of your brain to the center of your head. At the center of your head the tiny nerve makes a turn forward to the point between your eyebrows. With one slow, deep inhalation let your attention travel gradually inside the nerve from the perineum all the way to the point between the eyebrows. As you exhale, retrace this path from the point between the eyebrows all the way back down to the perineum. Then, come back up to the point between the eyebrows with the next inhalation, and down to the perineum with the next exhalation, and so on.

Begin by doing this spinal breathing practice for five minutes before your regular meditations. We don't get up between pranayama and meditation. Just keep your seat, and begin meditation when your pranayama time is up. Take a minute or so before effortlessly beginning the mantra, just as originally instructed. Once you get comfortable in the routine of doing pranayama and meditation, one after the other, increase the time of pranayama to ten minutes. You will be doing ten minutes of pranayama and twenty minutes of meditation twice each day. Continue with this practice.

In a week or so, or whenever you are feeling steady with the ten minutes of pranayama before your meditation, add the following features: On the exhalations, allow your epiglottis to close enough so that there is a small restriction of the air leaving your lungs. This is called "ujjayi." The epiglottis is the door in your throat that automatically closes your windpipe (trachea) when you hold your breath or swallow. By partially closing it as you exhale, a fine hissing sound will occur in your throat. Be easy about it. Don't strain. Keep the slow, deep rhythm of breathing you have become accustomed to as you add this small restriction in the throat during exhalations. On the inhalations, allow the throat to relax and open more than usual. Do not restrict the air coming in. Rather, allow the deepest part of your throat to open wide, comfortably. Do not change the slow, deep rhythm of breathing you have been doing. Keep your mouth closed during pranayama. An exception would be if your nose is stopped up and you can't breath easily through it. In that case, use your mouth.

While all of these mechanical actions may seem complicated at first, they will quickly become habit as you practice. Once the mechanical habits are in place, all you will have to do during pranayama is easily allow the attention to travel up and down inside the spinal nerve with your automatic slow deep breathing. When you realize that your attention has slipped away from this easy up and down procedure of traveling inside the nerve during spinal breathing, you will just easily come back to it. No forcing, and no strain. We easily come back to the prescribed route of attention in pranayama, just as we easily come back to the mantra in meditation.

This pranayama will quiet the nervous system, and provide a fertile ground for deep meditation. With this beginning in spinal breathing, we are also laying the foundation for additional practices that will greatly enhance the flow of prana in the body. Once we have stabilized the practices we have learned so far, we will be ready to begin gently awakening the huge storehouse of prana near the base of our spine.

The guru is in you.

Addition – Over the months, several have written and asked about a form of pranayama called "nadi shodana." This is alternate nostril breathing. It is one of the most basic breathing techniques, and is usually the first breathing method taught to beginning students in hatha yoga classes. These days it is also taught by mental health professionals due to its calming influence on the nervous system. Nadi shodana is done by breathing slowly out and then in with one nostril blocked by the thumb of one hand, and then slowly out and in with the other nostril blocked by the middle finger of the same hand. That is all there is to it. It is a well-known practice that brings almost immediate relaxation. Why is it not taught in the Advanced Yoga Practices lessons?

The reason nadi shodana is not used here is because spinal breathing includes the benefits of nadi shodana, plus it is a tremendously more powerful practice with effects extending far beyond those of nadi shodana. The calming effects of nadi shodana come primarily from a reduction of the breath rate by using one nostril at a time – restraint of breath. In spinal breathing, the breath is restrained on inhalation voluntarily with the lungs and on exhalation with ujjayi (partially closed epiglottis), while the attention is used in the particular way of tracing the spinal nerve discussed in this lesson. While spinal breathing does not include alternating nostril breathing, this is not a shortcoming. Otherwise nadi shodana would be included along with spinal breathing. It is possible to do both practices at the same time, but it would be complicating our practice for very little gain. That is one of the guiding principles in all of these lessons – Is there a substantial benefit derived through the addition of an element of practice? If there is not a significant benefit from an additional element of practice, we leave it out. That is how we keep the routine of practices as simple and efficient as possible. Otherwise we would be loading ourselves up with all sorts of supplementary things and risk losing focus on our main practices. There will be plenty of practices added as we go through the lessons that will have huge impacts on results. We want to save our attention, time and energy for those, so we can achieve the most with our yoga.

Still, if you are an avid nadi shodana practitioner, or are strongly attracted to it, it will do no harm to incorporate it into your routine. If you have time, you can do some alternate nostril breathing before spinal breathing. Or you can incorporate it into your spinal breathing session. Keep in mind that nadi shodana is not recommended if you are beginner in spinal breathing. There is plenty to learn in taking up spinal breathing – new habits to develop – and nadi shodana is not in the mix for the reasons mentioned. But, since it has been asked about by several people, and perhaps wondered about by others, it is covered here.

It should also be mentioned that nadi shodana is sometimes taught in combination with voluntary breath suspension. Breath suspension is an advanced practice and is discussed in detail later in the lessons. Nadi shodana with breath suspension is a different practice altogether, and can be hazardous if done without a good understanding of correct methodology and the effects. If you are a beginner and contemplating using breath suspension (holding the breath in or out) with nadi shodana or spinal breathing, it is suggested you wait until we get into it in these lessons, which is at lesson #91 and beyond. The Sanskrit word for breath suspension is "kumbhaka."

So, for now, it is recommended you develop a good understanding of spinal breathing and get the habit solidly in place, with as few distractions as possible. The following Q&As will help with that. Later on, there will be plenty more to add. One step at a time…

Lesson 42 – Is this Pranayama Natural?

Q: I am struggling to incorporate all the pieces involved in the spinal breathing, and am not getting much out of it so far. It seems contradictory to your repeated mention of how "natural" these practices are supposed to be. It is certainly different from meditation, which I find to be very easy and enjoyable. Is pranayama supposed to be easy and enjoyable too?

A: Yes, pranayama will become easy. And enjoyable is an understatement. Ecstatic is a better description for what pranayama becomes. It may take some time to get it together though. Take your time building up to it. Give it a fair chance in your regular practice, and you will not regret it. There will be help coming in the form of new elements of practice that will make pranayama much more pleasurable to do. You will learn how to light everything up from the inside. But first things first. Get the basic habits of practice in place. Over time, it gets progressively easier and more enjoyable. Meditation is easy and enjoyable from the start for most people. With pranayama, it might take a little longer.

Is pranayama natural? There is no doubt that pranayama, with all of its supplementary pieces, is a complex practice, and it may not feel natural at the start. However, as with meditation, pranayama is tapping a natural ability inherent in us. In the case of meditation, it is the mind's natural ability to become quiet and experience pure bliss consciousness. Just set up the proper condition in meditation and the mind becomes quiet all by itself. In the case of pranayama, we are tapping the nervous system's natural ability to refine and become ecstatically radiant from within. Setting up the initial conditions takes more doing. But once we have taken the necessary steps through pranayama, the condition of ecstatic radiance comes up naturally. Once it gets going, it is completely automatic. It is then that you know without any doubt that your body was designed to sustain divine ecstasy – quite a revelation. Just as inner silent bliss consciousness is our natural state brought up through meditation, so too is ecstatic radiance our natural state brought up through pranayama. Once stimulated through pranayama, ecstatic radiance deepens in meditation. Pranayama cultivates the soil of our nervous system to the point where meditation is capable of yielding a dynamic flowering of pure bliss consciousness. Pranayama enables the silent seed we are awakening in meditation to grow into ecstatic radiance, and this overflows generously into our daily life.

The objective here is to structure the advanced yoga practices to be as easy as possible, and be pleasurable and fun. Otherwise, not many will want to bother with it. Patient persistence will sometimes be required during formative stages of practice. With your ongoing commitment to daily practice, experiences will keep advancing. In time, you will be rushing to get to your meditation seat, because the ecstasy coming up there will be so great. Then, before you know it, the ecstasy will be everywhere. The whole world will be transforming before your loving eyes.

The guru is in you.

Lesson 43 – Relationship of Pranayama to Meditation

Q: I am having wonderful blissful feelings in my first pranayama sessions, and they are flowing over into my meditation period. I found myself swaying with pleasurable feelings coming up my spine, covering me with goosebumps. I found my attention drifting back into spinal breathing during my meditation. Is this okay? What is the relationship between pranayama and meditation? Is pranayama a kind of meditation? Can pranayama stand alone as spiritual practice without the meditation we have learned?

A: Your early experiences are beautiful, a wonderful taste of things to come. Let them inspire you to carry on along the path toward enlightenment. With regular practice of pranayama and meditation your experiences will go much deeper.

If there are movements during pranayama or meditation, don't mind them too much. This applies to either pleasurable movements, or unpleasurable ones. Just easily go back to the procedure of the practice you are doing, whether it be pranayama or meditation. If the movements persist to the point where you are unable to easily go back to your practice, then let your attention rest with the movements for a while, not favoring or resisting them. Once they settle down a bit you should be able to effortlessly go back to your practice.

Pleasurable movements, and pleasurable feelings without movements, can be tricky when they arise in pranayama and meditation. We tend to be attracted to these. It is natural. The tricky part is in not confusing the rise of pleasure with practice, and becoming unduly focused on the pleasure. Keep in mind that these experiences are rising due to correct practice of pranayama and meditation. In order to advance, we must continue our practices and not fall off them into excessive attention on the ecstatic experiences that will be coming up. This is not to say these experiences are not welcome. Certainly they are – we are doing advanced yoga practices so we can rise to a life in ecstasy! As we continue our daily practices, ecstatic experiences will overflow and become a regular part of our daily life. This is what we want. So, if they are coming up during our pranayama and meditation, we welcome them with joy and go back to our practice. This is how we promote the rise of ecstatic experience in life. We will be discussing the topic of maintaining the integrity of our practices during ongoing experiences of ecstasy in more detail later on. In time, ecstasy will become the predominant experience during our practices, and this presents a unique challenge on the road to enlightenment. It is a most enjoyable challenge.

It will happen sometimes that we will find ourselves doing pranayama during meditation, or vise versa. When this happens, we just easily go back to the practice we are supposed to be doing at that time. We should not attempt to do both at once. Both rely on the simplicity of attention, i.e., easily favoring the mantra in meditation, or easily favoring spinal breathing in pranayama. If we try and favor both procedures at once, we divide the attention and this detracts from both practices. So, first we do pranayama, and then we do meditation. This is the formula for maximum effect.

Meditation and pranayama are distinctly different practices with distinctly different purposes. Meditation instills in us the silence of pure bliss consciousness. Pranayama loosens the subtle nerves and stimulates the flow of prana in particular ways. This provides pure bliss consciousness the opportunity to flow dynamically in the nervous system. This is experienced first as the ever-increasing expansion of ecstasy, and later as the rise of universal, blissful self-awareness.

Pranayama is on the edge of meditation, but it is not meditation. Meditation is on the edge of pranayama, but it is not pranayama. You might say that they both come from opposite sides to the edge of the subtle boundary that exists between pure bliss consciousness and prana everywhere in us. By doing pranayama and meditation in succession we are dissolving the boundary from both sides. It is a double whammy. This is the great benefit of doing both practices.

Pranayama in its various forms has tremendous value, and we will make extensive use of it. It is one of the master keys to opening the human nervous system to divine experience. But, pranayama is not a replacement for meditation. Only through meditation can the nervous system be permeated with pure bliss consciousness. Pranayama and other techniques we will discuss aid greatly in providing the ground for pure bliss consciousness to come up, and they are means for its expansion outward, but they are not the primary cause of its coming up. Meditation is. For this reason, pranayama is not recommended as a stand-alone practice without meditation.

Meditation can be practiced as a stand-alone. It is a complete practice that will lead to a full flowering of pure bliss consciousness in a person over an extended period of time. This is why meditation was said to be enough for those who are not inclined to pursue other advanced yoga practices to speed up the journey. Meditation is the best single practice one can do.

On the other hand, practicing pranayama alone without meditation can leave the practitioner vulnerable in some ways. Imagine you plow a field, turning the rich soil over and over. It is exposed, fertile, and ready for the seed to be planted. What will you plant there? If you meditate deeply with an effective method, you will plant the field full with the seed of pure bliss consciousness, and it will germinate and grow strong, filling the field with joy. But what if you don't meditate, and you don't plant anything in particular in your fertile pranayama field? What will grow there? Something will. But what? Whatever happens to be around. Some desires, some thoughts, some emotions, whatever happens to be blowing over the field. To tell you the truth, a lot of weeds can grow there, because there is no crop of pure bliss consciousness filling up that field. This is why pranayama, practiced as a stand-alone over months and years, can lead to less instead of more. In some people this type of unbalanced practice can lead to increasing rigidness, egotism, anxiety, anger and just plain bad luck. Meditate every day after you do pranayama and you will experience the opposite of these things in great profusion – flexibility, compassion, peace, joy and lots of good luck. That's how it works.

The guru is in you.

Lesson 44* – Finding the Spinal Nerve

Q: I am having some difficulty imagining the spinal nerve. Does it look like a nerve or a tube? You mentioned both. Does it have a color, a taste, a feel, or any other sensory characteristic?

A: We effortlessly imagine the spinal nerve as a tiny tubular channel going from our perineum (the spot underneath, between the anus and the genitals) to the point between the eyebrows. During inhalation we trace it up the center of the spine to the center of the head, and turn forward to the center of the brow. On exhalation we trace it back down the same path to the perineum again, and so on, over and over, for our time of pranayama. If we realize we are not tracing the spinal nerve up and down during our pranayama session, we just easily come back to it. We don't force the mental image of the spinal nerve. We gently favor it. The details will come on their own.

What is the spinal nerve? What is this sushumna thing? Is it something we will just keep imagining in our pranayama forever, and that's it? Fortunately, not. Imagining the spinal nerve and tracing it up and down in pranayama is only the beginning. At first, it is like making a survey of the land where we have been told there is a rich vein of gold underneath. Then we are digging, and soon we are into the gold. Then the imagining, the tracing of the mental image of it, takes on a different quality. We find we are into the vein of gold and there is no more looking for it. We know where it is. It is shining in our face. Our imagination is supplemented by the growing reality of it.

So, imagining the spinal nerve is just a beginning, We have to start somewhere. As we trace out the path of it over and over again with the breath, something begins to happen. Something starts coming up. It may be feelings. It may be colors. It may be sounds. We will experience something. We just keep practicing, not detouring very much into the sensations that come up. All the senses operate in the inner realms, and we are gradually opening them up. How we first perceive the spinal nerve depends on our unique condition, our unique pattern of purification that is going on in both pranayama and meditation. However unique our pattern of purification may be, we are uncovering the same thing, the sushumna, the spinal nerve. In doing so, we are opening up our highway to the infinite.

What we are doing in spinal breathing is simultaneously finding the spinal nerve and opening it. We find it by opening it, and then we keep opening it. It will not be the imagination alone for very long.

Soon we will be adding powerful features to our pranayama practice that will aid in opening the spinal nerve more quickly. The breathing and imagination will get lots of help. When you are mining for gold, you may want to use some dynamite. There is plenty of dynamite available. It will soon be brought to you. Then you can be quickly uncovering something very real as you go up and down in spinal breathing. The spinal nerve will become tangible on the inside, palpable. There will be less imagining of it. You will be in it, experiencing the inner dimensions of yourself. Ecstatic radiance will fill you and start to stretch you from within.

At some point you will come to a realization that is both comforting and scary at the same time. You will realize that while you have been looking for the spinal nerve, the spinal nerve has been looking for you. In finding the spinal nerve, the spinal nerve has found you. Then the doing will shift. Before, you were the one doing the seeking, digging and digging. Finding the spinal nerve changes that. Now it is the awakened spinal nerve that is doing the seeking, spreading out everywhere inside you, and purifying every cell in you. You become a witness to a vast and glorious display of cosmic cleansing, and you are falling into an endless abyss of ecstasy. It is a humbling experience, and a gratifying one. Now you are witnessing first hand what has been recorded in the scriptures and truth writings of humanity for thousands of years.

This is what finding the spinal nerve is like. It is like being found. Then we move into a mode of surrender, accommodating the divine process going on inside, because we are no longer alone on this quest. We never were. We don't sit back and do nothing. There is much more for us to do – many more means that can be applied to facilitate the transformation. So we go on with our daily practices, and add more advanced yoga practices, as we are able to digest them. There is no resting on our laurels. We may be full with ecstasy, but there is more, and we will not stop.

The guru is in you.

Addition – This Q&A is provided to offer further clarification on the matter of visualization:

Q: For the last month or so I've been practicing the spinal breathing. Is it ok to visualize the breath ascending and descending in the "thin tube" in the spine as a light moving up and down?

A: Yes, your visualization for spinal breathing is good. Just be easy with it, and not embellish it too much. Spinal breathing is a simple process. When the energy becomes more lively going up and down the spinal nerve, that can be used instead of visualization. You might first notice cool and warm currents (lesson #63). There can be light also. That is the beginning of what we call "ecstatic conductivity." Because of the coming reality of the energy itself, a lot of elaborate visualization is not encouraged. Complex visualizations can end up distracting from what is really happening. We just use visualization to prime the pump. Once the water (inner energy) is flowing, we can go up and down the spinal nerve with that.

I wish you all success on your chosen spiritual path. Enjoy!

Lesson 45 – Breathing is Slowing Down in Pranayama

Q: Since I began pranayama, my breathing has undergone a change. At first I couldn't seem to find a rhythm, and I was behind or ahead of my need for air as I breathed slowly. But lately, it is smoothing out. I seem to have enough air, even as I slow down more and more. Sometimes my breathing seems to suspend at certain points in the cycle. Is this normal? Am I doing damage to myself when my breathing becomes so slow that it almost stops?

A: Your experience is very good. It demonstrates that much cultivation is going on underneath in your nervous system, and the life force is coming up from the inside to replace your reduced intake of oxygen. This is why you feel comfortable with your breath slowing down, and are without strain. This is a normal consequence of pranayama and it will not be harmful to you, as long as you don't force the process.

There is a great natural principle at work here. It is why pranayama is so effective for cultivating the nervous system. Recall that "pranayama" means "restraint of the life force." When we restrain the life force in a simple unforced way, something is created. The gentle restraint of breath creates a biological vacuum effect, a small suction on the life force in us. The body must deal with this gentle deficit of life force in some way. It does so by pulling from the vast storehouse of prana within the body, and this prana flows out from deep within the nervous system. This is a new dynamic in the nervous system, and the outflow of prana from within plays on the nerves with a great loosening and purifying effect. This process is at the heart of all the effects that come up from pranayama. Right behind the flow of prana coming up in pranayama is the bounteous flow of pure bliss consciousness, assuming we are practicing our meditation every day.

We are all familiar with the benefits of applying the principle of restraint in various areas of our life. If we gently restrain what seems to be our immediate need, we invariably benefit in some way. This is particularly true if we have been overdoing in terms of fulfilling our perceived needs, as we are prone to do in our consumption-oriented Western lifestyle. There is great wisdom in the saying, "Moderation in all things."

A very simple and obvious example is eating. If we gently restrain our food intake, we begin to burn the fat in our body to replace the reduction in food intake. This has an overall purifying effect in the body, and will improve our health as long as we don't take the process to an extreme and become anorexic.

The principle of restraint operates in many areas of life. If we restrain our spending, even a little, we find that we have more money. If we lose our job, which is not always perceived as a positive event, very often we end up in a better one. Life has a way of compensating for whatever is restrained, often with something better. There is no doubt that if we moderate our excesses, we find more in life. In many areas of life, we find that less is more.

This principle is also operating in meditation. As we easily favor the mantra, we are gently restraining the endless streams of thoughts that we are almost always immersed in. In meditation, we create a state in the mind where the attention is not focused on meaning. Yet, we are keeping the mind active with the mantra. We have not put the mind to sleep. So, with less opportunity for attention to cling to meaning there is a kind of vacuum created in the mind. What happens? Well, you know what. The attention goes to quieter and quieter levels, until the mind becomes completely still in the great silent expanse of pure bliss consciousness. By gently restraining the flow of mind, we create a vacuum that draws pure bliss consciousness into us.

It has been said, "Nature abhors a vacuum, and rushes to fill it." It is true. Much of yoga is based on the application of this principle to stimulate the human nervous system to a higher level of functioning and experience. We are not usually inclined to voluntarily restrain things that we consider basic to our existence. Yet, if we understand the principle of compensation that is operating everywhere, we will find opportunities to move forward in our lives with greater skill. Pranayama is one shining example of the application of this principle. As you will see, pranayama reaches far into the essence of what we are, and plays a major role in pulling us out, enabling us to become ecstatically radiant.

The guru is in you.

Lesson 46 – Which Way is Up in Spinal Breathing?

Q: Why do we go up the sushumna on inhalation and down on exhalation? Can it work just as well the other way, down on inhalation and up on exhalation?

A: In the beginning stages, pranayama can work either way. With basic spinal breathing, a case can be made for one approach or the other. However, later on, it becomes clear that learning spinal breathing going up on inhalation and down on exhalation is the preferred approach. It will become obvious when we get into new advanced yoga practices that involve deliberate suspensions of the breath when the lungs are full. At this time it is necessary for the attention to be near the top at the sushumna for performing yoga procedures in the upper part of the body. Also, there will come a time when the breath suspends automatically with the lungs empty in connection with the internal biology of prana being released from its vast storehouse near the base of the spine. This will manifest as an emptying of the lungs and then a drawing up from near the bottom of the spine. We will learn means to cultivate this automatic drawing up process that occurs when the lungs are empty, so the attention will be near the bottom of the spine then and not at the top. These two types of suspension of breath are primary determinants on which way we go in the sushumna with our attention during spinal breathing.

When our breathing stops, we know without a doubt which way is up. Ultimately, the direction our breathing takes us in the sushumna is not an arbitrary thing at all.

We will get into more detail on suspension of breath (called "kumbhaka") further down the road in these lessons (#91). By going up inside the sushumna with your attention during inhalation and down during exhalation, know that you are laying the right foundation for all that is to come.

The guru is in you.

Lesson 47* – Chakras?

Q: I have read about the importance of chakras in spiritual practice. What are they and how do they figure into the lessons here?

A: Chakras, also known as spiritual energy centers, are components of our internal energy anatomy corresponding to various aspects of our nervous system. They are vital internal mechanisms through which consciousness, as prana, functions in us. Philosophically, they are prominent in the religions of the East, and can be found in Christianity as well, for example, in the *Book of Revelations.*

How important are chakras in Advanced Yoga Practices? They are important, but not in the sense that they need to be intellectually understood for maximum spiritual progress to occur.

Think of your car for a minute. When you get into it in the morning, there are just a few things you have to do to get going on your way. You turn the key, put the car in gear, step on the gas and go. Then you have to steer, step on the brake, and so on. Driving a car is something that most of us can handle fairly easily. But suppose while driving we had to involve ourselves in every detail going on under the hood to make the car go. Suppose we had to pump the gas from the tank to the engine, fire the spark plugs, monitor the pistons going up and down and follow the torque through the crankshaft and transmission to the wheels. Suppose we also had to simultaneously supervise everything going on in the engine cooling system, lubrication system, air conditioning system, electrical system and so on. Could we drive the car then? Probably not. The reason we can drive the car as easily as we do is because we know how to handle the main controls. All the rest is automatically going on under the hood. We don't even have to think about it. The car was designed to be easy to drive, even though the technology inside it is complex.

This is just how it is in Advanced Yoga Practices. Spiritually speaking, we were designed to be easy to drive. We can use the main controls, and all the rest will go on automatically. We do not have to be involved in every detail. For the most part, the functioning of the chakras is "under the hood." There is a tendency we all have to get involved in the details of things. We are a curious species and we want to know how things work. We like to tinker. That's okay, but it doesn't have much to do with engaging in effective spiritual practice, i.e., driving the car. These lessons have to do mainly with driving the car, not analyzing the machinery under the hood.

Having said that, let's take a brief look at how the main controls we've learned so far affect the chakras.

In meditation, we are quickly calming all the inner machinery and going straight to the source, the silence of pure bliss consciousness. So, the effect of meditation on chakras is to calm them, to still them. In meditation, purification occurs according to the unique pattern of obstructions in the nervous system. The chakras are involved in this, but not in any predictable way. The purification goes the way it needs to, and all we do is follow the simple procedure of meditation.

In pranayama, we are tracing the inside of the spinal nerve up and down with the breath. The spinal nerve, or sushumna, is the main highway in the nervous system. Every other nerve is influenced by what is happening in the spinal nerve. It is the master nerve over the many thousands of nerves in our body. The chakras are rooted in the spinal nerve, spread along it from bottom to top. So, as we travel up and down, purifying the spinal nerve and increasing the flow of prana in the nervous system, we are also purifying and enlivening the chakras. It is automatic.

As we progress in our advanced yoga practices, we will be increasing stimulation of the spinal nerve in particular ways. In doing so we will be influencing the chakras. This will be done through practices that are both physically and mentally oriented. We will not be pondering the chakras as part of our practices. But we will influence them tremendously all the same as we utilize the master controls. We may mention a chakra occasionally in these lessons as we discuss the various experiences that are coming up. Too much focus on chakras can be a distraction to spiritual practice, just as thinking too much about the car engine can distract us from our driving.

We are doing quite a lot with chakras already in meditation and pranayama. It is going on automatically under the hood. So take it easy and enjoy the ride.

The guru is in you.

Addition – For information purposes, brief descriptions the seven main chakras are included here. Some of the comments here provide hints on practices to be covered further on:

- Muladhara – Means, "root or foundation." The first chakra, located at the perineum, where kundalini energy is first awakened.

- Svadisthana – Means, "dwelling place." The second chakra, located in the area of the internal reproductive organs. It is the dwelling place of the great storehouse of pranic energy, the sexual vitality. Once activated, vast energy flows up from there and spiritually illuminates the entire nervous system.

- Manipura – Meaning, "city of gems." The third chakra, located in the naval/solar plexus area, is associated with digestion, including the higher metabolism that produces enlightenment-promoting organic compounds in the GI (gastrointestinal) tract that radiate sparkling energy. Hence the reference to gems.

- Anahata – Means, "unstruck sound." The fourth chakra, located in the heart area. This is where the yoga practitioner first experiences the vastness of inner space, which is often filled with celestial (unstruck) sounds and other inner sensory experiences.

- Vishuddhi – Means, "purity." The fifth chakra, located at the throat. This is a gateway for pranic energy to rise into the head. It is also a key center for speech and communications. With daily yoga practices, purification and opening occur naturally in the throat, and the internal and external expressions of energy through this chakra open up simultaneously.

- Ajna – Means, "command." The sixth chakra, also known as the third eye. It encompasses the neuro-biology from the center of the brow to the center of the head, and the medulla oblongata (brain stem). The ajna is the command center controlling the ecstatic aspect of the enlightenment process, which is progressive and safe awakening of kundalini.

- Sahasrar – Means, "thousand-petaled lotus." The seventh chakra, located at the crown of the head (corona radiata). Awakening and entering it leads to the merging of individual consciousness with infinite divine consciousness. Awakening the sahasrar prematurely can lead to many troubles in a nervous system that has not been sufficiently purified beforehand. Awakening the ajna (third eye) first prepares the entire nervous system, while at the same time indirectly opening the sahasrar in a way that is compatible with a rate of overall purification the practitioner can comfortably regulate and sustain – progressive, yet safe. This is covered in detail later in the lessons (#199).

Lesson 48 – Pranayama and Health

Q: Does doing pranayama have any practical health benefits? It seems like it would.

A: Yes. As with meditation, pranayama promotes purification in the nervous system. Being a physical process, it also has direct effects in the body that we can readily notice as our practice progresses. It has positive effects on the lungs, the brain, the digestive system, the heart and the reproductive organs, just to name a few. It also steadies the mind and emotions. As prana flows increasingly in the body, a lustrous, palpable energy radiates from the skin, creating an "aura" of health and strength that can be beneficial to others.

But none of this comes overnight, or from irregular practice of pranayama. Neither does it come from "binge" practicing where nothing is practiced for days or weeks, and then excessive pranayama is done impulsively to try and take a big step forward all at once. It does not work like that. In this respect, pranayama is like any other kind of bodily culture. A little practice twice each day is far superior to a lot of practice days or weeks apart. The latter is not bodily culture at all, nor yoga, and can be hazardous to the health.

If you decided to become a long distance runner, would you begin by working out once a week, or whenever you felt like it, trying to run five or ten miles at a time right out of the box? If you did, your career in running would be short lived. For the best chance of success, you would start out running short distances every day, and gradually work up to your goal distance over a period of months. Physical culture requires regular, measured practice. This is how serious athletes train.

Spiritual practice is like athletics in that we are gradually training our body and nervous system to conduct and radiate a greatly increased level of pure bliss consciousness. This is a large undertaking that can be accomplished through many small, daily steps over a long period of time. The benefits of such an approach are cumulative, and noticeable along the way. Advanced yoga practices promote purification and balance deep in the nervous system, and some results will be noticed almost immediately after starting practice. One of the easily noticeable benefits is improving health. So, yes, pranayama continues the trend toward good health that we began when we started meditation.

It should be emphasized that pranayama is not a miracle cure that will instantly do away with the results of years of unhealthy living. In fact, if unbalanced living has seriously compromised the health, it may not be possible to undertake pranayama right away. A certain level of health, particularly of the respiratory system, is necessary to undertake pranayama. We never should overextend beyond our physical capability in pranayama. Our practice should be matched to the level of our capability. If we are weak, pranayama should be at a minimum, or not at all. If we are strong, we can do more. Always consider carefully before you commit to a level of pranayama practice. Meditation can be practiced by almost anyone in any health situation without putting an extra burden on the body. Pranayama is different. It requires a certain minimum level of health to be practiced safely and effectively. Be mindful of that and always gauge your practice of pranayama to your present physical condition so as not to put an undue burden on your body. For example, while meditation during sickness can be helpful, pranayama will not, especially if one is suffering from a respiratory illness. When the lungs are ailing, do not tax them. Neither would we go out and run a mile if we were sick.

If you combine good, old-fashioned common sense with your pranayama practice you will gain many benefits, including improved health.

The guru is in you.

Lesson 49 – Perspiration in Pranayama

Q: Pranayama before meditation is great. I can really tell the difference since we started pranayama. When I am doing spinal breathing, I feel like I am really sinking my teeth into something. After I breathe slowly for ten minutes, I am sometimes covered with perspiration. I don't get out of breath or hot or anything. My heart rate doesn't go up. I am just sweating like crazy. Is this a normal experience?

A: Yes, it is normal. It is a good thing. It is a direct symptom of purification going on in your nervous system as prana flows through in increasing amounts. You are not doing aerobic exercise, or anything physical that would cause such perspiration. It is the internal exercise of prana moving on the nerves that is driving the perspiration out through your body, carrying impurities with it.

The sweating will not last forever. Gradually, as the body becomes more purified, the perspiration will become less. Other experiences will be coming up that indicate purification also. These will be more subjective, internal sensory experiences. With pranayama, we begin with the physical and work our way inward, opening and enlivening the spinal nerve as the master control of the whole nervous system. With meditation, we dive completely beyond the body and mind and work our way back outward again as pure bliss consciousness. With these two approaches, we have the deep obstructions surrounded and are flushing them out in large quantities. Sometimes we can actually see it happening with our eyes. Hence the perspiration.

If discomfort, restlessness or irritability accompany the purification process, make sure to take an appropriate amount of time to rest when coming out at the end of meditation. The importance of adequate rest at the end of practice was covered in the meditation Q&As. Usually, pranayama will not lead to discomfort in meditation. It almost always has a calming and deepening effect. But anything is possible as the body is being purified, so be mindful about following the guidelines for dealing with the uncomfortable experiences that can come up from time to time. It is all the process of purification, and we each will experience it in different ways. So it is important that we each supervise our own practice. We should know our strengths, and take advantage of them. We should also know our limits, and work within them.

As a practical matter, if you are soaking wet at the end of pranayama, take a few minutes to dry off before meditating. Change your clothes if it helps you be more comfortable. It is not necessary to meditate in a puddle of your perspiration. But do not delay the start of meditation for more than a few minutes after completing pranayama. We want to carry the effects of pranayama into our meditation.

The guru is in you.

Lesson 50 – Managing the Time in Pranayama

Q: I love my pranayama and meditation, but there is so little time. I leave for work at 7:30 in the morning and don't get home until nearly 6:00 at night. It seems impossible. What should I do?

A: It has been said, "Where there is a will, there is a way." Near the beginning of these lessons we pointed out that desire is the essential ingredient. It is really the key. We can have all the knowledge in the world, but if the will to use it is not there, it is for naught. What we choose each day will determine our path, and the results. If we find ourselves in a situation where we are not able to act on our most cherished desires, then, sooner or later, the situation must change. With continuous desire, i.e., devotion, and a commitment to act, we will find ways to work around every obstruction.

How do we find a way to practice twice a day? There are lots of options. It requires flexibility to take advantage of the opportunities we have. The current routine is ten minutes of pranayama and twenty minutes of meditation. With the rest time at the end, it adds up thirty-five minutes or so, twice a day. With a long workday like yours, this may be too much. Not too much practice, but maybe too much time, particularly in the morning. You have the option to make it shorter. It's not the ideal thing, but much better than no practice, or getting frazzled trying to do too much in too little time. It is very important to do "some" practice twice a day – in the morning and in the evening. Two short sessions is much better than one long one. In the morning, time may be at the greatest premium, while in the evening you may have more time, but maybe you are tired then and don't feel like doing anything, even meditation.

Decide how much time you have in the morning, no matter how little, and work with that. Maybe it is twenty minutes, or maybe only fifteen minutes. Whatever it is, work with it. If it is twenty minutes, do five minutes of pranayama, ten minutes of meditation, and five minutes of rest. If it is only fifteen minutes, do a few minutes of pranayama, ten minutes of meditation and a few minutes of rest. A strategy that can work for you is to do your practice in bed as soon as you wake up, before you get up. That puts your practice first on the list in the morning, and not likely to be missed. When you wake up, just prop yourself up and begin pranayama. Then do your meditation. You can have your practice done before you get up and spring out of bed fully charged with pure bliss consciousness.

In the evening, you may have more flexibility on the time. If you are tired, know that pranayama and meditation will rejuvenate you. This will be especially true when we add on the next few layers of advanced yoga practices. Make it a habit to get to your meditation seat as soon as you can when you get home from work. If there is no time before dinner, do your practices an hour or two after dinner, or right before bed if you have to. This is not ideal, but much better than no practice in the evening. If you can, take a full thirty-five minutes in the evening. But don't try and compensate for a short session in the morning with an excessively long one at night, not at this beginning stage. It could create some discomfort. Later, when you have more experience, and your nervous system is more purified, you will be able to engage in longer sessions without creating discomfort. At this stage, in the current situation, do the best you can to get in as much of the thirty-five minutes of practice, morning and evening. If you don't have the time, design a shorter twice-daily routine for yourself. It is in your hands.

In the meditation Q&As, we discussed ways to do meditation while traveling, or otherwise stuck somewhere away from our regular meditation seat at home. These suggestions also apply with pranayama added on to the front end of our session. Pranayama can be done discreetly in public places. It looks the same as meditation – a person just sitting there with eyes closed. We are relaxed while doing pranayama. Our slow deep breathing is barely noticeable to an outside observer. So it is possible to do our entire routine in a public place. We probably won't be crossing our legs in a public place. That's okay. It's not a perfect world.

What about while driving the car? Many of us are spending an hour or more sitting in traffic going to and from work every day. It is a big slice of time out of our day. Can we be doing anything useful with it? Not with eyes closed. That's for sure. That leaves meditation out. But what about pranayama? It is best to do pranayama with the eyes closed. However, it is possible to derive some benefit doing pranayama with the eyes open, because it is a physical practice. Doing it while driving the car is far from ideal, but it can be done with some benefit. You may want to try doing some slow, deep breathing for ten minutes or so while driving home from work. You can also trace the spinal nerve up and down with the rising and falling breath, with your eyes open. Keep your attention on your driving. Be aware that pranayama is secondary. Be easy about it. Pranayama with the eyes open is less distracting than listening to the radio. It is your first responsibility to drive safely. There can be some pranayama there too; going on in the background.

If you are doing pranayama in the car, don't overdo it. When you get home, sit and mediate for at least ten minutes to sow the seed of pure bliss consciousness in your fertile pranayama field. We don't want any weeds taking root in those beautiful cultivated nerves of yours. If you are committed to your spiritual transformation, it will be your job to get in two sessions of practice every day. There are many ways to do this. Be creative, and always be safe in how you do your practice.

Of course, the ideal situation is to have all the time we need in the morning and evening. People who are self-employed or retired can give advanced yoga practices the time necessary to cultivate the maximum benefit. As they become experienced, they also have the option to gradually increase the time of practice to accelerate progress even more. Advanced practitioners who have a regular job also have the option for extended practice on holidays and weekends, and perhaps even on a daily basis before and after work. There are many ways to skin the cat. Later on, we will be discussing options for extended practice you can consider as you advance along the path.

Managing the time of advanced yoga practices is an important area of consideration, both for establishing regular twice-daily practice in the beginning, and for extending practice as more advanced stages of transformation are coming on. Be mindful about the time you have available in this life, and make the very best use of it you can.

The guru is in you.

Lesson 51 – Strange Gurglings in Pranayama

Q: Pranayama has been going smooth for me, and my breathing gets very slow. But something strange is happening. It feels like air is accumulating in my belly, and my intestines are making strange gurgling noises. That's not all. I've noticed a glowing mint-like sensation there too. What's happening?

A: This is an excellent sign of progress. It means that prana is being drawn up from your pelvic region into the digestive system, and air is being drawn into mix with the prana. You have food in there too, of course. Prana, air and food; these are the three elements that fuel a new process that occurs in our digestive system as our body transforms to a higher state of functioning.

Actually, it is the activation of the belly chakra. In Sanskrit, the language of the ancient wisdom of India, it is called, "manipura," which means, "city of gems," referring to the glowing sensation you described. The Chinese are less romantic about it; in Taoism it is called "the cauldron," referring to the mixing and cooking that goes on in the belly. By whatever name, it is a tangible process in the body that is stimulated by advancements in pranayama and meditation. As our body and nervous system gradually become purified, breath naturally begins to suspend, and a new kind of biology comes up in us.

But to what end? We know that mind and body are connected. The condition of our nervous system determines what we can experience. Advanced yoga practices work to purify and open the nervous system. This is not separate from our biological functioning. As we transform neurologically, biological transformations will occur also. In the ancient scriptures, there are references to inner alchemy and to magical substances such as "soma," "ojas" and "amrita/nectar" occurring in the body. These are biological substances that are produced as the body transforms to a higher state.

The process that comes up in the digestive system is one of the primary producers of refined biological essences in the body. From the digestive system, these essences go out and play a central role in further biological and neurological transformations throughout the body. We can readily observe these essences working in our body both during practice, and in daily activity. We witness the transformation going on within through our refining senses.

In time, the distinction between the body and the witness (our pure bliss consciousness) becomes blurred. They become one continuum. This transformation is as much biological as it is spiritual. The two are aspects of the same reality. So, we should not be surprised as biological transformations occur in us in connection with our journey. No stone will be left unturned as we enter our new life in yoga – union.

For thousands of years humanity has regarded enlightenment as something that is for a chosen few, as coming from somewhere else, or from someone else – a mysterious spiritual blessing that arrives like magic on the doorsteps of the anointed ones. This is an incorrect view of humanity and its capabilities. It is self-limiting. In this scientific age, we will come to know the process of spiritual transformation for what it really is – the result of a systematic application of specialized knowledge.

The truth is that we all have equal access to the divine life through our human nervous system. You can choose to be anointed if you are willing to do the work that goes with it – the work of applying the knowledge of human transformation, which is doing spiritual practices every day.

The guru is in you.

Lesson 52 – Big Little Nerve

Q: It is the strangest thing. I am doing spinal breathing, going up and down in the tiny little nerve, and the next thing I know I am in this huge blissful space, I think still going up and down, but I'm not sure. I'm not even sure I'm still breathing, but there is no discomfort. On the contrary, it feels fantastic. Am I still in the nerve when this happens?

A: Yes, you are still in the nerve. It is a very big little nerve. An amazing paradox. The inner dimension of it contains galaxies. Yet, you are sitting there on your seat doing this simple pranayama procedure in such a tiny channel in your body. If your breathing naturally suspends in that situation it is okay. Nothing to worry about. The breath will return to normal rate as you return to regular body functioning. We don't force the breath. It finds its own level according to the state of our nervous system during practices. Sometimes the breath may not settle down much in pranayama. That is fine. We just go with it wherever it is, breathing as slowly and deeply as we comfortably can. Other times it may settle down right away. It all depends on the cleaning out process that is going on inside at that time.

Be nice to yourself when doing pranayama. The benefits do not come from practicing heroically in a session. They come from practicing comfortably like clockwork in many sessions over months and years. Slow and steady wins the race.

It is a glorious mystery, this human nervous system we have – our doorway to the infinite. All we need to know is which levers to pull every day.

A couple of lessons from now we will begin to explore further means to systematically awaken that great realm within us. As we continue to practice, the play of pure bliss consciousness will become more and more dynamic inside. It will also become increasingly perceptible in our daily activities. That is when we might be seen singing and dancing down the street for no apparent reason at all.

The guru is in you.

Lesson 53 – Light and Sound in Pranayama

Q: Sometimes I see colored lights in pranayama, and hear sounds too. Yesterday I heard a crashing sound inside my chest and everything turned a glowing golden color. Then I was filled with a delicious humming sound. It was so beautiful. What am I supposed to do when these experiences come over me?

A: Such experiences are wonderful. In time they will commingle with us in daily activity for our constant enjoyment. During practice, we welcome them and then gently go back to our procedure of pranayama, our spinal breathing.

Keep in mind that we are engaged in a process involving causes and effects in our practice. If we favor the cause, the procedure, the effects will grow both in practice and outside it. If we favor the effects (the lights, sounds, and whatever else might come up), we will no longer be engaged in the causes, and further progress will be hampered.

In our current practices we are doing two things. First, in pranayama, we are purifying and opening the spinal nerve, which, in turn, cultivates all the nerves in our body. Second, in meditation, we are permeating our entire body with pure, silent bliss consciousness. From these two actions, everything else comes up. How and when it comes up is a function of the unique process of purification going on in our nervous system. It is unique because we each have our own distribution of inhibiting obstructions embedded in our nervous system. How it comes out is anyone's guess. But it will come out if we keep doing pranayama and meditation.

This is not to say that experiences of light and sound are bogus. Not at all. If they are of the nature of a "peak experience," you may consider them to be glimpses of truth you see as you are peeking between the clouds. In practices, you are in the business of removing the clouds. While you are doing that, you will get these glimpses. The more clouds you remove, the more common the glimpses will become. In time, there will be no clouds left, and the view of ecstatic beauty will be constant. Then all of life will be a peak experience.

The experiences that come up along the way to enlightenment should be regarded as milestones, indicators of progress that will inspire us to carry on with our practice. Once we zoom on past them, they have already served their purpose, and we are on to a new level. Maybe we will want to stop once in a while to enjoy the view. If we stop and look, that's okay. Soon we will be back in the car and on our way again.

Some traditions put much attention on experiences of light and sound, using them as objects of meditation. When they are not there, then they are imagined and meditated on. It becomes a goal to see certain visions. While this may be a valid approach for some, it is not the practice we are doing here in these lessons. Our goal is to keep it as simple and effective as possible. We want to be using as few levers as possible, the main ones that trigger the natural abilities within us that open the inner doors. There is only so much we can do at once, and do well. If we bog our attention down trying to do too many things, our progress can easily stall. This is why we first do the simple procedure of pranayama, and then do the simple procedure of meditation. If we do these correctly, everything else will happen automatically.

When the Wright Brothers were methodically going through the process of inventing the first successful airplane, one of their biggest challenges was in identifying the least number of levers necessary to control the airplane's pitch, roll and yaw. After much trial and error, they got it down to just a few controls that anyone could handle with some training. The principles the Wright Brothers mastered are still used today in modern aircraft. What we are doing here is the same. If we try and manage everything that is happening in pranayama and meditation, we will have no chance of success. If we identify the basic controls necessary to open the nervous system fully to pure bliss consciousness, and use them faithfully, well then, the sky will be the limit, and beyond!

The natural principles that govern human spiritual transformation have always been, and will always be. They exist in each one of us. Finding the levers has been a hit or miss affair for humanity for thousands of years. Now is the time for us, the human race, to get our collective act together on this.

Speaking of levers, next we will be adding a layer of new practices to our pranayama session. But before we do that we need to develop some understanding of what these practices are for. So, let's get a good running start, and take a flying leap into the deep end of the swimming pool. Ready?

The guru is in you.

Lesson 54 – Kundalini – A Code Word for Sex

"Kundalini" has become a buzzword in many of the innumerable spiritual communities that span the globe these days. It has within it all the elements that attract people – knowledge, power, mystery, intimacy, excitement, alchemy, romance, adventure, danger, ecstasy and more. But what is kundalini, really?

Put simply, kundalini is our connection between sex and spiritual transformation. There are a thousand ways to describe this, but in the end it boils down to the expansion of our sexual function into the spiritual arena, i.e., upward through our nervous system. Some say it is a "transformation" of sexual function, but that implies we are leaving our current sex life behind. "Expansion" of sexual function is a better description. As we consciously encourage the spiritual dimension of sex, maybe we will leave worldly sex behind, and maybe we won't. It is not for anyone to decide but us. It is our choice. Leaving sex behind is not a prerequisite for entering into advanced spiritual experience, not in these lessons, and not in life.

For thousands of years, the spiritual traditions of the world have tried to keep a lid on sex, usually to the detriment of their adherents, and sometimes with disastrous results. Why? Because sex is the greatest force in humanity. If it is not coaxed in a productive direction, it can be destructive. Lacking reliable means to enable sex for spiritual transformation, the tendency of spiritual traditions has been to try and squelch it. It is a fruitless endeavor, this attempt to squelch. The genie always finds her way out of the bottle. It is not possible to keep her in there for long. When she is not coming out to make babies, she is expressing in every other way through humanity – nurturing of the family, charity, the arts, philosophy, science, money gathering, politics, empire building, war, abuse, crime… You name it. Much of it is good. Some of it is horrible. For better or worse, it is all the expression of the life force in human beings, the expression of human prana. The great storehouse of prana in human beings is in the sexual anatomy. The key to spiritually managing sex is not in squelching it, but in giving it a natural channel to go in that will satisfy its evolutionary instincts. This takes some conscious doing. We need some more levers in the form of advanced yoga practices to facilitate the expansion of sex in a new and natural direction.

So far, we have skirted the issue of sex in these lessons. We have mentioned the "huge storehouse of prana" near the base of the spine. We have talked about prana being "drawn up from the pelvic region" during pranayama. We have described the beginnings of ecstatic experience as prana moves through the spinal nerve and spreads out through us. And we have talked about pure bliss consciousness brought up in meditation illuminating us with pure joy from the inside through our pranayama-cultivated nervous system. In all this we have skirted the word "sex." We could continue to skirt it as we move into advanced yoga practices that directly stimulate our sexual function upward into greater manifestation in the process of spiritual transformation. But of what benefit would this continued skirting of the issue be? Certainly not to your benefit.

We live in a highly scientific age. Above all, we want to know the truth of things, so we can apply it to better our lives, and the lives of others.

Jesus said, "You will know the truth, and the truth will set you free."

Don't we know it? Look what science (the systematic application of truth) has done for us in just about every field of human endeavor. It is spectacular what humanity has done with truth so far. We have lagged miserably in only one area – the systematic application of the spiritual truth inherent in our nervous system. Success in applying spiritual truth immediately addresses the ethical and moral problems of the world, and the widespread feelings of emptiness and insecurity that affect so many of us, even as we live in material comfort. The stakes are high, and we can't afford to skirt anything that has to do with applying spiritual knowledge in reliable ways.

So, will we be talking about sexual energy in relation to spiritual development? You bet. A lot is riding on it. We will do so in a dignified way. Consider it to be an extension of your original education about the birds and the bees. Now it will be about the birds, the bees and the angels. Along those lines. As we get into it, there will be some amazing surprises. It will be like entering a second puberty.

There is much more to be said about kundalini and the expansion of sexual functioning – about the inner dynamics of it. We will get into that as we review direct experiences. For now, let's focus on letting that genie out of her bottle in a direction she naturally loves to go in, up into our pranayama-cultivated nervous system. It is her home, her temple. There is so much for her to do there, and we will give her lots of help. Besides wanting to give us a good housecleaning, she is looking for her lover there, and we will bring her groom to her. We'd better. She will raise all kinds of hell if we don't. We will talk about that too.

We are speaking in simple metaphors here about a process that is embedded in our nervous system, an evolutionary process that is completely natural. As we do a few specific things in our daily practice, nature will take over. The metaphorical language of kundalini is about nothing other than the inner dynamics of your own nervous system. So it is with the metaphorical language of every spiritual tradition. It is always about the human nervous system. The nervous system is the common link, the one thing that transcends all differences, the one thing that gives everyone equal access to the divine regardless of race, religion, culture, upbringing, or station in life.

Everyone can sense the truth inside, how special each of us is. We are always on the edge of knowing who and what we are. It is so close, a part of us, but seemingly just out of reach. No more. If you really want to you can know the truth and be set free, just like Jesus said. The essential ingredient in this is your desire. You can open your gateway to the infinite if you choose to.

The guru is in you.

Lesson 55 – Mulabandha – Enlivening Sexual Energy Upward

Now we are ready to add some new elements of practice to our pranayama session. That is, in the writing and reading we are. In terms of your actual practice, it will depend very much on your time line. To review, you may want to go back and reread lesson #38, "What is your time line?"

Everyone is different, and you should only take on new practices according to your capacity. This means you should be stable and comfortable in your current pranayama and meditation routine before you undertaken new techniques. If you are borderline and go for it, you will find out soon enough if you are taking on too much. That's okay. If you find that you are taking on too much too soon, just go back to a comfortable level of practice and try again later. Design a more gradual approach for yourself. No harm done. The American president, Teddy Roosevelt, said, "A man's reach must exceed his grasp." That obviously goes for women too. That is how we progress. But don't lose your hand in the process. Use your common sense, and only take on what you can digest in a reasonable period of time. The knowledge will be here when you are ready for it.

It should be emphasized that the practices we will be discussing are not recommended without daily practice of both pranayama and meditation. If you try them without pranayama and meditation, you won't get much out of them. And you could end up going in the wrong direction, to boot.

So, with that, we will look at a practice called, "mulabandha." The translation for that is, "root lock." The words are much stronger than the actual practice. Everything we do here is gentle. "Gentle persuasion," you could say. We want to gently coax our nervous system to a higher level of functioning. Not force it.

Mulabandha is simple to do. Yet, it will take some getting used to. Just about all of the advanced yoga practices we undertake have to go through a clunky stage, where it feels strange until we settle in with it. It is like that with most things in life we try for the first time. We have to get through the clunky stage with just about anything new. Remember how it was the first time you cranked up a computer? Talk about clunky!

With mulabandha, we sit in pranayama like we always do. As we do, we lightly flex our anal sphincter muscle and hold it. That is, lightly. It is barely beyond the intention into the physical sensation. What we want to do is develop the habit of holding this light flex of the anal sphincter throughout our pranayama session. At the same time, while we do this, we lightly flex and pull up above the flexed anal sphincter, through the pelvis and into our lower belly. There will be little physical movement, just a little beyond the intention, just enough to create a physical habit with. Later on, just the slightest intention will be enough to send sexual energy flying upward. What we are doing now is beginning the development of a new sensitivity in the pelvic region. As discussed in earlier lessons, pranayama draws the prana up from the pelvis through a biological process having to do with the gentle restraint of oxygen in the body. We are now helping that rising prana with some direct stimulation, amplifying its upward flow.

Mulabandha is a physical maneuver that quickly becomes a habit. In the beginning, our attention will be drawn to the sexual sensations it produces. It can be distracting for a while. That is normal. The aroused sexual energy may want to go down as much as up at first. That is normal too. We just continue with our pranayama practice as always, easily favoring our spinal breathing. This brings the energy up and down in our spinal nerve. In time, we will feel pleasurable sensations higher up, and the event of sexual energy going down during pranayama will become a rarity, and, eventually, never. How much time? Days? Weeks? Months? It depends on the practitioner. It will happen with practice, and according to the unique course of purification occurring in the nervous system.

At times during pranayama we may notice that mulabandha is released. That is okay. When we notice, we just easily reestablish that flexed intention and continue spinal breathing. The occasional releasing and gentle flexing is normal, and has another name, "asvini mudra." We won't deliberately do that now. It will happen of its own accord. In time, a very subtle undulation will naturally occur in the pelvic region and above. Associated with it is much pleasure and inner luminosity. As sexual energy circulates up through the body, a new functioning arises on its own – a new biology. We are initiating it with these advanced yoga practices. Once it gets going, it is self-sustaining in the body both inside and outside of practices. This is how we come to experience continuous ecstasy.

The rising pleasure is good. It indicates the natural rise of the inner ecstatic biological functioning. We continue our practices as before, and we notice more and more pleasure coming up in them. That's how it goes.

Practicing meditation after pranayama is as important as ever. During meditation, we don't deliberately do any of the practices we are doing in pranayama. If we find ourselves in mulabandha in meditation, we don't favor it or push it out. We just easily come back to the mantra. We want to keep our meditation as simple and pure as possible – just that simple procedure of using the mantra. You may notice a change in experiences in meditation as more ecstatic energy is naturally flowing through the body after pranayama. Ecstasy is just one more thing that can be happening during meditation, like thoughts, feelings and physical sensations. We just easily favor the mantra, let it refine and disappear over and over again. This will make the rising sexual essences all the more pleasurable in the subtle nervous system. Meditation will be all the more effective as pure bliss consciousness rises, and permeates and expands inside the ecstatic energies coursing through the nervous system. Extraordinary joy!

Now let's go up to the other end of the spinal nerve, to the point between the eyebrows, and do something there. Believe it or not, this has to do with stimulating the rise of sexual energy too.

The guru is in you.

Note: Following this initial instruction in mulabandha, several people reported some difficulty maintaining and/or returning to the slight flexing of the anal sphincter without a more noticeable cue. So, a suggestion was made to coordinate the flexing with the breath during spinal breathing pranayama. This is an optional approach. Some additional exercises were suggested too. As long as some flexing is there during pranayama, the desirable effect will be produced. In time, the flexing becomes an automatic part of our internal neuro-biology, and much subtler. The suggestions are covered in detail in lesson #119.

Lesson 56 – Sambhavi – Opening the Third Eye

In the last lesson we discussed mulabandha, which is applying direct stimulation near the lower end of the spinal nerve (sushumna) to enliven sexual energy upward. Now we are going to the top end of the spinal nerve and begin to make a connection there.

A connection with what? This is one of the most amazing things about working with the spinal nerve. As the spinal nerve gradually becomes purified through pranayama and meditation, a new kind of experience becomes possible. We begin to awaken sexual energy in an upward direction near the root, and then we make a connection between the lower and upper ends of the spinal nerve. This connection is real and can be felt clearly by the practitioner as a kind of conductivity through the spinal nerve, an "ecstatic conductivity," if you will. The spinal nerve becomes a conductor of ecstatic experience. From there it spreads out through all the nerves in the body. This is perceived directly through all five senses operating inside the body. As the experience of ecstatic conductivity goes deeper into every cell in the body, the senses go inward with it. The experience is so pleasurable and captivating that the senses cannot resist following. It is a unique situation where the senses willingly go inward instead of outward. In yoga terminology it is called, "pratyahara" – withdrawal of the senses inward. It is a perfectly natural situation as the experiences of huge inner pleasure lead our senses inward. It is great fun too. Some say more fun than worldly sex. Well, you can be the judge of that.

With mulabandha we began the process of directly stimulating ecstatic conductivity in the body. When we first start this, it is sexually stimulating and a bit distracting. The vital essences gradually work their way higher, enlivening the higher energy centers in the body. Over time, the experience grows into something more expansive than worldly sexual feelings. To facilitate this process, we will employ more advanced yoga practices. Each level of experience comes up naturally once the door has been opened a little using the necessary levers. The body was designed for ecstasy, and even a small taste is enough to convince the skeptic. There is nothing like direct experience. The goal in these lessons is to enable you to have direct experiences, so you will be engaging in practices based on your own experiences, rather than by rote, or by blind faith. Your progression through the advanced yoga practices is designed to be experience-based.

So, what we will do now is stimulate the spinal nerve as it comes to the point between the eyebrows. This stimulation is called, "sambhavi." We will do this during our regular pranayama session at the same time we are doing everything else that has been given. Be sure you are stable in your pranayama practice as you consider taking on sambhavi. Things may still be a bit hectic with mulabandha. It is okay to introduce sambhavi with sexual energy bouncing around in the lower regions, as sambhavi will help bring sexual energy up higher where it will become more stable. Sambhavi and mulabandha work together that way – stimulating and stabilizing sexual energy traveling up and down the spinal nerve during spinal breathing.

There are two main components to sambhavi. First is a gentle furrowing of the brow, the point between the eyebrows. It is bringing the two eyebrows slightly toward the center. This is barely physical, mostly just an intention. It is only physical enough to allow feedback for a habit to form. Under normal circumstances it will not be visible to an outside observer. Maybe only a little in the beginning stage. With practice, you will find that this is really an internal movement reaching back into the center of your brain, pulling the center of your brain forward toward the point between the eyebrows. We begin this internal activity with the brow-furrowing impulse just described. It will evolve naturally after that, as ecstatic conductivity arises. You will feel it working inside your head.

The second component of sambhavi is a physical raising of the eyes toward the point where the furrowing is happening at the point between the eyebrows. The sensation of furrowing at the point between the eyebrows is where the eyes will go. This will involve some raising and some centering of the eyes. We keep the eyes comfortably closed as we do it. We don't force the eyes. In the beginning, they may not go as far up as we would like. That is okay. Do not force them. Just let them gravitate naturally toward the sensation of furrowing at the point between the eyebrows. Again, it is a subtle physical habit we want to cultivate. Once the habit in place, the attention is free for spinal breathing. All of pranayama is physical habit, except for the attention going very simply up and down the spinal nerve with the breath. As we become adept at it, everything will be happening automatically, with our attention completely free to be easily going up and down inside the spinal nerve, which will be transforming before our inner sight.

As we do these two things simultaneously, the slight furrowing of the center of the brow and the raising and centering of the eyes to that point between the eyebrows, we continue all the other elements of pranayama just as before. It should be pointed out that as the attention goes up and down in the spinal nerve with the breath, the eyes remain aimed up toward the point between the eyebrows. We are not looking through our eyes with our attention. Our attention is going up and down in the spinal nerve. We do not try and look at the point between the eyebrows with the attention through the physical eyes. The eyes are physically going there, but our attention is going up and down in the spinal nerve. In fact, our physical eyes aren't doing anything other than muscular. When they are going up to the point between the eyebrows, the eyes are physically stimulating the spinal nerve all the way back through the brain and all the way down through the spine to the perineum. We are using our eyes in a physical way to awaken the spinal nerve. Meanwhile, our vision (attention) is in and through the spinal nerve, easily going up and down inside. It is a new kind of seeing we are beginning, an inner seeing.

Depending on how far you have gone in purification of the spinal nerve so far in pranayama, when you do sambhavi you may feel a sensation all the way down in the pelvic region. Or you may not. Either way, the spinal nerve is being stimulated and purified by the combined effects of all the practices covered to date. It is only a matter of time before the ecstatic conductivity begins to occur and we start to "see," really see. When it happens, there will be more milestones we will observe on our journey home. First we will perceive the spinal nerve inside to be like an ecstatic thread. Then it becomes like an ecstatic string. Then it is like an ecstatic rope. Later on, like a big column of ecstasy filling our entire body. Finally, it goes out in all directions and gently encompasses everything we perceive outside our body. All this emanates out from the spinal nerve. So you can see how important traveling the spinal nerve and cultivating ecstatic conductivity is.

Even before advanced yoga practices, there is biological precedence for what we are discussing here. Perhaps at some time in the past you have noticed some pleasurable feelings in your pelvic region when you crossed your eyes. It is common knowledge that the eyes tend to cross and raise up at times during the sex act. There is an instinct there. Something in us knows how to raise the sexual energy up through the center of the nervous system. It is an inherent ability we have, a natural reaction that is observable even before undertaking yoga. With mulabandha and sambhavi, we are consciously promoting a natural ability inside us, just as we have been doing with all of the advanced yoga practices discussed from the beginning. And so it shall be with all the practices we discuss in the future. We are systematically awakening what we already have – our spinal nerve, our highway to heaven.

The point between the eyebrows is called, "the third eye." Why? What is it that we can see through there? In the language of chakras, it is called, "ajna," which means, "command" or "control." These two descriptions point to the importance of the energy dynamics that come up in our head as a result of advanced yoga practices. Not only do we begin to see something there, but we also are in command there.

Jesus said, "If your eye be single, your body will be filled with light."

This is usually taken figuratively to mean, if we are one-pointed in our devotion we will be filled with the light of God. This is certainly true. We have emphasized the importance of devotion on the spiritual journey. Without single-minded devotion to spiritual transformation, and action in the form of daily practice, not much will happen.

These words of Jesus also have a literal meaning – a very literal meaning. If your attention becomes centered in the single channel of the spinal nerve, taking it to the point between the eyebrows again and again, your body will become filled with light. This is how it happens. Sambhavi is one of the most important means by which the third eye is opened. In opening the third eye, all that is below is activated as well. Sambhavi has direct influence through the spinal nerve on sexual energy. As purification of the nervous system progresses, sambhavi gives us a great degree of control over the cultivation and rise of sexual energy. This, in turn, gives rise to the experience of increasing ecstasy in the body, which includes profound experiences of divine light surging through every nerve in us. Our body is "filled with light."

As this transformation continues, we also begin to see beyond the body. We find that the spinal nerve doesn't stop at the point between the eyebrows, but extends out far beyond it. As we observe this, our spinal breathing takes on a new dimension. The third eye opens!

The guru is in you.

Note: As with mulabandha, some people reported difficulty in developing the habit of sambhavi, particularly coordinating the eyes going toward the point between the eyebrows, while attention is going up and down the spinal nerve during spinal breathing. An exercise was given which helps to develop the necessary coordination for this. The exercise is in lesson #131. Sambhavi is discussed extensively in future lessons, because it is a primary influence in the rise of ecstatic conductivity in the body. In the topic index you can find a number of key lessons listed for sambhavi.

Lesson 57 – The Guru is in Me?

Q: You end every message with the phrase, "The guru is in you." Does this mean I am my own guru and don't need any outer guru or teachers?

A: No, it doesn't mean that. We all need outer knowledge to open ourselves to inner experience. The phrase is intended as a constant reminder that your enlightenment depends on you more than anyone, because it is only through your desire and action that divine experience can rise in you. It is only through your nervous system that pure bliss consciousness and divine ecstasy can be known. You cannot delegate it. It is only by you making a daily effort to purify your nervous system that anything can happen. It is you who are making the journey.

Maybe your journey means surrendering at the feet of an outer guru for your whole life. Or maybe it means purifying yourself by following a number of teachers over your lifetime. Whatever the outer relationships turn out to be, it is the divine expression coming from inside through your heart's longing that will lead you to them. What happens outside is a reflection of what is happening inside, not the other way around. This is the meaning of, "The guru is in you."

If we long deeply inside, we will attract the teachings we need. Then it is up to us to take advantage of the blessings we have attracted, and act. If we do, then there will be an expansion inside – an expansion of pure bliss consciousness and awakened divine ecstasy within us. We will find whoever or whatever ideal we have chosen expanding within us also. So, the guru is inside, even as we may be interacting with him or her in form (or forms) on the outside. Outer teachers and gurus are storehouses of spiritual knowledge and energy we attract and are drawn to on our journey to the infinite. Ultimately, our interaction with them is inside. Inside is where the rubber meets the road.

The guru is a flow of consciousness that begins in us, travels outward on our desire, connects with outer knowledge, and then expands inside us as the knowledge is applied.

There is the old saying, "When the student is ready, the teacher will appear." A question we should ask ourselves every day is, "What have I done lately to get ready?"

The guru is in you.

Lesson 58 – Step by Step

Q: My question relates to the effects of combining the methods recommended by you with the ones that I am formerly accustomed to. Will they enhance each other or will they be counterproductive? Relating to the most recent addition – sambhavi – all I can say is, Whoa! You could most definitely say I'm going through that "clunky" stage! The ability to hold anal sphincter tone, contract abdomen, breathe with a hiss on exhalation, cross your eyes to reach the third eye ... all simultaneously ... is really quite a task, much less to try to do it in a relaxed mode.

A: Of course, whatever you practice is your choice. If you are following an established teaching, there is no wish here to interfere with that. In that case, just consider these lessons to be "food for thought." If you are trying to piece things together yourself, then some definite advice is offered.

First, less is more in spiritual practice. Simplicity is the key. Trying to put together overlapping pieces from several sources is not going to help you, unless you are advanced and are filling in clear gaps in your current practice. You don't seem to be in that position yet, but you will be if you keep at it long enough.

It is suggested you simplify what you are doing. You will know you are practicing at the right level if you are having stability (and fun!) instead of knocking yourself out trying to do too much. The best measure of the stability of your practice is how you feel afterward in daily life. If you feel frazzled during the day, go back and stabilize your practice at a comfortable level. Always make sure you rest adequately at the end of meditation.

Remember that we are working with natural abilities inherent within our nervous system. The ways in are delicate, and don't work well if we muddy things up too much with divided attention. These natural abilities are:

- Our mind's ability to become still, opening our nervous system to the infinite field of pure bliss consciousness.

- The ability of our breath and attention to cultivate our spinal nerve, enabling our whole nervous system to become fertile ground for pure bliss consciousness to grow in us.

- The ability of our sexual energy to rise and enliven the spinal nerve to an ecstatic conductivity which expands throughout our nervous system, and beyond.

- The ability of the senses to refine and travel inward along the many roads of ecstatic experience.

- The ability of pure bliss consciousness expanding in us and beyond to reach a unified level of awareness encompassing all of existence. We come to know ourselves as that.

We want to stimulate all these abilities into their natural manifestation. This is the road to enlightenment. But we can't be successful by beginning with everything at once. Rome was not built in a day. We must develop each level of practice into a stable habit. It is like that in the application of any knowledge. We develop a stable habit at each level of knowledge. First we learn step one. We do that until it is well established. Then we can add on step two, stabilize that, and so on. If we try and do steps one through ten all at the same time, we will have little chance of success. It is like that with anything new we undertake. It is like that in academic education. We take class after class, working our way from the beginning gradually through to the end.

The difference here is that it is all being laid out fairly quickly, far faster than anyone can take on in practice. For some additional perspectives on building up practices, it is suggested you go back and reread the lesson #38, "What is your time line?"

If it is these lessons you want to use as your primary practice guideline, then, at this stage, it is suggested you don't muddy up your practice with other methods. Start slow with meditation. Get that down first. Then after a few weeks or months, add on basic spinal breathing. Get comfortable with that. Then, later, you can add on the practices in subsequent lessons. Take on practices one at a time, not all at the same time. This is mentioned over and over in the lessons.

The challenge used to be finding the knowledge. Now the challenge is applying it in an orderly way. It is in your hands.

The guru is in you.

Lesson 59 – Some Mantra Particulars

Q: I have some questions about the *I AM* mantra. What if I have been given a mantra from someone else for meditation? Does *I AM* have the same effect as *OM*? Can I use *I AM* for chanting? Can I use it during the day while I am at work? Can I use it as I go to sleep at night? You said don't use *I AM* during pranayama. What about using a mantra such as *So-Ham* with the breath during pranayama? Besides morning and evening, can I meditate using *I AM* in the middle of the day too?

A: If you are following another teaching or tradition, and it is going well, stick with that. That goes for any other mantra you have been given as well. In that case, just consider these lessons to be "food for thought." There is no wish here to interfere with existing systems of practice. These lessons are designed to present an "open system" of integrated spiritual practices that can be used by anyone to the degree desired. Beginners can start from scratch at the beginning and go all the way through with these lessons. Experienced practitioners can tap in anywhere and pick up a few pointers. Like that.

If you have decided to use these lessons as the primary source for your practice, then you would do best to discontinue any overlapping practices and follow the lessons precisely. There are only so many things a person can do at once. You can see there are plenty of practices here to digest. There will be many more advanced yoga practices coming. Keep it simple and go one step at a time. If this is going to be your primary source, there will be more than enough to do. We will leave no stone unturned.

The *I AM* mantra is similar to *OM*, but not exactly the same, so the effects are somewhat different. *I AM* has both linear and circular qualities contained within it, while *OM* is circular. "I" is the linear quality in *I AM*. "AM" is the circular quality in *I AM*. So you can see *I AM* has something extra. What is that something extra? It is a polarity. *OM* is well known to be the sound of kundalini moving through the body, the nervous system becoming enlivened as sexual essences circulate higher up and a new biology emerges. Many can hear it. *OM* is the sound of Mother Nature in us, and she is ecstatic bliss. Ahhh...

OM is Mother. But where is Father? As we become enlightened, a divine romance occurs in us. A joining. In the *I AM* mantra, "I" is the Father vibration, and "AM" is the Mother vibration. Recall that yoga means "to join." This happens on many levels in many ways. In meditation, we are refining the vibrations of the mantra every day to stillness, to silence, to pure bliss consciousness, over and over again. Using *I AM* as mantra, we are cultivating pure bliss consciousness fully through the nervous system, permeating the natural polarity that exists within us. We are enlivening both divine masculine and divine feminine qualities within us at the same time. This has a direct relationship to the dynamics in the spinal nerve, and to the dynamics of kundalini. More on that later. The thing to understand here is that *I AM* has some special characteristics. This may sound theoretical, but it becomes very experiential in time. As your experience advances, you will find that the vibrational quality of the mantra has a direct correspondence with inner ecstatic experiences that constitute a consummation of polarities going on in the nervous system. It is a complex, but automatic, process we stimulate with our daily practice.

Continue to be relaxed and easy in your meditations. All this theory means nothing compared to the simple process of meditation. Forget the meanings when you meditate. If all this meaning comes up in meditation, just treat it like any other thoughts. Easily go back to the mantra. Just meditate every day, and everything will come naturally. In time, you will experience inside what has been mentioned here.

Chanting *I AM* is not recommended if you are using it in your daily meditation. The reason is that we use the mantra for going inward to stillness of mind and body. Chanting is an outside activity. We want the habit with the mantra to be going in. In time, you will think the mantra once and be gone into pure bliss consciousness. Your nervous system will become habituated to dive into the meditative state at the drop of a hat – a wonderful ability to have in this hectic world. If you love to chant, find something else to use. Chanting has its own benefits and is wonderful, especially in groups. Stick with using the *I AM* mantra for going in with the simple but powerful procedure of meditation. If you like to use *I AM* at bedtime as you go to sleep, that's okay, but keep it inside. Keep in mind it can be very stimulating for some people, especially as we further awaken kundalini. That could keep you awake. Of course, it is okay to use "I AM" in regular conversation. That is fine. That is on the level of meaning. Meditation is beyond verbal meaning, on levels of inner refinement of the vibration of thought where there is much more power.

Thinking the mantra during the day while in activity is not recommended. When you are in the world, be in the world. When you are in meditation, be in meditation. Your activity will stabilize pure bliss consciousness in your nervous system. That will happen naturally if you meditate twice a day. In general, keep meditation and activity separate. Both have their purpose. Likewise, we don't deliberately use the mantra while we are doing pranayama, or vise versa.

The reason we don't use the mantra in pranayama is because we are already building many other habits of practice relating to spinal breathing. Spinal breathing is an advanced practice, and becomes more advanced as we add on the other things that we do during pranayama. There are breathing mantras like *So-Ham* that people use during pranayama. That is fine as a beginning practice when the attention is not going up and down the spinal nerve and also building the other habits that are necessary for advanced yoga practice. Because we begin with spinal breathing in these lessons, we skip the beginning practice of breathing mantra. Instead, we do pranayama first and meditation second. In these lessons we don't do both at the same time.

Twice a day is the formula for meditation. If morning and mid afternoon are best for you rather than morning and early evening, then do it. Take a good rest when coming out so activity will be smooth. Meditation three times a day may make you cranky. If you have a weekend or holiday, and are removed from responsibilities, you can try three meditations for a day or two. But keep in mind you are using a powerful practice that releases obstructions/impurities in your nervous system. If they come out too fast, it can be uncomfortable. That is why we rest after meditation, and then go and be active to stabilize the pure bliss consciousness in our nervous system. Find your steady pattern, and make it a routine. Regularity in practice over time is how to progress. Short intense practice for a day here and there won't make much difference. It is what you do day in and day out for months and years that will make the difference. Then the silence of pure bliss consciousness will come up and permeate every part of your life.

The guru is in you.

Lesson 60 – Unexpected Interruptions

Q: What do I do if my practice is unexpectedly interrupted?

A: If someone yells, "Fire!" or your mother-in-law walks in on you, do what must be done.

When you get done with the interruption, then, if possible, go back and pick up where you left off in the session time-wise. Don't start over. If you are out of time, then just meditate for a few minutes, rest, and go. If you feel irritable due to the disruption, then lie down and rest until you feel smoother. Don't meditate anymore then. Then go be active, and look forward to your next regular session.

If you can't go back and finish, then you will have to make the best of it. Know that resting quietly is the best cure for irritability. You can also use the procedure in lesson #15, "Restlessness in Meditation," for dealing with uncomfortable sensations that may occur in the body. The good news is that, after a long time of practice, the obstructions in the nervous system will become much less and the process will be much smoother all the way around. Then, if you are interrupted, it is not such a big deal. You will be in pure bliss consciousness every minute of every day.

But, even then, we aim for privacy during our regular practice. It is a very important habit to have. Our success in yoga depends on it.

The guru is in you.

Lesson 62 – Duration of One Spinal Breathing Cycle?

Q: How long is one spinal breathing cycle supposed to be?

A: It varies from person to person, and even in one person at different times. It depends on how the nervous system is operating at a given time. This varies as the cycles of purification are occurring. When the breathing is slow, there are few obstructions being released, but the preparation for release of obstructions is happening during the slow breathing. When obstructions come loose and are released, the breathing will not be so slow. The instruction is to breathe slowly and deeply with comfort during pranayama, not to press beyond the present natural limit. That limit may change from day to day, or even within a single session.

With the above points for basic understanding, we can say that a spinal breathing cycle (including both inhalation and exhalation) can vary from fifteen seconds to half a minute. It can be shorter or longer than this range. Don't set goals. Let your body tell you what is right. Sometimes we may need more air. Other times our breath may suspend completely during pranayama. It is a natural process. We just go with it and follow the procedure.

Likewise, we may notice changing patterns of breath in meditation, where there is no direct supervision of breath at all – just using the mantra. The body will purify itself when given the opportunity. Changes in breath are an indicator that something good is happening. Advanced yoga practices are working for us. We just stay with the program.

The guru is in you.

Lesson 63 – Cool and Warm Currents in Pranayama

Q: I think am getting it together with spinal breathing, mulabandha and sambhavi. My breath is going very slow, stopping by itself sometimes. I am getting strange sensations of coolness coming up from my root on rising inhalation and warmness going down there on falling exhalation. What is this? Is it a good sign?

A: Yes, a very good sign. A real milestone on the way to enlightenment. As sexual energy comes up it has that coolness to it, and the warmness going back down. So you are having a direct experience of awakening kundalini. It is one way the beginning is experienced. There are other ways. Not everyone has it begin the same way. But most everyone will have some form of the cool and warm currents sooner or later.

We can amplify those sensations of coolness and warmness to enhance our practice. It is kind of like pulling ourselves up by our kundalini bootstraps. This is accomplished by using the inductive power of the breath. We already are using the breath to induce the flow of prana up and down in the spinal nerve. Now we can latch something else on to that. The rising and falling breath has its own sensations of coolness and warmness built into it. This is a handle we can use in going from imagining the spinal nerve to actually feeling it. For those who are not feeling coolness and warmness rising and falling in the pelvis, adding this sensory awareness in breath can help it come up. For those who do have the feeling of cool and warm currents already, it can be enhanced. Here is how it works.

Purse your lips and suck air into your lungs. Do you feel the coolness of the air passing through your lips, through your mouth, and down your windpipe into your lungs? Now go the other way and push the air out. Do you feel the warmness coming up and all the way out through your pursed lips? Now try it with your mouth closed, just as you would breath in pranayama. The coolness and warmness is still going in and out your windpipe, isn't it? Now, let that sensation of coolness coming in the windpipe on inhalation go along with your attention as you come up inside the spinal nerve. You begin at the perineum and end at the point between the eyebrows, coolness all the way up. Don't forget the turn forward in the middle of your head. As you exhale, let the sensation of warmness that occurs as air comes out the windpipe go along with your attention as you go all the way back down inside the spinal nerve. And so on during your spinal breathing session. Like so much of what we do in pranayama, this is a habit that can be easily built into the routine. With a little patience you will get through the "clunky" stage fairly quickly. As with all practices we discuss, don't take it on until you feel reasonably stable with everything else you are doing. There is no rush. Too much too fast is not a help.

If you don't feel the coolness and warmness being induced in the spinal nerve, don't worry about it. It will come at some point as your sexual energy begins to noticeably stir upward. In the mean time, you are helping it along with all the means we have presented. There will be more means too.

Over time, the coolness of sexual energy coming up and warmness going down will change. It will begin to spread out and develop a mind of it's own. It can get fiery and expand into a column of swirling energies. This is kundalini coming awake inside. In our spinal breathing, we just continue easily, not trying to force any particular sensation on the energy moving inside us. At some point we will realize we are not directing what is happening so much any more. Instead, we are partnering with the energy inside, accommodating its needs. Spinal breathing is important in this, because it provides the balance of polarities necessary for kundalini to fulfill her destiny inside us. Spinal breathing balances the masculine and feminine energies inside. The *I AM* meditation also balances masculine and feminine energies, as discussed two lessons ago. Without that balance, things can get a little dicey. Kundalini can go a little crazy when she can't find her husband. Even in the smoothest kundalini scenario there will be some symptoms. If there is imbalance between the masculine and feminine energies inside, the symptoms can become uncomfortable. We will talk about kundalini symptoms, imbalances and remedies in subsequent lessons. The goal is to make the journey as smooth as possible.

Know you are on a great and wonderful adventure – a journey of destiny, homeward to your divine self.

The guru is in you.

Lesson 64 – The Ecstatic Silver Thread

Q: I think I have gotten a little carried away with the mulabandha. It just feels sensually very good to do it, especially moving it around, pulling it up and so on. Well, I don't want to stop doing it. I noticed after practices yesterday while I was walking outside that the energy I have been playing with in mulabandha is coming up in a very fine line, like a thread of pleasure coming up in my pelvis and lower spine. In my mind's eye it looks silver, a searing silver feeling, and is both hot and cold at the same time. Is this kundalini? My heart is swooning before this new experience.

A: Yes. A very good experience. A milestone. It is another way kundalini can manifest in the beginning stages of awakening. It gives clarity to the spinal nerve too. So be sure and take advantage of that added definition in your spinal breathing practice. You will soon find the thread going all the way up to the point between the eyebrows, and a direct connection with sambhavi will emerge. This is the rise of ecstatic conductivity in the spinal nerve.

As for the desire to engage in mulabandha for the pleasure of it, there is nothing wrong with that. Actually, if you are moving rhythmically with it, it is asvini mudra, and that is okay too, as long as you are responding to a natural urge. Was it ever said here that spiritual practice is not supposed to be pleasurable? Just the opposite. If it is pleasurable, it is just right. The path to enlightenment is a path of pleasure.

Having said that, make sure you do not completely disrupt the structure and procedure of practices with your ecstatic reveries. Remember, you are going for much more than beginning experiences of ecstasy. If you stay true to your practices, the experiences will steadily advance.

Spiritual practice can evolve into a wonderful ecstatic party twice a day. It will, and it will spread out into every corner of life. But make sure it remains a party with a plan. Continue to follow the easy procedures for pranayama and meditation. Remember that engaging the attention excessively in experiences will be at the cost of spiritual practices. As for what you do with it as it expands into your daily life outside practices, it is entirely up to you. Enjoy!

So party on, but do it responsibly. There is much more in store if you keep your practices intact no matter how good the experiences get.

The guru is in you.

Lesson 65 – The Pineal and Pituitary Glands

Q: When I do sambhavi as instructed, I can feel a pull coming forward in my brain, and a sexual sensation down below like you said. Does this connection have something to do with the pituitary or pineal gland?

A: That is great you are feeling the connection between sambhavi and below. Something good is happening. There is no doubt the pituitary and pineal glands are involved in the process of human spiritual transformation. The spinal nerve passes near both of them, and sambhavi affects them both directly. Later on, we will learn another advanced yoga practice called, "kechari" which also acts on the pituitary and pineal glands, as well as many other aspects of our biology and neurology.

The pineal gland is located in the middle of the head near where the spinal nerve turns forward. If you point your fingers into your head above the ear holes at the level of the temples, you will be pointing right at it. The pituitary gland is located between the temples, sitting in a bony structure above the nasal pharynx, the large cavity going up above your soft palate.

Awakening ecstatic conductivity in the spinal nerve awakens the connection between the pineal and pituitary glands, and this corresponds to the opening of the third eye, the opening of inner sight. It is a complex process involving the entire nervous system. Someday science will unravel all the chemistry involved in the human transformation to enlightenment.

For now, we will do best to consider such intricacies to be "under the hood," much the way it was suggested we regard the chakras in an earlier lesson (#47). Otherwise, we risk getting too involved with the internal details and lose focus on the simple procedures of practice that promote the opening of the nervous system to divine experience.

Our concern in Advanced Yoga Practices is with the main controls that influence the complex machinery inside, coaxing the nervous system and all the biology to a higher level of functioning – naturally giving rise to sustained pure bliss consciousness and ecstatic experience in daily life.

If you are a doctor, biologist, neurologist, or just plain curious, all of this will be fascinating stuff. If you decide to do some research on the internal workings of the enlightenment process, it would be best to avoid doing it during practices. Better to stick with the main controls during flight. Then, feel free to reflect on the machine's inner functioning to your heart's content after you have arrived back at the landing strip.

The guru is in you.

Lesson 66 – We are Arriving, Not Leaving

Q: I am a bit afraid that the pranayama practice may feel soooo good that I may lose complete interest in sexual contact with my spouse. Does this happen; and if it does can it be prevented?

A: The rise of divine ecstasy is an expansion, not a leaving. Sex is always a matter of choice. While it is true that the attention will naturally be attracted to inner ecstasy, it is also true that outer sex is turned radiant by this, becoming a blossom of the divine rather than an end in itself. This is what pure bliss consciousness and inner ecstasy do to all of life – illuminate it from the inside. Then pure joy is found everywhere. That is an improvement, yes?

The lessons will get into more on yoga and sex down the road – the enlightenment process as it relates to relationships, marriage and sex – not necessarily incompatible things at all. Key tantra practices will be covered also, so that outer sex can become a part of the process of divine expansion rather than a drain on it. Of course, all advanced yoga practices are at your option. That goes for everything here. It is up to you to decide what makes sense for you, and what doesn't.

If you really want to make the journey, you will find the way through. If you decide to make the trip, you will find that you are arriving, not leaving.

Your desire will lead the way, which brings us to further consideration of a very important topic: Bhakti.

The guru is in you.

Lesson 67 – Bhakti – The Science of Devotion

Devotion is the most commonly practiced yoga technique around the world, though it is rarely called "yoga." Devotion, the continuous focus of desire for a particular spiritual ideal, is so common that the world's great religions are called "belief systems" or "faiths," as if nothing else but that exists in spiritual practice. What is this thing called devotion? Why is it so important?

The importance of desire was discussed early in these lessons, and has been mentioned often ever since. At first we looked at the purely logical aspects of devotion. If we have an idea about something, a vision of it, and an ongoing desire to attain it, then we have a mental and emotional vehicle that will enable us to act in order to get there. Considering a trip to a beautiful place called California was given as an example. If we never were able to imagine the place, had no knowledge of it, how could we ever decide to go there? So, first comes an image. Then desire merges into that image. Then action. Or maybe we have desire surging up first, undirected. We don't know for what. For something more. It latches on to one thing, then another, and then another. Finally it latches on to something big, a big idea: "Enlightenment." Then we set out for that, knowing it is the most we can attain. Desire is always looking for more. Desire is always looking for the biggest, the best, the most. All the desires that come up in us are divine in their origin, and seeking the greatest possible thing in life. Desire is the primordial form of the guru. Obviously, desire alone is not enough to get us there. It must be aimed in certain ways.

Devotion is more than the simple psychological mechanism of placing an ideal in the heart and mind which we can then strive for. There is much more to it than that. Directed emotional energy, desire, has great power. The act of devotion, the act of desiring the highest ideal we can imagine, is a transforming power itself. It creates changes deep in our nervous system. If we have devotion for a high ideal, this alone will be changing us inside before we ever sit to do any pranayama or meditation, or any of the rest of the advanced practices. Devotion is the first yoga practice, the main yoga practice, and the fire that lights everything on the path. Without it, everything else we do is just going through the motions. Devotion to our highest ideal is the guru in action in us.

Like all of the other abilities we have discussed here, devotion is a natural manifestation in our nervous system. It is the one that is most obvious, coming up in everyone in one way or another. Yoga methods work to stimulate and open up the natural abilities in us to full functioning. There is a branch of yoga called, "Bhakti" that is concerned with optimizing desire and devotion to the highest level of spiritual effectiveness. Having a basic knowledge of the methods of bhakti yoga, and applying them, can have a huge effect on the course of our spiritual life.

Bhakti means, "love of God." If "God" is not the right word for you, use a phrase like, "love of highest ideal" or "love of highest Truth." Whatever represents the greatest attainment you can imagine. Whatever it is, loving it will change you, and inspire you to do all that you can to merge with that. We all know that love changes us. When we care about something or someone more than our own self, we are being changed. As the Beatles sang, "All you need is love…" Ah, if it were only that simple, the earth would be paradise by now and every religion would be producing saints by the millions. We are not there yet, but we are on the way. Love was the right start then, and it is the right start now. That is not love of anything and everything – scattered all around with no particular focus. That kind of universal love comes later, as the natural outflow of pure bliss consciousness and divine ecstasy come up. The kind of love that drives human spiritual transformation and all the yoga that brings it up is love of your highest ideal.

What is the highest ideal? Who decides what it is? Your guru? Your priest? Your rabbi? Your mullah? There will be plenty of suggestions. Everyone wants you to love their ideal. That's okay. It is a game that we humans have played for thousands of years. Love my ideal, will you please? Or else!

But only you can choose. Only you know what burns brightest in your heart. That is your highest ideal, that which burns like a beacon in your heart. Maybe it is Jesus. Maybe Krishna. Maybe Allah. Maybe your guru. Maybe the light inside you. It can be anything. Only you can know. Whoever or whatever it is, it is yours. It is personal. You will know it when you see it because it will burn like a beacon in you. It will be all goodness, all progress, projecting no harm toward anyone. It is that which leads you home to pure bliss consciousness and divine ecstasy.

In the language of bhakti, it is called "ishta," which means, "chosen ideal." You choose it. If nothing comes up burning bright like that, it is okay. Guess what? You are reading these words, and therefore you are moving toward your highest ideal, your ishta. Your highest ideal is in your movement to study, and perhaps an inclination to practice yoga methods. Your ishta is in you somewhere. Your desire is leading you to something. This is as much ishta as having a clear vision in your heart. Your journey is your ishta.

Bhakti begins with that very first question: "Is there something more?" The amazing thing about the process of bhakti is how it clarifies over time. At first, there is some fuzzy notion. Some desires coming up. A sense of mystery. That opening alone brings knowledge in. Who knows from where it will come? Then we grab on and start doing something. Some practices. Then some inner experiences start, some blissful silence, and then there is some clarity. Then we read the scriptures, and words that were just words before come alive with radiant meaning. After a while, our ishta becomes clearer. We find ourselves in a relationship with what is happening inside. All the while the bhakti is getting stronger, and we are falling deeper into the divine game. Somewhere along the way we will find the techniques of bhakti, and falling into the divine accelerates. Maybe we will read about the techniques. Or maybe we discover them naturally.

So what are the techniques of bhakti? Well, there is really only one. It manifests in a thousand ways. It is not a practice we do while in our daily sessions of pranayama and meditation. It is something that gradually rises in our daily activity. There are always desires coming. We want this. We want that. We want money. We want food. We want a lover. We want a new car. Even anger and frustration are desires – desires that have hit a wall, so the energy goes haywire in our nervous system. So many desires are flying all over the place, sending us hither and yon, crashing into each other. You name it. The technique of bhakti is in redirecting our desires, harnessing them. Some people naturally find this ability. For others, it comes up over time, as there is more silence in the mind and heart from meditation. The inner silence cultivated in meditation is underneath the desires bubbling up, so we can see them like moving objects. Then we are a bit detached from the emotional energy in us, and we can nudge it toward our highest ideal. Just a very easy nudging. No forcing. No big campaign. It is just an easy favoring of our ideal when we notice some emotional energy surging up. It does not matter if it is positive or negative energy.

For example, suppose we are stuck at a traffic light and getting frustrated because we are late for an appointment. A lot of emotional energy is there getting frittered away. So we are frustrated. Take that frustration and redirect it. With your attention you can easily let the red light go as the object of the frustration simmering there. Easily bring in your highest ideal as the object. It is much like meditation. You easily favor one thought object over another. So now you are frustrated about your highest ideal. "God damned ishta! Why am I not merged with you yet? I am very frustrated!" Now you have a real motivation not to miss your daily meditation. Not only that, your emotional energy directed in that way produces spiritual changes inside your nervous system. It opens your nervous system to your ideal. It is ironic that we can't change a red light with our emotions, but we can open our nervous system to the divine with them. It seems like a worthwhile thing to do, doesn't it?

This kind of procedure can be done with every emotion, positive or negative – with our feelings about everything we do. Does it mean we stop doing the things we are doing and run off to meditate instead? No. We meditate when it is time to meditate, and in activity we do the things we have chosen to do in our life. Redirecting emotional energy to our highest ideal will animate our actions, whatever they may be, and it will turbo-charge our practices whenever we sit to do them. When in practices, we do the procedures of the practices, not the bhakti procedure. To the extent bhakti is simmering in us from the redirection of desires during the day, our practices will be enhanced. What we want is to quietly cultivate a habit of bhakti in life. We will look the same outside, but inside the wheels of bhakti will always be turning. We will experience a rise in our spiritual intensity. It is called "tapas." Tapas is bhakti that is a habit and never stops, like an endless flame burning in us. With that kind of bhakti, all of life becomes spiritual practice.

Mother Theresa of Calcutta said she saw Jesus in the eyes of every disadvantaged child she helped. That is non-stop bhakti. That is tapas.

It won't always work for us like that. It isn't supposed to. Don't judge yourself on whether or not you were able to transfer your frustration at the red light into a frustration for getting enlightened. Just remember this procedure from time to time as you go through your daily life, especially if you catch yourself in a whirlpool of emotional energy. That is prime time for bhakti. Just an awareness of this principle of bhakti will set things in motion inside when emotions flare up.

The great nineteenth-century Indian saint, Ramakrishna, was a master at creating huge outpourings of bhakti. He would writhe around on the floor at the base of the statue of Mother Divine he worshipped, sobbing and sobbing for the slightest touch from her inside. The more upset he got the more he would direct it toward his ishta, the statue. He seemed like a crazy man. All the while his bhakti was working like a laser beam, slicing through every obstruction in his nervous system. By bhakti alone he merged with the divine.

The extremes of bhakti are not necessarily what we are aiming for here in these lessons, though it is up to you. Even a little bhakti goes a very long way. There is great power in it. So much so that we have to remind ourselves that intense bhakti can have a big effect on the rise of our kundalini, both directly through the emotional energy, and in the turbo-charging effect that bhakti brings into all of our practices. As with all yoga practices, we can overdo bhakti, so we must be mindful about that. Our experience is the best measure of whether or not we are overdoing it. Everyone has their own time line, their own pace for the spiritual purification process. Let your experience be your guide.

Because the method of bhakti produces predictable results over and over again, we can say that it is a systematic application of knowledge. Bhakti is the science of devotion – a powerful science indeed.

The guru is in you.

Lesson 68 – Relationship of Traumatic Experiences and Bhakti

Q: Four years ago my bother and I were in a car crash. I survived and he didn't. After that my life was hell, filled with grief, guilt, anger and despair. Then something happened. I just couldn't take it anymore. I longed for an answer, and something let go inside me. Immediately, spiritual knowledge started pouring into my life, and I knew what I would do for the rest of my days. Your lesson on bhakti rings true with me, though my experience with it has not been gradual. It came suddenly out of my traumatized state, and my emotional state continues to move me forward rapidly. What are your thoughts on this?

A: Traumatic experiences can often lead us to an awakening. While the sudden loss of a loved one can never be fully rectified by anything, if we are able to open, the process of bhakti will certainly try. The emotions are so huge that the slightest letting go, the slightest redirecting of emotional energy will have dramatic results. None of us would volunteer for such a mission, but in life it happens.

When trauma happens, whether it is the loss of a loved one, a loss of health, or other serious dislocation in life, a cycle of grief will occur. It begins with disbelief, then can go into denial, then anger, and then down a long emotional slope into despair. For most of us, there is little control while this is happening. Then, at some point, there comes a letting go. It can be months later, years later, or decades later. Maybe a letting go doesn't happen at all for some. Everyone is different. When it does happen, this is a crucial point in the process. Crucial in the sense that emotionally we may gravitate back to some semblance of the way things were before the trauma. It is normal to try for that. Or, we may let go into a divine space, as you have done. That point in the grieving process is a kind of crossroad.

Again, it comes down to the first impulse of bhakti, that question: "Is there something more?" If that question is there in some form, emotional energy will rush into it. That question is a letting go, and the beginning of the manifestation of our ishta inside, our highest ideal. It is also the beginning of the manifestation of the guru, and responses are stimulated in our outer environment by it.

It is an opening, a receptivity, a letting go that enables the bhakti effect. As soon as we surrender our emotions to a higher purpose, they become divine energy rushing in. Traumatic experiences put us in a position where we may have little choice but to surrender, or face many years of misery. It is a much more clear-cut choice to make than considering the divine quest while engaged in the smaller ups and downs of mundane life in the work-a-day world. The truth is, every emotion is an opportunity for bhakti – the very small ones, the very big ones, and every emotion in-between. The emotions will be there. The letting go may or may not be there. That is up to us. It is we who choose.

Having embarked on the spiritual path with a strong and continuing bhakti surge, you have found something sacred in your tragedy. Keep in mind that bhakti is powerful spiritual practice. Make sure to balance your practices to give the best chance for a smooth unfoldment of pure bliss consciousness and divine ecstasy.

The guru is in you.

Lesson 69 – Kundalini Symptoms, Imbalances and Remedies

Q: I am new to this group. I have been experiencing various symptoms of kundalini awakening including but not limited to burning sensations at random places on my body. Before beginning regular meditation (similar kind from another source) a year and a half ago, I was experiencing an intermittent aching at the third eye. I undertook some other practices as well from yet somewhere else. Now the third eye has an almost continuous burning sensation. At times I have felt prompted to focus on moving the energy upwards and circulating it in a systematic manner through my body. I have an almost continuous burning sensation at the base of my spine, however at the moment if I release the energy I experience "devastating" emotions such as despair, isolation and emptiness. Yet, I feel the need to continue and refine this practice. Any suggestions, comments, feedback would be appreciated.

A: You are wise to be taking a measured approach, gauging your practice to your experiences. The most important thing is to find a stable platform of daily practice that brings balance to the inner energies. Once you have that in place, then you can facilitate the expansion of kundalini in a more comfortable and pleasurable way, while being more aggressive at the same time. Finding this stable platform may involve doing some things outside your regular sitting practice as well.

First off, if you have not already, it is suggested you begin a light session of spinal breathing before meditation, only five or ten minutes. See if that brings some balance. See if you can find a platform of practice with only pranayama and meditation that is smooth. Don't do any mulabandha or sambhavi yet. Make sure you take plenty of rest coming out of meditation. It is suggested you suspend the other things you are doing for the time being, as they may be exacerbating the kundalini energies. If you are heavy into bhakti, having intense spiritual emotions, you should consider tempering that also. That means lightening up a bit for the sake of building a stable, effective spiritual practice. Bhakti is great until we hit a wall. Then it can become problematic. It can surely test us.

After all that, if you don't notice an inner balancing, consider backing off on your meditation time a bit for a while, keeping the spinal breathing at the same level, unless the spinal breathing adds instability. It shouldn't, but anything is possible. See if you can find a routine with just pranayama and meditation where you come out into your daily activity feeling smooth, with less intensity in the symptoms you described. From that stable platform, you can begin to add things on, step by step.

All of this may seem limiting, given your desire to continue even in the face of some difficult obstructions. There's no doubt the racecar can go, and there's no doubt you want to get on with it. However, it is a good idea to make sure the wheels are on straight before you put the pedal to the metal. Once you have done that, much greater speeds will be possible, and it will be a faster, safer and more pleasurable ride.

Let's look at some of the principles involved in rising kundalini and how imbalances can occur. As we do, we will look at some other measures you can take.

The metaphorical mythology of kundalini describes a union between Shakti (a name for kundalini in motion) and Shiva (pure bliss consciousness). As you know, Shakti starts out near the base of the spine in the huge storehouse of prana there, i.e., sexual energy. In the mythology, Shiva is located at the top of the head. So the way it is described is Shakti awakens, goes up through all the chakras until she reaches the top of the head, and there she finds union with Shiva who is waiting there for her. He is just hanging out there doing nothing, you know. They make love, and nectar (amrita) overflows downward, enlightening the practitioner. Very romantic, isn't it? Especially for Shiva, who sits up there doing nothing while Shakti fights her way upward (through your nervous system!) to find him.

While it looks great on paper, this scenario does not work very well. In practice, most of the time this approach is a flop because it assumes that Shakti will do all the work, and find Shiva at the crown. She will surely try, and tear up your nervous system in the process. Hence the excessive kundalini symptoms. Things can get so uncomfortable that practices can't continue, and then it goes into a long slow burn from then on.

The answer to this is to get Shiva off his butt and doing something. He has to get off his lofty perch and "get down" with Shakti wherever she may be in the body, which is everywhere once she is awake and coming up. While their union may finally end up somewhere "up there," Shiva and Shakti must be brought together everywhere in the body first. If this is done, some craziness may still be there, but it will be the craziness of the ecstatic union of Shiva and Shakti going on in every nerve and cell in the body, rather than the blistering chaos of Shakti's energy alone burning through everything it meets, all of which is in your body. In short, which do you prefer, ecstasy or agony?

This is why spinal breathing is the first recommendation. It directly activates both masculine and feminine energies, and it brings them together in a balanced way. The ascending breath brings Shakti to Shiva, and the descending breath brings Shiva to Shakti. It is a balanced relationship. Then, in union, they go out together to every nerve and cell in the body. With this approach, much more energy can be moved with far less stress to the system. It opens the possibility for much more aggressive spiritual practice than is possible using the Shakti-only approach. And it is a lot of ecstatic fun too.

It should be mentioned that with the *I AM* mantra, the balancing of masculine and feminine energies is taken into account also, as was discussed in lesson #59, "Some Mantra Particulars."

The rest of our advanced practices are also designed to be dual-pole in nature. We introduced mulabandha at the root and sambhavi at the third eye. In the future we will continue to take this approach of introducing new practices in a dual-pole way. Balance. The rise of ecstatic conductivity in the spinal nerve is a manifestation of this balance, the ecstatic union of Shiva and Shakti in the sushumna.

What about the crown? We have deliberately left that out of the lessons so far. It is called the sahasrar, the "thousand-petaled lotus." Later we will deal with it. It too must be addressed. But to do so prematurely can lead to the kind of "devastating emotions" you mentioned. First we want the third eye to root spinal nerve cleaned out and ecstatic conductivity fully established. Then, the crown comes into play naturally. It has its own connection to the sushumna. If we go there too soon and try to make a shortcut, we will pay the price. The surest way to approach the crown is via a sushumna that has been well purified beforehand. Going to the crown first and then purifying the sushumna is a formula for unpleasantness – lots of excessive kundalini symptoms can happen. Even in the smoothest kundalini awakening there will be some symptoms. There can be some aching and/or heat around the extremities of the spinal nerve, just as you described – third eye and root. With easy spinal breathing and meditation they should not become extreme. If they do, back off practices somewhat, as recommended, and try some of the further measures mentioned below.

Many other things can happen: Light burning sensations here and there. Some lurching of the body or sudden movement of air from the lungs during practices. Buzzing sounds in the head and elsewhere. The feeling of insects crawling on the limbs, or little pricks like they are biting occasionally during the day. Strange feelings in the feet that are both pleasurable and itchy at the same time – this can be smoothed by walking regularly. It can happen in the hands too. There can also be a varied assortment of goose bumps, occasional shivers, hot pinpricks, slight headaches and other weird sensations. All of this stuff settles down in time. To the extent any of it remains, it is overshadowed by the experience of pure bliss consciousness and divine ecstasy coming from inside. You will find things like these in a normal kundalini awakening. All of them are symptoms of obstructions coming out, making way for a new life in unending ecstasy.

If symptoms become extreme and we cannot smooth them in pranayama and meditation, even by reducing times of practice, then more measures are necessary. These can also be considered by anyone doing spiritual practices for prevention of kundalini difficulties.

There are three factors affecting the way kundalini energy moves in us – bodily constitution, lifestyle and practices. These factors determine our tendencies for kundalini energy to be balanced or unbalanced.

First is the bodily constitution. This is what we are born with. We each have certain tendencies in us that determine how energy (prana) will flow through our body. These are delineated well in the Indian system of medicine called "Ayurveda," which is all about balancing energies in the body. There are three aspects to our constitution, and we can have too much or not enough of any of them:

- Vata – Is our nature flexible, or moving around too much?
- Pitta – Is our nature focused, or fiery and angry?
- Kapha – Is our nature steady, or stuck in inertia?

These are the three "doshas" (aspects) of our constitution. We are each a different mixture of the positive or negative traits mentioned. Much can be done to balance the doshas. Ayurveda has many means for compensating for imbalances in the constitution, and this can help with excessive kundalini symptoms. Particularly helpful are diets and herbal supplements designed to pacify too much fire (pitta) and/or movement (vata) in the body, mind and emotions, which are classic for kundalini symptoms. You can check out the writings of Deepak Chopra, and others, for more on Ayurveda. See the AYP links section on the web site for these resources, plus Ayurvedic diet guidelines that can help reduce dosha imbalances.

The second factor affecting the way kundalini moves in us is our lifestyle. Are we doing too much spiritual practice and not getting enough activity? Are we working too much, or not enough? Do we keep enough of the right kind of company that is supportive of our spiritual commitment? Things like this are important. If we are having excessive, or even minor kundalini symptoms, activities that are "grounding" can be helpful. Taking long daily walks with a relaxed mind is one of the best therapies for smoothing out surging kundalini energies. Tai Chi, practiced regularly, is very grounding also. Yoga asanas (postures), which we will get into in the next few lessons, can help. Physical exercise in general is good for grounding the energies. A heavier diet during periods of excessive kundalini energies can help ground them. Grounding activities do not do away with kundalini. Rather, they bring in the Shiva component that helps integrate the kundalini energy into our nervous system. Such activities are good to do in addition to spinal breathing, meditation and other advanced yoga practices.

The third factor affecting the way kundalini moves in us is our practices. We have covered that up and down and sideways, but can always say more.

The trick is to look at your life from all these angles and determine where the root of an imbalance lies, and then deal with that. We started out on the high level of balancing the masculine and feminine energies inside our practices of pranayama and meditation. This is where we'd like to find the balance first, built right into our practices. If this works, then we can charge ahead, adding on more practices and going into constantly expanding experiences of pure bliss consciousness and divine ecstasy. If there is something else somewhere in our constitution or lifestyle causing an imbalance, then we will have to deal with that. Once we have, we can also go at a good rate of speed with our practices without unnecessary discomfort.

For those who don't have kundalini symptoms, just keep practicing as always, following the procedures of practice given, adapted for your personal capacity and timeline. Keep this lesson handy for a rainy day. Maybe everything will go as smooth as silk, and you will glide blissfully into enlightenment without a hitch. That would be wonderful. If there are a few kundalini symptoms here and there along the way, you will not be surprised after reading all this. This lesson will give you a way to review what is happening, and to consider making some adjustments, as necessary.

The guru is in you.

Lesson 71* – Yoga Asanas – A Wonderful Billion Dollar Industry

A billion dollars is only a guess. Maybe it's more. Maybe it's less. No one can deny that the teaching of yoga asanas (bodily postures) is a huge worldwide business. It is a good thing.

The important thing is that yoga has caught on with the public and become very popular. So much good comes from it. It doesn't matter which branch of yoga caught on in a big way first. All the branches of yoga are connected. If you do asanas, you will be drawn to pranayama and meditation eventually. If you do meditation, you will be drawn to asanas eventually. That's how it goes. Our nervous system knows a good thing when it sees it. Wake up the nervous system a little and it wants more. All of the branches of yoga are, after all, expressions of the natural ways that our nervous system opens to divine experience. In truth, our nervous system determines the practices, not the other way around. They come to us when we need them. It is amazing how that happens. It is the power of bhakti. In time, all of the practices come together automatically. We just have to give a nudge here and there. A little bhakti is enough to put us in nudging mode. See how simple it is?

It is no surprise that yoga asanas are so popular. We live in a world where human experience is based mainly on physicality. Our senses are yet to be drawn inward to the point where inner experiences will become as real (or more real) than experiences in the external world. So we are always looking for a physical solution. Yoga asanas begin to take us from physicality to more subtle experiences of divine energy in the nervous system. This is why asanas are so relaxing. It is their main draw. People do asanas for relaxation, for some inner peace. Yoga asanas are very good for that. They are also very good for preparing the body and mind for pranayama and meditation. This is the way we will look at them in these lessons – as a preparation in our daily routine for pranayama and meditation.

There are exceptions to the "relaxing" mode of asanas. Nowadays, you can go take a class in power yoga, aerobic yoga, and get a good workout. That is okay. It is not suggested for right before meditation though. We are going the other way in that case, to less activity in the nervous system, not more.

Asanas in the traditional sense are for quieting the nervous system. But more than that. They are designed to facilitate the flow of prana in the body, particularly in the sushumna, the spinal nerve. So you can see that this makes asanas an excellent preparation for pranayama, for spinal breathing.

Asanas are part of a broader system of yoga called hatha yoga. Other yoga systems include asanas too. No one owns them. In hatha yoga there are some additional practices that are more direct approaches to moving prana in the body. There is an Indian scripture called the *Hatha Yoga Pradipika* that goes into these additional practices. They can also be found in other systems. For example, kundalini yoga and tantra yoga use them.

It all comes down to what we were talking about in the last lesson dealing with balancing kundalini – the joining of feminine and masculine energies in the nervous system, the joining of Shakti and Shiva. Hatha yoga means "joining of the sun and the moon," masculine and feminine energies. We will run into this theme in every tradition, because it is an essential characteristic of the human nervous system. The Taoists call it yin and yang. The Christians call it the Holy Spirit (or ghost) and God the Father. The Christian patriarchy has tried to make the Holy Spirit androgynous, but it doesn't matter what they say. It does not change what she is inside us.

There is some overlap between asanas and the more advanced practices of hatha yoga. Some of these advanced yoga practices keep the name "asana," while others carry the name "mudra" or "bandha." Whatever you call them, they are mainly physical practices facilitating the movement of prana and pure bliss consciousness inside us. We have discussed a few of these methods already – mulabandha and sambhavi mudra. We are about to take on some more.

But first, let's talk some more about asanas. If you live in or near any town or city, the chances are good there is a yoga studio close by. If you have not already, go and take a yoga class. This will give you a basic routine to do at home, if you are so inclined. About five or ten minutes of gentle asanas before pranayama and meditation is an excellent way to start your session. If you are not inclined to do asanas, or don't have time, it is okay. Review the lessons on "finding the time" (#18) and "managing the time" (#50) back where we covered keeping up a daily practice of meditation and pranayama. These same time management procedures apply when adding asanas to your schedule. When time is short, asanas are last in the pecking order. If there is time for only one thing, the best choice is usually meditation. If two things, then pranayama and meditation. If three things, then asanas, pranayama and meditation. Like that. This is not to say that one practice is better than another. You may be naturally inclined to do asanas and leave pranayama and meditation behind. That's okay. It may even be necessary if you are having some kundalini imbalances. Asanas can help smooth out the inner currents. But if you do not have a strong urge one way or the other, you will usually do best to pick meditation if you have time to do only one thing. It is the deepest practice. It puts us directly in touch with pure bliss consciousness.

If you know nothing about asanas and live out in the wild somewhere, and are inclined to learn, there are plenty of good books and videos on yoga asanas. Any of them will do. (Also see the lesson addition below for an "Asana Starter Kit.") For our purposes here we are looking for some very simple bending and stretching before our pranayama and meditation. What you do is up to you. If you want to do more than five or ten minutes of asanas, that is okay. Some people love to do yoga asanas. It can become an end in itself for some. That's okay too. Whatever practices you choose to do, make sure you build a stable daily routine that you can keep up without undo strain or discomfort. If it feels good after practices for the rest of the day and night, you are in the right ballpark. Then you are in the best position to consider adding more advanced yoga practices at some point.

In upcoming lessons we will look at several additional advanced yoga practices that add stimulation to the flow of prana in the body.

The guru is in you.

Addition – Since this lesson was offered, and even before, many have written wanting to know what asanas they should do. Practitioners have even asked about the minute details of postures, where attention should be while doing them, etc. With thousands of hatha yoga teachers around the world, and dozens of systems of practice, the possibilities are practically endless.

However, there is something we can add to the asana discussion here. You know from this lesson that in Advanced Yoga Practices we regard asanas as a warm up for our sitting practices of spinal breathing, meditation and so on. Therefore, asanas are not the primary focus here. After all, in Patanjali's eight limbs of yoga, asanas are one limb, or one-eighth of the total of yoga practices.

You'll find more on the eight limbs later on in the lessons.

Quite a few beginners have written just wanting to know where to start with asanas. You know, starting from scratch with a few basic postures. That we can help with, at least until you can get to a class. Let's call it our "Asana Starter Kit." It is the least we can do. It will be very simple.

First we will cover a starter routine that can be done in about ten minutes right before pranayama and meditation. Illustrations for these are included. We will also provide an abbreviated starter routine of just a few minutes for those with little time, the rationale being that, when there is a pinch, it is preferable to spend most of our limited practice time doing meditation and pranayama.

Asana Starter Kit

We will look at a dozen or so basic postures here, which are done on the floor. If you have a mat, great, but there's no need to run out and buy one. A soft carpet with a large towel or blanket laid out will do just fine for this routine. Make sure you have your comfortable meditation clothing on before you start.

It is important that you not force any of these postures. If the posture calls for a toe touch and you can only reach your shin comfortably, stop there. That is the perfect posture for you. Never strain in a posture. In fact that is the rule for everything in Advanced Yoga Practices. It is the essence of self-pacing, and of all progress in yoga. Here is the routine:

1. **Heart Centering Warm-up** – Sit on the floor cross-legged. Gently massage your head with both hands as you move your hands down toward your heart – first down the front of your face and neck to your heart, and then down the back of your head and around your neck and down the front to your heart. Those two movements can be done in 15 seconds or so. Not too fast and not too slow. Now do the same thing with the left arm, starting with the left hand, using the right hand to gently massage all the way back to the heart – first along the top of the arm, over the shoulder and down the chest to the heart, and then along the bottom side of the arm, through the arm pit and to the heart. The left arm is done with the right hand like that. Now switch to the right arm and do it with the left hand the same way. Now do both legs from the toes all the way up to the heart – just a gentle moving two-handed massage on each leg. As you come up from each leg press in gently on your belly and solar plexus region with both hands on the way up to the heart. Finally, reach in back with both hands and do one moving massage from the buttocks, up your back and around to your chest and heart. All of these heart centering warm-up movements can be done in a minute or so. If you are wondering what to do with your attention during this heart centering, just let it be easy, going with your hands as they gently massage your energy toward your heart. Let your breathing be easy also. This is how we handle attention and breathing in all these basic postures, easy and relaxed with whatever we are doing physically, unless instructed otherwise.

2. **Knees to Chest Roll** – Lie on your back and bring your knees up far enough so you can grasp each upper shin with each hand. Or, if you can reach, clasp you fingers together around your upper shins, near the knees. Let your knees come toward your chest. Now roll from side to side, about five times each way, right to left, letting your head roll from side to side on the floor along with your torso. Roll as far to each side as is comfortable.

3. **Kneeling Seat** (Vajrasana) – Get up straight on your knees with legs nearly together. Put one big toe over the other behind you, and then sit down on your heels, keeping your torso up straight. Let your hands rest on your thighs or in your lap. Sit like this for about 10 seconds. (Use a mental count until you get a good feel for the 10-second hold on all of these postures.) Then go up straight on your knees again for a few seconds and back down into the seat for another 10 seconds. Go up again, and then relax. Sit on the floor with your feet in front of you.

4. **Sitting Head to Knee** (Janushirshasana and Paschimottanasana) – While sitting, put your left leg out straight and bring your right foot in toward your crotch. If it will go comfortably all the way, then let your right heel rest against your perineum. If the right foot won't go all the way in to the crotch, then just let it rest however far inward it will go with comfort. Now lean forward while extending your hands toward your left foot. If you can reach, then grab your left big toe with both hands. If you can't reach your toe, then just let your hands rest on your left shin however far you can comfortably go. Let your torso and head come down as far as comfortable. If you are very limber, your head may end up resting on your left knee. If it won't go that far, then just stop at your comfortable limit as you lean forward. Hold that position for about 10 seconds. Now reverse the whole thing and do it with your right leg extended and your left leg in toward your crotch. Hold it again for 10 seconds. Finally, do it with both legs out straight. This time, grab your left and right toes with your left and right hands, respectively. Or, if you can't reach, just let each hand rest on its corresponding shin at your comfortable limit of stretch. As with the other head to knee positions, let your torso and head come down toward your knees to a comfortable limit, and hold for about 10 seconds. Then relax. A more advanced version of the left and right head to knee posture involves sitting up on the heel, putting more pressure on the perineum, and holding a full breath inside (kumbhaka) while doing the posture. The breath is taken in and expelled using spinal breathing, and sambhavi, mulabandha and abdominal lift (see below – done while full with air in this case) are used during the posture. This advanced version of head to knee is called "**Maha Mudra.**"

5. **Shoulder Stand** (Viparitakarani or Sarvangasana) – Lie on your back with your hands at your sides. Bring your knees up and roll your buttocks up in the air, while bringing your hands under your upward curling back. Keep going up and straighten your legs and back out above you. Use your hands to support your back by propping them up with your elbows on the floor. Find a comfortable balance in this posture, and hold for about 10 seconds. It doesn't have to be straight up. The idea is to achieve inversion of your body. That is the main purpose of the shoulder stand. Before you come back down, go to the next posture.

6. **Plow** (Halasana) – While in the shoulder stand, let your legs and torso come down over your head, going toward the floor. Continue to support your back with your hands with elbows on the floor, as necessary. If you can, let your feet come all the way down to the floor with your legs straight, and let your arms down to lie flat on the floor behind you. Hold this posture for about 10 seconds. If the legs and back will not come far enough to let your feet touch the floor, then stop at your comfortable limit. In that case you can let your knees bend toward your shoulders for comfort, as if you are curling into a ball while propped up on your shoulder

blades with your arms supporting your back as in the shoulder stand. If you end up in that curled up position, hold it for about 10 seconds. Whichever degree of the plow you come to, after the 10 second hold, uncurl yourself gently back down to lying flat on your back with your hands at your sides.

7. **Seal of Yoga** (Yoga Mudra) – Sit on the floor cross-legged. Clasp your hands comfortably behind your back with arms hanging loose. Lean forward with your head and torso to your comfortable limit. If you are limber, your head may touch the floor. Hold this posture at your comfortable limit for about 10 seconds, and then sit back up.

8. **Cobra** (Bhujangasana) – Roll over onto your stomach, lying flat on the floor. Put your hands under your shoulders as if you are going to do a push-up. Lift your head and shoulders up using your upper back, with a little help from your arms. Your belly should not leave the floor. You will have a good arch in your back. Hold this posture for about 10 seconds, and come back down gently.

9. **Locust** (Shalabhasana) – Still on your stomach, lying flat on the floor, extend your arms with both hands, palms up, under both sides of your pelvis. Keeping your legs straight, lift your knees up using your lower back. Hold this posture for about 10 seconds, and come back down gently.

10. **Spinal Twist** (Ardha Matsyendrasana) – Sit on the floor with your right leg out straight. Place your left foot on the floor just outside your right knee. Your left knee will be sticking up in front of you. Reach with your right arm past the left side of your left knee and use your elbow against the knee to twist your torso to the left. With your left arm, reach around behind you, further twisting your torso to the left, and touch the floor behind you with your left hand. Turn your head to the left also, looking as far around to the left as you can. Hold this twist for about 10 seconds. Don't strain in the twist. Only twist as far around as is comfortable. Now, switch legs and do the same posture the other way, twisting to the right, again holding for about 10 seconds. Then relax.

11. **Abdominal Lift** (Uddiyana Bandha or Nauli) – Stand up, with feet shoulder-width apart, leaning with your hands on your knees. Take a deep breath and expel as much air from your lungs as you can. With air expelled, suck your belly in and up using your diaphragm. Hold your belly in and up like that for about five seconds, and then release your belly, but do not breathe in yet. Pull the belly in and up again for five seconds. And again for five seconds more. Now relax and take a deep breath. This posture is called uddiyana bandha. It can be advanced to be nauli when you have reached it the lessons. Nauli is covered in lesson #129.

12. **Standing Back Stretch** (Urdhvasana) – Standing with feet a little apart, reach with your straightened arms over your head and back as far as you comfortably can. Bend back with your spine as you do this, being careful not to fall over backwards. Hold this posture for about 10 seconds. Then stand up straight again and relax.

13. **Standing Toe Touch** (Padahastasana)– Standing with feet a little apart, reach down toward the floor with your hands while keeping your knees straight. Touch or grab your toes if you can without discomfort. If you are limber, you can let your palms rest flat on the floor. In doing this posture, your head may come close to your knees, or even touch them. If you can't reach, that is okay. Let your hands and head come down to whatever your comfortable limit is. Hold this posture for about 10 seconds.

14. **Corpse Pose** (Shavasana) – Lie down on your back with arms and legs spread a little, and relax. Let your mind relax completely. Remain in this posture for about one minute. Longer if you like. Now you are ready to take your seat for pranayama and meditation.

All of these postures can be done in about 10 minutes. If you are in a hurry, you can do them in less time, but that is not recommended.

These are basic asanas, and most of them can be done in more advanced versions. Nauli, an advanced version of uddiyana, is mentioned because it is already in the lessons further on from here (#129). Maha mudra is covered for those who want to incorporate the principles and practices of pressure at the perineum (siddhasana effect), spinal breathing, breath retention (kumbhaka), sambhavi, mulabandha and abdominal lift (uddiyana) into a single asana. Maha mudra is the posture for doing that, and it is an excellent way to loosen up the sushumna before pranayama and meditation. There are many additional postures that are not mentioned here. This is a basic routine – a starter kit. It is good enough to prepare the nervous system for sitting practices.

Abbreviated Asana Starter Kit

For those who are short on time, there is still the opportunity to do some limbering up before sitting practices. The trick is to do some twisting, abdominal lift, backward bending, forward bending and inversion. These are the essential elements that lie at the core of most asanas. Together, they flex and manipulate the spinal nerve, preparing it for spinal breathing and deep meditation. For that purpose, the following abbreviated all-standing routine is offered that can be done in a couple of minutes.

1. **Standing Spinal Twist** – Stand with feet shoulder-width apart and reach around behind you to the left as far as you can with both arms wrapping around your torso in that direction. Let your torso and head twist in that direction as far as comfortable. Hold this posture for about 10 seconds. Relax, and then do it in the other direction.

2. **Abdominal Lift** (Uddiyana or Nauli) – Stand with feet apart and do this the same as above.

3. **Standing Back Stretch** – Stand with feet a little apart, and do this posture the same as above.

4. **Standing Toe Touch** – Stand with feet a little apart, and do this posture the same as above. Besides flexing the spinal nerve forward, this posture also provides inversion, though not to the same degree as a shoulder stand.

From here you can go straight into your sitting practices. If you have the time and space to lie down for a minute (corpse pose) before beginning pranayama, that is good too. These four postures can be compressed down into a minute or so if time is very short, or stretched out to several minutes. If there is not enough time for a full set of asanas, this abbreviated session will be much better than no asanas. It does not require getting down on the floor, and can be done in street clothes just about anywhere.

Time is our most precious commodity in this life. Often, we find ourselves with too little of it. The topic of time management in our practices is visited periodically throughout the lessons, culminating with lesson #209, "Fitting Daily Practices into a Busy Schedule." There you will see how asanas fit into the pecking order in relation to all the other practices when time is short. We would like to do a full routine twice each day. This is how we speed our way along on the road to enlightenment. In this busy world, we are sometimes faced with having to make compromises. So we try and be as efficient about it as we can, prioritizing our practices and reaping as much spiritual benefit as possible from the time we have available.

See the illustrations for the Asana Starter Kit on the following pages. In time, you may tend toward more advanced versions of these, and add more postures into the mix. Or you may stick with this routine. Either way, you have this starter routine and can do some good bending and stretching that will aid you in settling into your sitting practices. Enjoy!

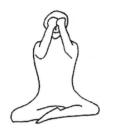

1a. Warm-up, head to heart

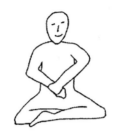

1b. Warm-up, arms to heart

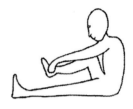

1c. Warm-up, legs to heart

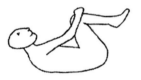

2a. Knees to chest

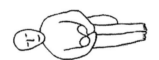

2b. Roll, right then left

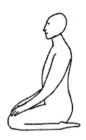

3. Kneeling seat

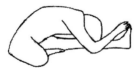

4a. Sitting, head to one knee

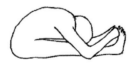

b. Sitting, head to both knees

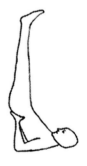

5. Shoulder stand

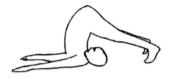 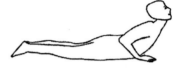

6. Plow   7. Seal of yoga   8. Cobra

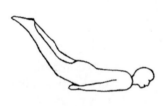 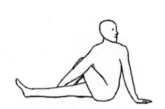 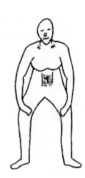

9. Locust   10. Spinal twist   11. Abdominal lift

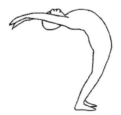 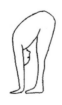 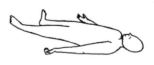

12. Standing back stretch   13. Standing toe touch   14. Corpse pose

Lesson 72 – Please Tell Me Exactly What To Do

Q: If I give you all the particulars in my life – my lifestyle, my habits, previous and current spiritual practices, my experiences – can you tell me exactly what to do with these spiritual practices you are describing so eloquently?

A: I am sorry, I cannot. With this approach, that has to come from you. The goal here is to provide everything you need to set up a good routine of spiritual practices, and evolve to higher levels of practice and experience over time under your own responsibility and supervision. General guidelines for practice are provided, along with the necessary precautions – plenty of precautions. It is not possible for me to individually guide every person, particularly since everyone has different tendencies, a different background in spiritual practices, and different manifestations of experience from past practices.

These lessons are being written for the masses. If they prove to be worth their salt, I hope they will eventually reach the masses. That is in the hands of all the readers, you, for it is mainly by word of mouth that good information is transmitted. My job is to make these lessons as good as they can be for a public audience. Maybe it is an impossible task. Time will tell.

Someone once said, "The difficult we can take care of straight away. The impossible will take a little longer."

This approach is not for everyone. Some (maybe many) will need the personal assistance of an outer guru or teacher close by. If you determine that this is your need, then by all means go and find a guru or teacher. In that case, consider these lessons to be a general resource. They are designed for that too. They are designed to crank up your bhakti (spiritual desire), and that may inspire you to go find an outer guru. Or, one may be attracted to you by your increasing longing. That would be perfect. Others will do fine with these lessons alone, utilizing the guidelines given. It is up to you – and that light perking up in your heart.

Of course, feedback and questions are welcome. All emails are answered to the best of my ability. I am happy to make suggestions, but I am not in a position to design a customized program of practices for everyone. Many sincere inquiries have come in and I am honored to receive them and respond. Inquiries and responses of general interest are posted to the lessons. Like this one.

The guru is in you.

Lesson 73 – More on Chakras

Q: As a healer I have always understood that the chakras should be in balance and that yoga is one way to help bring about a balance in these energy centres. I have, however, recently found a supposition that only the base, sacral and solar plexus chakras should be open and that the heart, throat, brow and crown chakras should be closed. This seems rather strange to me and I would appreciate some feedback on this matter.

A: If you go to lesson #47, "Chakras?" you will find a review of the approach taken in these lessons in relation to chakras. It is not a direct supervision of chakras, but allowing them to come into function naturally as pure bliss consciousness and ecstatic experiences come up in practices, particularly in meditation and spinal breathing.

Having said that, all of the practices act either directly or globally on the chakras, but not with attention on the inner mechanics of them. Because of the approach being practices-oriented rather than chakra supervision-oriented, there has not been much consideration on which chakra should open and which should not. The one exception is the crown, which can lead to problems if opened prematurely, as discussed in the recent lesson on kundalini symptoms and remedies. There are many unpleasant stories out there on this. Gopi Krishna's book, *Kundalini – Evolutionary Energy in Man*, many years ago is one example. It is a good book on how to get enlightened the hard way. So the crown is one that we don't want to open too soon. But we do want to open it when appropriate, and the later lessons here deal with that.

The supposition you mention about opening the bottom chakras and not the top ones does not seem to be consistent with a balancing of feminine and masculine energies in the body, and not conducive to enlightenment, if that is the goal. It certainly leaves out both meditation and spinal breathing, which both have global effects on all the chakras, and the sushumna (spinal nerve) in particular going between the root and the third eye. It also leaves out sambhavi at the third eye, and a boatload of further measures we will be covering here working in the upper body and head. The supposition implies stimulating only the bottom half of the sushumna and chakras, and relying on the energy finding its way upward by itself, with no provision for a downward flow to marry the upward flow. This seems to be a Shakti-only approach. It would certainly avoid the problems at the crown mentioned above. But it avoids, or at least greatly delays, the activation of the entire sushumna. It seems a one-sided approach. Then again it must be working for someone, or why would it be written down? Unless, or course, it is just a theory. Experience is the final arbiter of all theories.

We may be talking about two different things here. These lessons are about facilitating the enlightenment process in the human being, and there are many proactive methods being presented for use in every corner of the body, mind and heart. "Chakra balancing" and different approaches to that may be concerned mainly with restoring health, rather than going great guns into an enlightenment transformation, which is a much more ambitious course to take. Either way, it seems that balancing of feminine and masculine energies would be essential, not to mention bringing up pure bliss consciousness everywhere from within with meditation, which is a prerequisite for both good health and enlightenment.

The goal in these lessons is to avoid theoretical approaches to yoga as much as possible. The approach is experience-based, and therefore, hopefully, practical. In that sense, what you see here is what you get. That is the scientific approach, or, at least, as close to scientific as we can get when dealing with the subjective side of ourselves.

In healing, you are no doubt dealing with experience as well, which may be why you wondered about the supposition about opening lower chakras only. It seems to not make much sense to either one of us.

The guru is in you.

Lesson 74 – For This Life, and the Next One

Q: I am 73 years old and live alone, so I thought I would have plenty of time to learn to meditate, but I was told that it could take a lifetime to reach the state of bliss that meditators are reaching for, and I don't have much of a lifetime left. Do you have any suggestions?

A: It is very inspiring that you want to make the best, spiritually speaking, of the time you have left. The rest of us should all be in that mode too, no matter what our age.

Yes, the party line is that it takes a long time. But it is a relative thing you know. In the *Bhagavad Gita*, the great Indian scripture, it says that just one dip into the infinite erases lifetimes of mundane struggles in the future. So whether we are 23 or 73, if we can start dipping into pure bliss consciousness, there will be big progress. If you can entertain the possibility of reincarnation in that vein, it can be a great motivator. It is a form of bhakti, you know. We all have much to work for spiritually, no matter how young or old we are. No one should delay a minute.

One thing I can tell you for sure. Whatever you accomplish in spiritual practices now will not be lost. Later on, you will pick up where you left off and continue somewhere else, carrying on with your journey to enlightenment. Not only have I heard and read this from every sage I have encountered over many years, it is also my direct experience. I was born doing spiritual practices. Why? It had to come from somewhere. Maybe I was a 73 year-old man who kept up spiritual practices sometime in the past. Who knows? All I know is that I was born with this stuff singing inside. The fact that you are interested indicates you are not new to spiritual practices either. We have all been here before. What we do in practices now brings us closer to enlightenment. It will not be lost.

As you get further into the lessons, you will find things getting more aggressive in terms of practices. It is not recommended you try and tackle all that is in here, not at your age. Too much stress and strain. Aggressive yoga is for the younger folks. But there is still plenty you can do. Twice-daily meditation is the best foundation. That alone accomplishes huge things. It is your daily dipping into the infinite, as mentioned above. Some light spinal breathing before meditation can help, and maybe some daily yoga postures if you are willing and able. There are yoga (postures) classes for seniors available almost everywhere. Those three things are more than enough. If there is any discomfort with pranayama (or anything), scale back or stop immediately. See if you can find a steady, comfortable routine. The most important thing is to have a comfortable daily routine with no strain in practices. Then, doing that each day, you will know you are making a big contribution to the future in both this life, and the next one.

I am honored by your presence here. I am honored by everyone's presence here. It is a sacred thing for me. Thank you so much.

I wish everyone on earth could be here. Not for my sake, but for the sake of all the sincere longing that is out there.

The guru is in you.

Lesson 75 – Siddhasana – Living in a Fountain of Ecstasy

Okay, we are ready to move on to some more advanced yoga practices. We are crossing over here into practices that are decidedly more aggressive. Before taking on any of these, it is essential that you be stable in the practices previously undertaken. If you jump right into these new practices without meditation, pranayama and the rest very comfortably in place, not much good will come of it. Make sure you are in tune with your unique time line. You may spend years in the other practices before you feel ready for these very advanced yoga practices coming up, and that is perfectly all right. Rome was not built in a day.

By "aggressive," we mean more focused on stimulating prana in the body. While this means more pure bliss consciousness moving and more ecstasy coming up in us, it also means more purification in the nervous system. More purification means more stuff loosening and coming out from inside, and discomfort is possible. Always gauge your practices and lifestyle to keep at a stable rate of purification. We are always looking to balance our routine so it results in maximum spiritual progress while maintaining smoothness in daily life. How we feel outside practices during the day is the best measure. This has been said over and over, and can't be said enough. It is a fact of life for anyone seriously treading the path of yoga. You could call it the fine art of housecleaning without making a mess.

Having said all that, let's delve into it.

If you are still bright-eyed and bushy-tailed after all we have been through so far, you will be a natural for what is coming up. And you will love every minute of it. Either that, or you will be crying, "This is outrageous!" Maybe you will be doing both at the same time – loving the outrageous.

Siddhasana is the next step in our integration of practices. It means, "seat of the perfected ones." You will recall way back in lesson #33, we talked about "a new way to sit in meditation." You may wish to go back and review that lesson now.

We are going to take what was discussed in lesson #33 a step further. We said there that it would be good to become comfortable using a cross-legged position while meditating, tucking the toes under the opposite legs a bit with the feet turned partially upside down. This is best done on a soft surface, like a bed, and with back support. This applies in both pranayama and meditation.

Now we are going to bring the inner foot further under and put our heel under our perineum. We will be sitting on our heel there with the top of our foot lying almost flat on the bed. It is not a good idea to try this while sitting on a hard surface.

It is not necessary to put all of our weight on the heel. If we are using back support, as recommended, we can lean back a bit and find a reasonably comfortable position where we are sitting with our heel firmly against our perineum. Not too firm, not too light. We can use either foot underneath, and can switch them for comfort as necessary, as discussed in lesson #33. As with all new practices we take on, there will be a "clunky" stage, where it feels a bit awkward. This one may feel a lot awkward. Don't let that stop you from learning. It should not take long for you to find that this position is sexually stimulating, and that will add to the clunkiness of it. In the beginning, it will probably be clunky and sexy combined.

We will keep the other foot where it was, tucked under the shin of the leg going under, or we can leave that second leg out straight on the bed at times if this is more comfortable. This is a simplified form of siddhasana. The formal version has the second leg up on top of the first, as in half-lotus, with no back support, and maybe sitting on a hard rock somewhere. It is not necessary to do all that to get the correct effect. That effect is a constant stimulation of sexual energy upward from the perineum during our sitting practices of pranayama and meditation. We want that, and we sit with pressure at the perineum in such a way to deliberately foster it. It is supposed to feel good.

"How can I ever meditate while doing this?" you say. You can. Maybe not in the beginning without some distraction, but it is something you can work into gradually over time. Maybe at first you will only want to be in siddhasana during pranayama, and leave it out during meditation. In time, you will become completely comfortable in siddhasana and even forget that you are doing it throughout practices. It is a training that you are embarking on, a gradual buildup of a habit. There are two kinds of training going on at once, which is what makes learning siddhasana tricky.

First is the physical part of culturing the body into it to the point where it is completely comfortable physically to be in siddhasana. We all know that we can gradually coax the body in a particular direction. If we have managed to get comfortable in crossed legs before now, we know it can be done. If we have not gotten into crossed legs, this form of siddhasana won't be happening easily right now, not in the way just described. But there are other ways to do it. More on that below.

The second kind of training that is going on can be more challenging. That is riding through the sexual feelings that siddhasana creates. What we are doing in siddhasana is training our sexual energy to be comfortable flowing up, opening previously dormant pathways in our nervous system. We do siddhasana during our spiritual practices for two reasons. First is because we are sitting there for our time of pranayama and meditation, and that is automatically a certain amount of time of being in siddhasana as well. That makes siddhasana a regular daily practice like everything else, and we don't have to add any time to our practices to do it. Second, pranayama and meditation interact with the effects of siddhasana to greatly expand the flow of prana and pure bliss consciousness in the nervous system. In addition, we are also doing mulabandha and sambhavi. The integration of all these practices supercharges the process of evolution going on inside us.

Think of sexual energy as being like a wild horse. We want to use this horse for a useful purpose. So what do we do? We get on the wild horse and ride it. It jumps all over the place at first – the proverbial "bucking bronco." But pretty soon, the horse figures out who is in charge, and begins to settle down. It finds a new way of being within the conditions we have created. Then the horse becomes very useful for whatever our purpose has been in training her. This is exactly what siddhasana does. It creates a condition that sexual energy has to accommodate itself to for our spiritual benefit. Our purpose in yoga with regard to sex is to expand its use upward, adding something more in addition to the externally oriented reproductive function. We want to train sex to support our inner spiritual transformation. We have covered this principle in the lessons before when we first discussed kundalini and mulabandha (lesson #55). Now we are taking it a step further. When we cover tantra yoga methods, we will add other things, also leading in this same direction.

As the bucking bronco of sexual energy in siddhasana begins to calm down, our experiences in pranayama and meditation will change dramatically. What was before crazy sexual energy going this way and that, becomes a smooth upward flow of delightful energy, much like a fountain coming up from our root. It is peaceful luminous energy, ecstatic energy that we can sit in indefinitely with comfort. No more bucking bronco. When we get up and go about our daily activities the energy will still be there, even when we are not sitting in siddhasana. Our inner biology relating to prana flow inside will be changing to something much more. We will feel natural with it, being filled with divine light. We will become more self-sufficient in every aspect of life. Then we are in the best position to give to others, because our basic needs will be filled by an overflowing bliss from inside.

So, siddhasana is a very important practice. A tricky one to get established, but well worth climbing the learning curve for.

How long does it take to train the bucking bronco? It depends on the person. It is gradual for most. The first week or two can be crazy. In a month things will be settling a bit. In three months, it will be getting comfortable. In six months to a year there will be stability, and it will become a natural part of everyday life. After a few years, we are used to being bathed in ecstasy all the time, but never taking it for granted. We can sit in siddhasana anytime we want without any distraction – just normal ecstatic bliss. It is normal life with a spiritually awakened nervous system.

All of the effects of advanced yoga practices that have been discussed in these lessons are greatly enriched by siddhasana, and we can go on to more and more. That is the important thing, for there is always more progress to be achieved. A true yogi or yogini never stops, no matter how terrific the experiences get.

During all of this change brought on by siddhasana, we will be keeping our daily pranayama and meditation going just as before. The feelings that come up in siddhasana are treated just like other thoughts and feelings that come up in pranayama and meditation. We just easily favor the practice we are doing, as always. We also keep our practices of mulabandha and sambhavi as before. Siddhasana has a huge effect on the opening of the spinal nerve, and the rise of ecstatic conductivity in it.

For those who are unable to get into crossed legs for any reason, there can still be siddhasana, with the effects created by different means. You can use a prosthetic object of your choosing wherever you sit for pranayama and meditation. Maybe a rubber ball, or a hard little pillow, something that will approximate the pressure of your heel pressing up on your perineum. This is perfectly adequate. You can do it that way. You can avoid having to train your body in the physical bending and so on. You will still be training your sexual energy, which is the point of siddhasana. Everything else will be the same as discussed above. You will just be using a different method to achieve the same results.

If at any point the stimulation is just too much, and it is not possible to meditate or do anything comfortably in practices, it is important to back off. That goes for all advanced yoga practices. We back off when we know we are overdoing, because this is how we avoid falling off the wagon of practices completely. We don't try and be heroic and suffer though excessive difficulties. Always retreat if it gets to be too much. Find your best stable platform of reduced practice, and relax there before trying to move ahead again. You can always come back and pick up where you left off another day.

The guru is in you.

Lesson 76 – Siddhis – Are Powers Real?

Q: Are the famed siddhis real? ... in your experience, of course! If they are, could these practices lead to experiences of them? I know that many teachers warn that they are merely a distraction and a trap for the ego, but for me it would be evidence of human ability beyond what we have been taught.

A: Are you from Missouri, the "show me" state? Only kidding. It is a good question. If you believe the New Testament of the *Bible*, and numerous other accounts, powers are real. But I will not be flying through the sky or walking through walls any time soon for you. Nor will I be feeding the 5,000, or raising the dead. There is no claim of guru status here, so I don't have to do any of those things. I'm just an ordinary bloke like anybody.

It is important to note that we ordinary folks can cultivate constant miraculous experience in our lives. There is a relationship between this and siddhis in terms of practice.

As you may know, in Patanjali's *Yoga Sutras*, a procedure known as "samyama" is identified as being the source of siddhis. Samyama is systematically initiating particular intentions within pure bliss consciousness. But samyama isn't done for siddhis. It is done for the purification it produces in the nervous system on the way to siddhis. Samyama is a spiritual practice that can be integrated with all the other spiritual practices we are discussing. The primary effects of samyama are moving pure bliss consciousness and expanding ecstasy within and beyond the body. Samyama is an expansion of everything else we are doing in Advanced Yoga Practices. It was mentioned in the very first lesson, in the list of things to be covered, that we will be "cultivating silent inner awareness outward in powerful ways." This is samyama.

We will get into samyama a little later in the lessons. It will be for the further expansion of pure bliss consciousness and divine ecstasy, not for manifesting siddhis, though moving in that direction naturally. By the time siddhis come, will we care? Life will be permanent ecstatic bliss long before. Now that is a real miracle.

I understand your question and why you ask it. Will you settle for pure bliss consciousness and endless ecstasy? That we can have in abundance if we are willing to put in the effort. These lessons are about that. You can get on the road to siddhis if you want to by taking up advanced yoga practices. But you will probably not be very attached to them by the time you get them. The ego will long since be merged with the infinite.

The guru is in you.

Lesson 77 – Still More on Chakras

Q: This is about the recent query on closed and open chakras (lesson #73). I too am a healer, and what I have found both in teachings and experience, is that the chakras are naturally open. The degree to which a chakra is closed, or inactive (or over-active), and depleted or congested, is what determines dis-ease in the being – that is, things are not in sync in the etheric body, and the effect of it manifests on the physical body.

Also, as I understand it, the heart chakra is what enables us to give, to love, without restraints, without pre-conditions. As a healer, it is my belief that the heart chakra, more than any chakra, needs to be open, active and healthy for a healer to pass on the divine healing energies, to the patients. That is my belief. Hope I am not upsetting anyone.

And I also found your point on the opening of the crown chakra a little confusing, to say the least. When we do any pranayama, exercise or meditation, the kundalini energy gets stirred into activity. Depending upon the etheric condition of the sushumna, the ida and pingala, nadis, as well as the health of the chakras, the kundalini energy starts rising upwards. In most of us, needless to add, the etheric condition of these chakras and nadis is usually abominable!

When this happens, the kundalini energy goes haywire, and rushes into different nadis, wherever there is space. In the case of Gopi Krishna, for instance, it went up all the way to the crown by the way of the ida. And on the very verge of insanity, he managed to force some of it up via the pingala, and restore the balance, which is what saved him.

What I am trying to say is, the balance between the yin and the yang, as well as the Shiva and the Shakti energies, is extremely necessary for a balanced and safe meditation practice. The Shiva energy comes down from the crown – how can we afford to not open it? And if the kundalini and Shiva energy enter the sushumna from bottom and top respectively, they meet at the heart chakra – how can we keep that closed?

Please shed some light on this.

A: Thank you for your comprehensive note on chakras. You raise some good points.

Forcing the sahasrar early in the process of yoga is the main caution that has been raised, as kundalini under those conditions can go anywhere, as you point out. As you say, this applies to every other chakra and nadi as well. Many make the mistake of thinking yoga is just about chakra concentration going up, and get into trouble. More than a few have written with serious problems from this, and it breaks my heart.

The recommendation is not to keep anything closed (sahasrar included), but to let everything open naturally during advanced yoga practices. We really don't think about the chakras at all during practices in this approach. They are considered to be "under the hood" of the car as we use the main controls in the driver's seat. This is not to say other more direct approaches to chakras are not valid. It is just not the approach here.

So, this is why we start with global practices of meditation and spinal breathing to ease everything open as smoothly as possible, naturally from the inside. In this approach, meditation comes first as the balancing influence, rather than trying to balance the chakras first before meditation. We trust the rise of pure bliss consciousness in meditation and spinal breathing to do the right purification and opening, which it does when we follow the simple procedures. Then, after some time, with some global purification of everything inside us, we can go to more aggressive methods, and eventually to more focus on the crown. Shiva is brought down most smoothly in the beginning using the ajna (third eye) for awakening, which is an essential part of spinal breathing and the gradual rise of ecstatic conductivity in the sushumna and in all the nadis (subtle nerves). Again, this is the approach in these lessons. Other approaches may be very different, and that is okay. In the end, all methods must stand up to the scrutiny of their practitioners. Experience is the best arbiter of our practice. That is the scientific method. Sooner or later we will arrive at optimal yoga, just as we have in many applications of technology.

I agree with you 100% about the heart. This is why emphasis is placed on desire, devotion and bhakti all the way through. It is the opening heart that leads us home. Advanced yoga practices coming up in future lessons will place more direct emphasis on the heart. Even so, we rely on the global effects of meditation and pranayama to do most of the spadework in the heart. The rise of bhakti is dependent on this spadework. How can we be devoted with the heart not opened? How can we find the motivation to meditate without devotion? This is a great "Catch 22" in yoga. Which comes first, devotion or practices? We cannot have one without the other. One is the cause of the other. We need both, and sooner or later we will grab on to one or the other somehow. Once we do, we are on the way to having it all.

The nervous system knows what to do once we start nudging it a little with effective practices.

The guru is in you.

Lesson 78 – Pleasure and the Path

Q: I have formulated a theory that the sensuous pleasures of kundalini are connected with purifying the channels and that later they diminish and things behave more normally.

A: Yes, I agree that pleasure is one of the main avenues of awakening. Enlightenment is the rise of ecstatic bliss. And, yes, it does become quite normal. It is our natural state. That is the natural progression of experience when we undertake siddhasana, as discussed in the recent lesson. Your theory is well on the way to being proven. These experiences are real for those who have the prerequisite purification and have successfully tackled the sexual connection. In time, there will be increasing evidence of this among the people. It is the truth. Maybe humanity is mature enough now to enter into ecstatic experiences without superstition or guilt. We'll see.

In all of our ecstasy, let us not forget our daily meditation. It is the core practice. Pure bliss consciousness is the prerequisite for all spiritual progress.

The guru is in you.

Lesson 79 – Mantra Reminders

Q: I tried this out, the mantra kinda turns, for me, into something less sharp in my mind, something mores like *AHHHHH MMMMMMM* ...and seems to work naturally with the in-breath and out-breath ... without making it that way intentionally. Sometimes it gets meanings attached to it too.

This is a curious experiment for me. I am not new to mantra meditations, having done several kinds of meditation for many years. I never did experience much. I'm told this lack of experience is attributed to "bad karmas." Your comments would be welcome.

A: It is okay for the mantra to change, lengthen, shorten, etc, if it does so naturally during meditation. If meanings get attached to it, that is okay too. We just easily favor the procedure. We always easily come back to the original *I AM*. But there is a trick to that, mentioned in the lessons. You may be very settled and the mantra may be a very unclear pronunciation, very fuzzy. We will know that is it, and that is what we come back to, not forcing a clear pronunciation when it is naturally fuzzy. It is the easiest level to come back too, because that is where our attention left off. So we are starting a deeper cycle coming back to it that way, coming back to where it is, instead of trying to force it to a clear pronunciation.

Remember, losing the mantra again and again is the game. We can't make ourselves lose it. It goes by itself. This is the mind's natural ability to become still. We just keep creating the right condition with the procedure for using the mantra. The mind does the rest. At first, the experience of a quieting mind and nervous system may be subtle – a little silence, some peaceful feelings, some relaxation. We take that into activity with us after meditation. Gradually it can become profound feelings of deep bliss in meditation. This is pure bliss consciousness taking up residence in our nervous system. And this goes with us into activity too. This is the path.

On the breathing, if you find the mantra going with the breath, just favor the procedure for using the mantra. Don't push the breath awareness out or hang on to it. Treat it just the same as thoughts that come up. As was covered in detail in previous lessons, trying to have the attention on both mantra and breath divides the mind, and takes away from the effectiveness of simple meditation. If it comes, okay, but it is not to be done deliberately as dual practice. It is not the approach in these lessons.

Maybe some of the other advanced yoga practices, in addition to meditation, will help open things up for you. All karma will dissolve eventually. No effective practice you do to enter the infinite is lost. You obviously have strong bhakti, or why meditate all these years? The curtain shall part, and what you find in there will be good. In time, your divine inside will be blossoming outside.

The guru is in you.

Lesson 80* – Physical Fitness and Yoga

Q: What is the relationship of physical fitness and yoga? I would think the muscle building that is so popular is not very compatible.

A: There are many definitions of fitness. As they say, "Beauty is in the eye of the beholder."

For purposes of spiritual practice, fitness means keeping the body in good tone and flexible externally and internally, which can be done with daily walking or other light aerobic-style exercise, light calisthenics and isometrics for all muscle groups, and, of course, yoga asanas. Something like Tai Chi is also good, which builds a good connection between the physical and spiritual dimensions of us in a grounding way.

For the body builder (or any physically oriented athlete) that is not enough. He or she will want to do much more with the muscles. The practices must be aimed at the goal.

For spiritual practice, the things mentioned above are enough. For other definitions of fitness it will be something else.

By the way, there is no rule that says a body builder or any other kind of athlete cannot become a yogi or yogini. There is nothing that says one can't do both if so inclined. It is just a question of what one's interests are. I believe in free choice and in each taking personal responsibility for their life. I try to keep that idea out in front in all these lessons.

That's why every lesson ends with,

The guru is in you.

Addition – As mentioned above, light aerobic exercise for the cardiovascular system, as well as some calisthenics and isometrics for toning all the muscle groups, are good to help maintain the body in suitable condition for yoga practices. When these are done in addition to daily asana practice, then a good blend of strength and limberness can be achieved. For those who do not have an exercise program, some suggestions are being added here. Even if you do have an exercise program, maybe a few of these suggestions will be helpful.

Aerobic Exercise

So, what comes first in exercise? Cardiovascular conditioning is fundamental to good health, so let's start with aerobic exercise. What is aerobic exercise? It is activity that causes the body to process more oxygen. Doing such activity on a regular basis strengthens the cardiovascular system (heart and blood circulation). Aerobic exercise is engaging in activity that causes the heart rate to go up for a period of time. Somewhere between 10 and 30 minutes of elevated heart rate is considered to be a good aerobic exercise session. With this, the lungs, the heart and the circulatory system will be moving more oxygen to the muscles, tissues and organs. That is what "aerobic" means – processing oxygen. The more conditioned our cardiovascular system is, the better we feel, and the better we are for yoga too.

What are some good aerobic exercises? Walking is an effective way to get aerobic exercise. Not only does it give the cardiovascular system a workout; it also grounds the inner energies. That is why taking long walks is recommended to help stabilize kundalini imbalances. Other aerobic exercises are jogging, biking, swimming, stair climbing, rowing, lively dancing, or anything that requires constant physical movement producing an elevated heart rate (not too much) for at least 10 minutes.

As with a yoga routine, an exercise program is only good to the extent that we can maintain regular practice. Taking a long walk once a week will do some good, but it will not condition our cardiovascular system significantly. If we want the benefits of conditioning, exercise at least every other day is very important. Daily is even better.

Once we get started with an exercise program, the trick is to keep going, keeping to a schedule of daily (or every other day) aerobic exercise for a set time and/or distance. The goal is to get our heart rate up 20-40 beats per minute above normal and keep it there for the time of our exercise.

Make sure you don't have any health limitations before undertaking an aerobic exercise program. If in doubt, check with your doctor first.

Muscle Toning

Whatever aerobic exercise we are doing, we will get some muscle toning out of it. But the chances are it will be limited to our legs or arms, depending on the type of aerobic exercise we are doing. The main benefit from aerobic exercise is cardiovascular conditioning, which is what we want. What about the rest of our body – all those hundreds of muscles that enable us to function in daily life? Having them in good shape is an important support to yoga as well.

We live in the age of the "gym." Everyone goes to the gym. Well, almost everyone. But do we really have to go that far to get a good muscle toning all over our body? And do we really need all that equipment? When we don't have a gym in our house, and don't have time to go to one, what can we do to keep in shape? It is possible to keep all of our major muscle groups in good tone without exercise equipment, and without even going out of our house. The way to do this is with a concentrated routine of light calisthenics and isometric exercises. You will be amazed to see how much can be done in only a few minutes.

Let's talk about a streamlined routine of light calisthenics and isometrics that can be done at home in 5-10 minutes covering all the muscle groups. If you do these every day (every other day, at least), you will feel dramatically stronger within a few weeks, With this exercise routine, your muscles will become firm and toned, without the huge bulging physique. Before all the machines came along, methods such as these were used to build large muscles too, and still can be.

So here is a streamlined muscle toning routine for you to try:

1. **Easy Push-ups** – Everyone hates push-ups, present company included. But there is a way to do them without the pain and anguish, or like feeling like you just joined the football team or the military. They are very good for the chest, arms and back muscles. Here is the trick. Get two chairs, or anything about that height, and hold yourself up with your hands on those in push-up position. Not too bad? Now come down a little, not too far, and back up. That's one. Now do 25 of those, coming down just enough to put a little tension on your arms and chest muscles. Only come down far enough so you know you can finish the 25 repetitions, even if it is only

dipping an inch or two. If you are in good shape you can come down further, and do the 25 repetitions that way. In other words, this is "self-paced." Once you get comfortable doing 25 repetitions, maybe in a couple of weeks, raise the repetitions up to 50. Maybe you will not be going deep on each push-up, but you will be doing 50. Then you can work with that over time, and see how it goes, never putting yourself in the position of over-exerting. Just an easy 50, that's all. You will be amazed what that will do in a few weeks, and you will never have to strain like you are in army boot camp.

2. **Isometric Curls** – Stand up with feet about shoulder-width apart. Place the heel of your left hand on the heel of your right hand. Now lift your right hand up toward your chest with a curling motion, resisting firmly with your left hand as you go, and then all the way back down. Do 50 of these curls, resisting enough so you will get a good muscle toning, but not so much that you can't make it to 50 repetitions. Now do the same thing on the other side. This is a dynamic isometric for toning the arm and shoulder muscles.

3. **Easy Knee Bends** – Still standing with feet about shoulder-width, clasp your hands behind your head. Do a small knee bend, and another, and another, all the way up to 50. Don't go to too deep – just deep enough so you can make it to 50 without overdoing it. If your legs are in good shape go a little deeper. Self-pacing. This gives the upper legs a good toning. If time is short (as it often is), you can do the knee bends at the same time as the isometric curls. If you do knee bends with curls (one bend for each curl) all the way through while doing both arms, that will be 100 knee bends. You can stop the knee bends at 50, or go for the whole 100. You are standing there anyway, right? If you don't go too deep with the knee bends, 100 should not be a problem. Self-pacing. It is up to you.

4. **Neck Toning** – Now we will work on the neck muscles in four directions. First, place the fingers of both hands on your forehead and push your head forward and down against firm resistance from your hands 20 times. Now, place your fingers on the back of your head and push your head back and down against firm resistance from your hands 20 times. With the heel of your right hand against the right side of your head above the ear, push your head to the right and down 20 times against firm resistance. Then, on the left side, do the same thing. With these four isometrics, you will gain a lot of neck toning and strength.

5. **Foot and Calf Toning** – Take one of those chairs and put it against the wall. Step up onto the edge of it, with your heels hanging over the edge. Place a hand on the wall for balance. Now, lower your heels and lift them back up as high as you comfortably can, standing on your toes on the edge of the chair. This can also be done on the bottom step of a flight of stairs. Do 50 repetitions of this, using the same method of self-pacing so as not to overdo it. The key is to do 50. This is very good for toning the foot, ankle and calf muscles.

6. **Easy Sit-ups** – Lie on your back on the bed and anchor your feet in some way, like under the head-board or foot-board. Sit up and clasp your hands behind your head. Now go back down about half way, and sit up and lean forward toward your knees. Each time you come up, twist your torso so one elbow goes toward the opposite knee. Reverse the twist coming up each time.

Do that to 30 repetitions. These are sit-ups, only we are regulating the amount of tension placed on the abdomen in a way so anyone can do these. Only go back down far enough so you can easily do the sit-ups for the 30 repetitions. The toning is mainly in the upper abdominal muscles. Those with abdominal muscles not in good shape can just lean back a little to do easy sit-ups. Those with strong abdominal muscles can go all the way down, as long as the 30 repetitions can be completed. It should be easy for everyone, with good upper abdominal muscle toning occurring, no matter what level one is working at.

7. **Easy Leg Lifts** – Now lie on your back, anchor your hands over your head and lift your legs straight up, keeping the knees fairly straight. Let the legs go down toward the bed, and then back up straight in the air. Do 30 of these leg lifts, keeping in mind that you should only go down as far with your legs as you can comfortably lift them back up for 30 repetitions. Self-pacing. This tones the lower abdominal muscles.

That is just seven exercises. They can all be done in 5-10 minutes. Don't be fooled by the simplicity of these. This is a sophisticated, streamlined routine of exercises that will tone all the muscles in the body. It took years to refine it down to this level of efficiency. As with all the practices in AYP, these exercises are optimized for simplicity and power. The effective use of self-pacing allows anyone in any condition to begin toning the muscles.

For those who are in excellent physical shape, the exercises can be taken much further than the minimums, including increasing the repetitions, as comfortable.

Exercise, both aerobic and muscle toning, should not be done right before yoga practices. Doing them right after sitting practices and rest is good, or at any other time during the day. If you do the exercises at least every other day, you will find great benefits for both the short term and the long term.

Of course, all of these are suggestions, and you can use them how you see fit in your overall routine.

Lesson 81 – Charging Ahead Too Fast?

Q: I want to first thank you for your teaching! I am finding with your lessons that I am actually feeling the process of yoga, the beauty of all. My question regarding sambhavi is that I am finding my eyes are sore and my third eye feels a dull ache/sore. Am I trying too hard? Is this natural kundalini activity? I have also been helped along with spinal breathing by utilizing your comments about getting Shiva off his butt, and am visualizing Shiva going down to meet Shakti on the exhale, and Shakti coming up to meet Shiva on the inhale. I usually let them stay together for a short pause on inhale and exhale, and mingle. I am also finding I am getting distracted more often now though – is it because my silly little ego senses a little divine romance happening? Thank you again for your lessons. I look forward to them every day, and am religious in doing practices! Thank you …
PS – Is it okay if I do the meditation portion longer than the suggested 20 minutes – sometimes I go for 45 minutes or more depending on when I feel like coming out of union – for that is how I picture it – union with my soul, allowing the soul nourishment.

A: You are doing terrific. It's wonderful.

Discomfort around the third eye (or anywhere) can mean some forcing in practice. It can also be kundalini pressing through there. It can be both at the same time. You know what to do, right? Back off on practice to something more comfortable. If excessive symptoms are still there, then look at the lesson on kundalini imbalances and remedies and explore the many avenues there. Don't press too much ahead until you have stability. You are a spiritual athlete in training. You should build up gradually. That is the best approach.

Yes, I think you answered your own question about visualizing the romance of Shiva and Shakti in spinal breathing. It is mixing bhakti too much into what is a very simple procedure of spinal breathing. It divides the attention too. The same goes for doing long meditations for the "experience." Keep in mind that we do these practices for results outside them in daily life. We are moving mountains of obstructions inside, though we may not notice if we are in an ecstatic reverie. These enthusiastic undertakings of more and more practice can contribute to kundalini imbalances, while at the same time reducing the effectiveness of the practices. So be systematic in your practices. The guidelines are there for good reasons.

Ice cream is very good, but is eating two gallons all at once good?   All of these practices are very powerful, especially when integrated as we are doing, and should be done easily and precisely. If you are inclined to extend the time of your practices, do so very sparingly to see what happens at each step. Limiting yourself to not adding more than five minutes of anything in a month is a reasonable approach. Even then you could creep yourself into an unstable situation. So use your common sense. If activity outside practices is smooth, you are doing okay. If it isn't, then chances are you are pressing too hard or too long. Be sure and keep active in your regular daily life. That is as much a part of it as the practices. Activity stabilizes the pure bliss consciousness and divine ecstasy we gain in practices. You are doing fabulously, like the proverbial kid in the candy store. You are just the kind of person these lessons are designed for. It is very exciting. Please be responsible in applying the knowledge, and then we will both be glad that all this is being revealed.

The guru is in you.

Lesson 83 – There She Goes – Kundalini, that is

Q: Namaste! I took to heart your advice and dropped back to 20 minutes for meditation. However, during pranayama, heat and tingling came up. Thought nothing of it, but as I continued in meditation, heat arose from my sacral area, and continued up my spine. A high pitched buzzing rang through my ears and then a tremendous surge of energy pulsed through me. I ended meditation with a prayer, and actually kept working with breath prayer, then did a 7,7,7 breath to calm down – the energy was so intense. I went out to see my husband to have him help ground me, and he could feel the energy pulsating through my hands and back as I was sitting against him – this lasted for about an hour or so. Now my question – is this the bucking bronco you spoke of, or is this kundalini making herself known? I backed down in this morning's pranayama and meditation, taking out sambhavi, mulabandha, and siddhasana. I just did spinal breathing and *I AM* meditation, I still felt energy pulsating and high pitched buzzing but not as intensely. My inner vision prompts me to continue in this way for 4 days, then adding on sambhavi and mulabandha 2 days after the 4 day rest and see reaction, continuing on to siddhasana after I feel a balance. My quandary is this. Should I continue on with the advanced practices and try to train the bronco, or should I let the bronco relax and then try to gain control slowly? Also, FYI: walks outside, yogic breath, belly breath and restorative poses are what I am going to use today as well as nervine herbs such as skullcap, oatstraw, and chamomile. I have eliminated coffee all together – who needs that artificial stimulation when you have this dynamo inside yourself?

A: There she goes. Kundalini, that is. The thing to do is be very intent on integrating all this into your daily activity. You are very wise not to blindly push practices ahead. Find that stable platform of practices and lifestyle that goes around the clock, 24 hours. Very important. You will know when it is time to press ahead again. The tools will be there when you need them. Your job right now is to stay on the rails. Or, as they say in rural Mississippi, "Keep it between the ditches."

The "bucking bronco" referred to in siddhasana is sexual energy jumping around in the stimulation of the siddhasana seat. Over time, it changes and becomes very smooth and ecstatically blissful energy flowing up in the body like a fountain all the time. You seem to be making a sudden transformation, with sexual energy lurching upward into kundalini manifestation rapidly. It won't be that sudden for everyone. Everyone's nervous system is in a different condition according to past actions and practices – that means way back before this life. You are right to stay out of siddhasana for now. And the other stimulative methods too. Don't hesitate to back off on pranayama and meditation also, if your symptoms make it necessary. You have plenty going on. Focus on stabilization. You can go back later and add stimulation into your routine when it is obvious you can use it.

Right now it is obvious you have enough to integrate. Make sure you keep physically active. This is essential for integration of kundalini energies into the nervous system. If necessary, you can also eat a heavier diet for a while to help smooth things out. Review the kundalini remedies lesson (#69) and see if there are other avenues you are inclined to explore. It will get smoother as you continue on a course of "grounding" activities. Let your experience be your guide. The key to success in this stage is learning how to accommodate kundalini, and working with her. The yogi/yogini's role goes from instigator to partner. In time, you will find there is only one of you in there, and everywhere.

Keep in mind that this transformation is not an overnight thing. It is a long drawn out process that will take years to evolve. The nervous system has a lot of purification and evolution to go through. So, be prudent, patient and settle in for the long haul. Slow and steady wins the race. We'd like to avoid having it turn into an ongoing roller coaster ride. Live a full and active life, and let your growing enlightenment live it with you. The journey can be so much fun.

The guru is in you.

Lesson 84 – The Art of Doing Nothing

Q: Krishnamurti and other interesting people say that it is wrong to focus on techniques because there is no technique for meditation. Meditation is all the time, here and now. Doing a mantra and using pranayama is using a technique. And I reason it is to raise my energy level and tune in so that I can experience bliss and the world in its deepest levels. But why do some teachers say that techniques are wrong and that they will mislead you – and they give then no instruction but saying be aware, or maybe not even that. Why? Does that fit into the yogic understanding?

A: It is only a theory, but perhaps people like Krishnamurti are like successful mountain climbers who have lost their memory. They stand on top of the mountain and say to everyone down in the valley, "You don't have to do anything. Just automatically wake up on the top of the mountain like I did. You are here already."

They were born at or close to enlightenment, and apparently have no recollection of all the work they did in previous lives to produce that situation. If we do nothing, we will eventually reach enlightenment a kazillion years from now. If we do something, it will be much sooner. There are certain methods that are known to advance the enlightenment process. That is what yoga is.

Each chooses their own path, to do or not to do. Even a path of consciously doing nothing (or "being aware") is a doing. In a real sense, the meditation we do here is doing nothing. We just set a condition in the mind, and the mind does the rest. It goes to stillness. We don't do anything. The nervous system does it all once we set the initial condition. So, technically, I agree that doing nothing is the way. But doing nothing effectively is an art. It is the art of meditation. All of the other advanced yoga practices are also arts of doing nothing. We set initial conditions, and the nervous system takes over. We don't have to do anything once the natural abilities of the nervous system take over. Yoga is the art of nudging the nervous system in certain ways and then doing nothing.

Ramakrishna said yogis are like well diggers, and there are three kinds. The first kind finds the tools, digs the well (to enlightenment) and then jumps in, taking the tools with him. No one knows how he did it. The second kind of yogi finds the tools, digs the well and jumps in. But this guy leaves the tools behind lying around on the ground where others can find them. The third kind of yogi finds the tools, digs the well and hangs around for a while, showing everyone who comes around the tools and how to use them.

Maybe there is a fourth kind of yogi – one who is born enlightened, has no recollection about the tools he used in past lives, and tells everyone, "You don't need tools. Just be enlightened. It is easy. See? Here is the well. Just be aware and you will see you are in it already." Like that. Who knows? One thing is for sure. While yogis like Krishnamurti are inspiring, they can't offer much practical help to most people. Maybe a few high souls can benefit from them. It is a pretty exclusive club. The rest of us need a more comprehensive approach. Yoga! We need to do something in order to do nothing.

The guru is in you.

Lesson 85 – Enlightenment Milestones Revisited

Q: I would like to thank you for the lessons which I feel are very beneficial, and the program you are putting out seems to be a good one as it covers everything. I am following another yogi's teachings which I'm happy with, but forgot his kundalini meditation which I'm meant to do weekly so your priceless teachings are well and truly fitting the gap that had left in my spiritual program. (I was working on my heart and crown in a way that raises kundalini but not focusing on my kundalini directly.)

I'm taking your exercises very slowly. I have only been doing the first couple of things and only once a day, as I had a kundalini incident a few years ago which nearly killed me – very erratic heart beat, breathing problems, nearly knocked me out with each surge and also partly paralyzed me during surges which lasted almost an hour with the energy building up more and more each time. It was like a raging river surrounding me. Weirdly, it was running also outside my body, and right through my body raging upwards from the spine level. A master helped, saved my life in that incident by somehow pulling the energy out of my body during and between the surges (he may of been somehow converting the kundalini energy into a different energy), and then he tried to do some kind of complete energy drain thing as a last resort. Luckily, that instantly stopped the surges. I believe I would be dead if it wasn't for him and his hasty help. I was in big trouble. So, needless to say, I'm more wary than I used to be.

My question is about a dream I had last night, which I'm now wondering if it was a warning for me to slow down with my practices. Should I just ignore this (I wonder if it was maybe triggered by kundalini)? I dreamed a had kundalini surges going right up my spine but the kundalini was running into the inner top part of my crown (like the inside of the top of my head), it hit against it each time it surged up. In my dream it got rather tender on that part because of that.

Do you think I need to be concerned and cut back a bit?

A: Thank you for your generous sharing. Yes, given what you have been through, I agree you should be very conservative and measured in your practices. Any sense of foreboding should be taken seriously. Not that you should be "running scared" about your enlightenment process, which you clearly are not. For each of us it is a matter of knowing ourselves, our limits, our opportunities for stable progress, and gauging our approach to that. "Experience-based" is the watch-phrase around here. We will have tools galore, and how we apply them will make all the difference. Each must travel along their own time line, within their own capacity. It is a big responsibility.

The goal of these lessons is to give each person the opportunity to sit in their own driver's seat on their spiritual journey. Who else can sit there? It is an unorthodox approach to the transmission of spiritual knowledge. It is in the spirit of the rapid expansion of the practical applications of scientific knowledge over the past few centuries. So much good has come from practical applications of science, as we can see all around us. Is it absolutely safe for everyone? No, it isn't. There will always be some who will be at risk with the availability of powerful knowledge. Does this mean we should not have cars, airplanes, electricity, or the Internet? Do the occasional risks involved in knowing advanced yoga practices mean they should not be available to everyone? I hope not. How can the whole of humanity learn to travel the inner roads to pure bliss consciousness and divine ecstasy other than by doing it? This is the challenge. Astronauts will eventually go to

Mars and beyond. All of us will eventually join with the infinite within us, and bring that experience out into every day living. It is the journey of the human spirit to more – always to more. We know intuitively that we are infinite. There is no limit to what we can experience.

Now, what about these kundalini experiences we have been focusing on lately? Some have been pretty extreme. Are these necessary to reach enlightenment? Can we get through without having to endure such extremes? Let's step back for a few minutes and try and develop some perspective on kundalini experiences, why they come about, and how they fit into the overall journey to enlightenment. To do this, let's go back and revisit the lesson #35, "Enlightenment Milestones."

In that lesson, we talked about three stages of enlightenment, sometimes overlapping in our experience, each with its own particular characteristics.

The first stage is the rise of silence in the nervous system. Deep silence is the essential nature of pure bliss consciousness. It is absolute stability. Nothing moves it. It is like a solid rock foundation that is under everything we are and do. It is the essence of who we are. It becomes known primarily from meditation, and is the source of the inner peace and unshakable security we experience as we advance along the spiritual path. It is our immortal being, and its rise in our nervous system serves as the foundation for all other spiritual development.

The second stage is the rise of ecstasy. This is prana going into a greatly expanded mode of functioning in our nervous system. It is sexual energy going up. It is kundalini. It is also pure bliss consciousness, deep silence, in motion inside us. It is the expansion of sensory experience into the ecstatic realms. This change is promoted by pranayama and other techniques designed to stimulate prana into a kundalini awakening mode. It is usually enjoyable. But sometimes the experiences can be extreme, i.e., kundalini problems. Why? More on that in a minute.

The third stage is the rise of the experience of unity, where we see all as an expression of the One that we have become. This is the joining of the individual ego, pure bliss consciousness, divine ecstasy, and all that exists in temporal existence. It is brought about as our center in pure bliss consciousness is systematically encouraged to move beyond the body. It is enlightenment, realization, the fruit of yoga. Then we live the reality of "loving our neighbor as ourself." It becomes experientially obvious that our neighbor is ourself. This has a big effect on our behavior, of course – a positive effect with far reaching benefits.

There are advanced yoga practices associated with each of these three stages. And there is a logical sequence in the evolution of these three stages. At least in these lessons there is. Stage one, stage two, stage three. Like that.

It is all about purification. If our nervous system was entirely pure, somehow cleared of all the "seeds of karma" accumulated in our innumerable past lives, we would be born enlightened. Then we'd be like Krishnamurti, sitting around saying, "There's nothing to it. Just be aware." No meditation, no hair-raising kundalini, no journey at all. Just bliss, bliss, bliss!

Well, most of us still have a lot of house cleaning to do. And it is not an overnight job. It is not like hiring a cleaning service to come in for a few hours and the job is done. Even with the best spiritual practices, it takes years and years. Maybe lifetimes. No cleaning effort is ever wasted, as has been discussed before (lesson #74). It's the one thing we can take with us when we leave this earth.

So, it is the process of house cleaning that determines our spiritual journey, our experience. How we go about it makes all the difference. There are some approaches that seem to start in the middle of the enlightenment process. They start with methods for directly raising kundalini. What happens? Kundalini sometimes moves. Sometimes she doesn't. If she does, it can be up into a nervous system that is usually not ready, not purified enough. This is premature awakening, and is the cause of most of the extreme kundalini experiences. It is a tricky business, because someone may not have done any kundalini stimulation in this life and still be susceptible to premature kundalini awakening. Their nervous system seems to be wired for it. Maybe they did these practices in a past life and now have to stabilize it. Who knows? But there is no doubt that some are susceptible to premature awakening of kundalini. You will know soon enough if you are. If you are, you will have to be careful. Some others will zoom right through without a hitch. We should all be so blessed. For most people it is a gradual unfoldment, and Advanced Yoga Practices are designed for that, not to create an overnight wonder. Just steady progress.

The approach here is to do gentle "global" house cleaning first. That means meditation, bringing up the silence, the pure bliss consciousness. Bathing the whole nervous system in it. It is very effective cleaning of the whole nervous system, and usually very gentle. Working on the first stage of enlightenment, you know. Even so, if someone is susceptible to kundalini problems, even gentle meditation can stir things up. Then the practice should be moderated to shorter meditation times, more physical activity, more grounding methods. For some people, just meditation is plenty. Experience is the best guide.

If meditation is good and bringing in silence and peace, then spinal breathing can be added. This focuses the purification more in the spinal nerve, the sushumna, and a gentle course toward bringing up ecstatic conductivity can be taken. This is a very gentle way to stimulate kundalini, keeping her in the right channel, keeping her in touch with her polar opposite, the masculine energy coming down from above on every exhalation.

Then if meditation and spinal breathing are smooth, more can be added. This process of adding can take many months, years, or decades, depending on the person. The experience will be the determining factor, not some arbitrary schedule. And it should certainly not be directed by a reckless ambition to find a super fast short cut to enlightenment. That is like going out on the road with a car for the very first time and going 100 miles an hour. The outcome of that kind of approach is well known to all of us.

Whatever the past has been in practices, that is the past. For better or worse we have to live with the results of that. Today we can start anew, making sure we have taken care of the beginning before we try and rush to the end. If we cultivate the silence of pure bliss consciousness inside until it is stable within us, we will have the best chance of a smooth awakening of kundalini. That is, an ecstatic awakening instead of a horrific one. Awaking kundalini is a step along the path, somewhere in the middle. Raising kundalini is not the whole path. It is just the middle part. Bringing up the silence of pure bliss consciousness is the whole path, the beginning, the middle and the end. Everything else depends on that. This is why it was said early in the lessons that meditation will be enough if that is all one is inclined to do, and it should always remain at the center of our practices. For those who are ambitious, aiming to get the job done in this lifetime, the other means are offered. But it is not recommended that meditation be skipped, ever. It can make for a very difficult journey trying to do the other things without a firm foundation in deep silence, in pure bliss consciousness.

How long should one clean house with meditation before stimulating kundalini directly? It depends on the person. If the inner silence and stability are good, maybe soon. For others, meditating easily each day for years or decades will be a good route. It is a combination of your capacity and your desire (bhakti) that will determine your course. Some will be conservative. Others will be very aggressive. Just remember that Rome was not built in a day. Find your time line, know your capacity, and take it one day at a time. It is a long journey. There is no need to knock the wheels off the car on the first lap around the track, or on the one hundredth lap either.

The guru is in you.

Note: The most common cause of premature activation of kundalini of the extreme variety discussed above is a premature opening of the crown chakra. This has been mentioned in previous lessons #69 and #77, and is detailed further in later lessons (see "crown opening – avoiding premature" in the topic index), including the means for opening the crown safely while minimizing the risk of excessive kundalini energies.

Lesson 86 – Finding your Meditation Routine

Q: I have just recently begun following your practices (went back to the beginning). I have been involved with yoga and meditation for several years. I wonder is it all right to continue to use background music and aromas to enhance my meditation, or am I distracting from it? What about mala beads? Also, right now, I only seem to be able to get in about 10 minutes – how important is it to meditate for the full 20 minutes every day?

A: Of course, it is not for me to upset your established comfortable environment for meditation. If you are most comfortable with incense, aromas, background music, or whatever, it is your choice. However, I do suggest you carefully read all the lessons and Q&As on meditation for comments on external environmental things while meditating. Remember, meditation is for going in. If we are vibrating with music or other sensory inputs, this is not part of using the mantra, and there is the chance that our attention will be divided. This can take away from our attention settling naturally and deeply into pure bliss consciousness. Of course, as pointed out in the lessons, it is possible to meditate easily in airplanes, busy waiting rooms, or practically anywhere. So what is a little background music? It may not hurt, but it is not part of the meditation either, and it is something else besides thoughts that you will be easily letting go as you favor the mantra. You decide what works best for you. You are in charge.

Ten minutes is much better than no minutes, and ten minutes twice a day is much better than twenty minutes only once a day. There is a natural cycle of meditation and activity that is optimized by meditating twice a day. The "twice" is at least as important as the length of meditation.

If you are smooth in activity after twenty minutes of meditation, then do your best to build it into your daily schedule. You will accomplish so much more inner purification if you can get in the habit. On the other hand, try not to be erratic about it – twenty minutes this time, ten minutes next time, then fifteen ... The more regular it is, the more like clockwork it is, the better your nervous system will like it. Once the habit is in place, the nervous system will practically meditate itself. You will close your eyes and be in pure bliss consciousness immediately, and the peace and bliss of that will stay with you throughout the day and night. Meditation habituates our nervous system to be in pure bliss consciousness naturally. It really does work like that. It takes regular daily practice over a long time. As the obstructions are gradually removed, the experience of pure bliss consciousness steadily rises. It is like watching a tree grow. I wish I could say it is like watching a kudzu vine grow (much, much faster). Maybe for a few advanced souls born with pure nervous systems it is.

Mala beads are for a different kind of approach to meditation, and to pranayama as well. They are for counting. Malas were around long before clocks, and the number of mantra repetitions and breathing cycles were counted to have a measured approach, so as not to overdo or underdo practices. This produces a small restriction, especially in meditation, because it ties the mantra to an outer activity, ticking off the beads one by one with the fingers. It becomes an unconscious habit, yet still we are regulating the mantra with an outer activity. With the clock, we can let the mantra (and the breath in pranayama) go naturally according to the unique purification need of the nervous system. We have talked a lot about this already. Using the clock is a flexible approach to measuring the amount of inner practices. Of course, we will peek at the clock now and then, but in time we find that our automatic inner clock is nearly as good as the outer one. The outer clock then becomes an occasional confirmation of the inner one. There is a lesson (#23) on this in the meditation Q&As called, "Watching the clock in meditation."

Malas may also have a sentimental value, a bhakti value, and that is an okay reason for wearing them. Whatever stimulates your bhakti is good, as long as you are not blasting off the planet in a kundalini overdose. A mala may be part of your ishta (ideal) if it connects you with your chosen ideal. And maybe your meditation and pranayama learned elsewhere are mala-based. That is okay too. The mala has not been outdated, not going the way of the buggy whip any time soon. It has been around for thousands of years. But keep in mind, the mala is for measuring how much we do in practices. In these lessons we use the clock for that. That's the difference.

I wish you the best on your journey homeward.

The guru is in you.

Lesson 88 – The Magic of Bhakti

Q: Practices are good. I have a rather strange inquiry however; I am finding that in just reading some of your posts, my state automatically changes into an almost ecstatic one – excitement! It's like my very being resonates with what I am reading. Having done some NLP training, I am aware that anything can trigger any state within a person depending on their particular make-up, and that words have a hypnotic effect; but this does feel different. I wonder if can shed some light on this from your perspective. I look forward to seeing what effect your response will have. I am a very hungry being ... Hot for IT!

A: Yes, it is amazing how bhakti works. Something in us is quickened when we are exposed to an expression of truth. It is in us already. Even just someone's attempt to write down truth can do it. It doesn't have to be perfect, just in the right direction. The nervous system knows it when it sees it. A few lessons back I mentioned that part of the purpose of these lessons is to stimulate bhakti in folks. I hope that revealing all of this practical knowledge, accumulated and utilized over a lifetime, will help others be inspired to practice according to their own inclinations.

Go for it, with prudence of course. Follow your blossoming bhakti wisely, and you will arrive home straight away. I am honored to be offering some extra stimulation to what is in you already. You will find that "IT" is everywhere.

The guru is in you.

Lesson 89 – The Caduceus – A Snapshot of You and Me

Q: I know you advocate an approach of simplicity and working too much "under the hood," but I am most curious about ida and pingala at any rate. To your knowledge, are these two related to any known spinal tract pathways in "Western" medicine/neuro-anatomy? If so, could you please direct me toward those references?

A: A great question. Thank you. I am sure there is a correspondence in the neurology, but not being a physician, I can't give you a definitive answer. However, the symbol of the modern medical profession, the caduceus, is a staff with two snakes spiraling up it, biting the wings of a glowing orb on top. It is easy to see that this represents the sushumna, ida, pingala and more. So, the Greeks (or whoever came up with the caduceus) clearly understood that there is a connection between medical science and our spiritual anatomy. Whether modern medicine has any recollection of this is another question. Maybe it is time for a renaissance? If we all do our daily practices and awaken the glorious ecstatic truth stirring within, there will have to be one. Who could ignore it then?

The guru is in you.

Lesson 90 – Caduceus Correction and Ida/Pingala Review

It has been pointed out to me that, while the caduceus is of ancient spiritual origins, it was adopted as a symbol of Western medicine only about a century ago. This indicates that perhaps Western medicine does not come from such enlightened roots as mentioned in the previous lesson. So, instead of a "renaissance" (revival) of its spiritual connection, medical science will perhaps be discovering the relationship between our physical and spiritual anatomies for the first time. It is likely this will come as more holistic systems of medicine, like Ayurveda, merge with Western medicine in the coming decades. The focus will shift more toward balance and prevention, and hopefully the medical profession will come to enjoy an existence that is not so crisis oriented. Humanity deserves a break, and so does the medical profession. The master key to good health is in the lifestyle we adopt. It gets down to what you and I do with our lives. And, of course, the medical profession has an important role to play in inspiring and supporting that.

Speaking of inspiring, the reason the caduceus has been mentioned in the lessons has been for the purpose of bhakti – devotion to a high ideal. Whenever you see the symbol of the staff with two serpents rising up around it to that glowing orb, I hope you will be inspired to keep up your daily practices. The caduceus can be used to generate useful bhakti like that. It is a quiet reminder of the reality of the human spiritual anatomy for the medical profession, and for all of us.

Now, let's open the hood for a few minutes and take a look at the ida and pingala.

As we lift the hood, we see a wondrous tangle of glowing nerves, chakras and ecstatic energy surging outward. My first impulse is to slam the hood shut and take us all back to doing practices. Enjoying being behind the wheel of the car, you know, watching the beautiful scenery going by, instead of being lost under the hood. But here we are staring at the inner workings, so let's take a closer look.

By now, we should be very familiar with the sushumna, the spinal nerve, as we have been using it in spinal breathing. Or at least thinking about using it. For some it has become palpable, as ecstatic radiance has begun to stir in the long thread-like nerve running between the perineum and the point between the eyebrows. We can play with it using the practices we have learned so far. It is quite pleasant – ecstatic, we can say. Others have experienced the expansion of the ecstatic radiance to a much larger dimension. This is when we begin to experience the ida and pingala. As kundalini energy expands the sushumna outward, the ida and pingala are first in line for illumination.

Traditionally, the sushumna, ida and pingala are considered to be the three main highways of an awakened kundalini. These three nerves regulate the flow of prana through the entire nervous system. This regulating effect is there even before kundalini is awakened. As the awakening occurs, the flow of prana in the sushumna dominates, but the ida and pingala are awakened too. The ida runs up and down through the nerves on the left side of the spine, connecting the perineum with the sensitive tissues high up in the left nostril. The pingala runs up and down through the nerves on the right side of the spine, connecting the perineum with the sensitive tissues high up in the right nostril. Just as the sushumna expands ecstatically to encompass much more than the tiny channel in the spine, so too do the ida and pingala expand ecstatically to encompass much more than the limited physical dimensions of the nerves running up and down the outside of the spine.

This is a key thing to understand about the nervous system. We begin with the limited physical dimensions where the nerves are located in our body. Then, as kundalini awakens and ecstatic radiance rises, the physical dimensions are left behind. So, a nadi, or spiritual nerve, only corresponds with physical nerves in the beginning. As it is awakened, a nadi expands, radiating energy far beyond the physical location of the nerve. There are two ways of looking at this. We can say we are "going within," traveling in an expanding inner dimension. It feels like that as the sensory experience expands inside. The other way of looking at it is to say we are "expanding outward" in the physical dimension. In other words, expansion on the inner plane is the same as expanding outwardly in the physical dimension. We have to go in to go out. Those who have had kundalini experiences have described the energy going beyond the body as they are expanding inwardly at the same time. Anyone who comes to deep silence in meditation feels this expansion also – going in, but also radiating something peaceful out into the physical world. Whether the experience is the expansion of an awakened kundalini or the expanding silence of pure bliss consciousness in meditation, this is the nadis expanding. Both are different levels of the same thing. It is all the expansion of pure bliss consciousness.

So what does this mean in terms of experiencing the ida and pingala? As these two nerves are awakened by the expansion of the sushumna. They also expand beyond the physical nerves, and are seen to be like whips of ecstatic energy moving out in loops around the spine. They are not doing this statically in one place. They are moving, swirling, so one can barely tell left from right. One is hot (pingala), the other cold (ida), and this gives rise to the sensations of heat and cold coexisting in the body. There is a helix-like effect. Imagine a swirling column of ecstatic energy emanating from the center of your spine expanding outward. This is the sushumna. Now imagine it being surrounded by swirling whips of ecstatic energy. These are ida and pingala.

At certain locations along the spine, these three energies converge into whirling vortices in their ecstatic dance. These locations of convergence are the so-called energy centers, or chakras. The sushumna, ida and pingala are the main energy conduits connecting the chakras. As the nerves awaken, the chakras awaken. It begins as the spinal nerve awakens to an ecstatic radiance. But before any of this, it begins with gentle purification of all the nerves through meditation.

The sequence of awakening in these lessons begins with global purification of the nervous system through meditation, then to gentle awakening of the sushumna through spinal breathing, and finally to more targeted practices aimed at expanding ecstatic radiance to infinite dimensions. Not all approaches to yoga are like this. Some aim to awaken the sushumna straight away, before any significant amount of meditation is done. Others work to balance the ida and pingala first, and then enter the sushumna after that. Others work directly on the chakras first. Whatever the particular approach may be, the final outcome will be the same, a fully awakened nervous system, expanding in radiant ecstasy far beyond the confines of the physical body. All roads lead home, though the routes taken can vary considerably, as can the speed and comfort of the journey.

Okay, let's shut the hood and climb back behind the wheel. There are some more controls (advanced yoga practices) we will discuss now that can help speed us along on our way.

The guru is in you.

Lesson 91* – Yoni Mudra Kumbhaka – Purging the Third Eye, and More

Now that we have gotten everyone cautious about directly stimulating and awakening their kundalini energy, we will dive straight into the granddaddy of all the kundalini stimulators – kumbhaka (breath retention), with a full array of bandhas and mudras. Why not? When you are ready for it, you won't have to go hunting. It will be right here. Until then, I trust you will be wise and not push your practices to excess.

We will approach kumbhaka under the auspices of a practice called "yoni mudra," which means, "seal of the goddess." You can substitute the name of any female deity you want for "goddess." We all know who she is, even if by different names.

Before we get into yoni mudra, be reminded that all the same cautions apply here as detailed at the beginning of the recent lesson on siddhasana. You should be reasonably stable in all of your practices, and not experiencing internal energy instability in your everyday activities. You will find that much of what we have already been doing is part of the expanded style of yoni mudra we will be discussing here. We will be tying a group of practices together into a whole that is greater than the sum of the parts. This will give our nervous system the opportunity to evolve more quickly to a broader and more integrated style of natural functioning relating to the flow of pure bliss consciousness and divine ecstasy inside us.

There is an extra caution we should mention. We will be holding our breath here, and adding some gentle targeted inner pressure in the body. Nothing extreme will be recommended – certainly nothing more than the equivalent of jumping in a swimming pool and holding our breath voluntarily for a short while. If you have a heart condition, respiratory problems, high blood pressure, or any other condition that could be aggravated by holding your breath, then, either skip this advanced yoga practice, or get your doctor's permission before getting into it. In other words, if you know your doctor would not approve of you holding your breath and swimming underwater in a swimming pool, then you should stay away from yoni mudra kumbhaka. Safety first.

The practice of yoni mudra we will be discussing here is optimized in such a way so as to cover the entire sushumna by bringing in several other simultaneous practices.

It will be performed at the end of spinal breathing and before meditation. Right in-between those two well established practices.

Let's begin by sitting as we do in pranayama. This means sitting in our chosen version of siddhasana. We are at the end of spinal breathing when we do yoni mudra kumbhaka, so we have been going up and down inside the spinal nerve on our inhalation and exhalation for our allotted time.

Now, to go into the yoni mudra phase we will begin by placing the tips of our two index fingers close to the outer corners of our closed eyes against the lower lids. Then we gently push the eyes up and to the center in the direction of the point between the eyebrows. This should not be done with any strain or discomfort. Just a gentle nudge of the eyes toward the point between the eyebrows. If you have long nails on your index fingers, you may have to trim them for this part of yoni mudra.

Now, with our closed eyes in third eye nudged mode, we go up inside the spinal nerve with our inhalation from the perineum to the point between the eyebrows. When our lungs are full and our attention is at the top of the spinal nerve at the point between the eyebrows, we close our nostrils on the outside with our two middle fingers pressing from either side of the nose. At the same time we keep the index fingers in place pressing the eyes gently toward the point between the eyebrows.

Also, at the same time, we lift our tongue to the roof of our mouth, sealing off the mouth inside so no air can escape through there. Now we are holding our breath. But we are not holding it with the epiglottis in our throat, as we normally would. Instead, we allow the air pressure from our expanded lungs to come up easily into our nasal passages and sinuses. This is not a big pressure, only a small one. We don't push it up there. We just let the natural pressure of our filled lungs be up there. Our middle fingers and tongue block our nose and mouth, so no air can escape.

Try that and see how it works. Pretty easy, isn't it?

What we do now is hold our breath for a comfortable duration – not too long, not too short. Depending on your capacity it could be thirty seconds, a minute, or maybe longer. If you are a professional sponge diver, it could be several minutes. It doesn't matter exactly how long it is. What matters is that we hold our breath inside for a time that is both comfortable and going a bit toward the edge of our capacity. Not to the point of straining. Not to the point of gasping for air when we are done. When we are done and ready to exhale, we let our middle fingers go from the nostrils, but not the index fingers from our eyes or our raised tongue. We should have enough composure left to do a nice smooth exhalation through our nose going back down the spinal nerve with our attention to the perineum. When we exhale we should not be desperate for air. We can go a little faster than in normal spinal breathing, both on inhalation and exhalation, but if we are in a big rush to get air, we have held our breath too long. Find a balance. It will be a bit clunky at first, as all of these advanced yoga practices are. But it will smooth out quickly to a comfortable practice. The idea is to spend quality time with the breath suspended inside. It should not be an exercise in heroics.

Starting out, we will do only three of these yoni mudra kumbhakas between pranayama and meditation. So it is only a few minutes we are adding in the middle our practice of pranayama and meditation. But there is more to yoni mudra kumbhaka than just mentioned. There are some other things we want to be doing during our kumbhaka to produce the most positive results. So let's get into more detail.

Having just come out of spinal breathing, we will have been doing mulabandha and sambhavi already, as well as sitting in siddhasana. In yoni mudra kumbhaka we continue with mulabandha. Sambhavi is modified during yoni mudra because we are nudging the eyes toward the point between the eyebrows with our index fingers. With our index fingers doing that, we do not do the lifting and centering of the eyes part of sambhavi. However we do continue with the furrowing of the brow, gently bringing the eyebrows together toward the center. So sambhavi in yoni mudra is a combination of lifting and centering the eyes with the index fingers and gently pulling the eyebrows together with the muscles in our head. Also, in yoni mudra kumbhaka, our attention is brought to the point between the eyebrows for the entire period of retention of breath, until we go back down the spinal nerve on exhalation. In fact, we may find our attention being draw out in front of the point between our eyebrows during yoni mudra kumbhaka. This is natural. As the spinal nerve begins have some ecstatic conductivity, it becomes quite pleasurable to do sambhavi. Nudging the eyes toward the point between the eyebrows with the fingers while pulling the eyebrows together in yoni mudra can fill the whole body with pleasure as the ecstatic conductivity rises in the spinal nerve. ("If your eye be single, your body will be filled with light.") The pleasure naturally increases as the attention goes out beyond the point between the eyebrows. There is something out beyond the body that calls us with ecstasy. We find that the sushumna keeps going, and it is okay to go there as we are naturally attracted. What will we find there? Oh, we will find out. It is all good. If this extension of the sushumna is occurring it is okay to let our attention go the full distance of it out in front during our normal spinal breathing as well. It is a natural evolution of the sushumna, and spinal breathing. It is promoted during yoni mudra, and is only one of the many benefits of this advanced yoga practice.

The maneuver with the tongue going to the roof of the mouth is the beginning stage of an advanced yoga practice called "kechari mudra." The tongue has a very important role to play as our practice advances. For now, we just want to comfortably seal off the air from escaping through the mouth during yoni mudra. Maybe that means the tip of our tongue is placed behind the front teeth. Or maybe further back. If we can comfortably reach the point where the hard and soft palates meet on the roof of the mouth, that is a good place to park the tip of the tongue. It does not have to be there though. Whatever works most comfortably now is what we want. There will much more on kechari in future lessons.

There are two other components we'd like to add to yoni mudra. First is something called "jalandhara bandha," which means, "chin lock." We will take a less stringent approach than what is implied. All we will do during breath retention in yoni mudra kumbhaka is let the head come down as far as it comfortably goes toward the chest. During inhalation and exhalation we lift it up again. That's all. We just let the head hang down during breath retention, and let our fingers, placed on the eyes and nose, stay in place as the head comes down. If our chin goes comfortably half way down to the hollow of our throat, that is fine. If our chin goes all the way to the hollow of our throat that is the full chin lock. Either way is fine. Jalandhara stretches the spinal nerve in the upper part of the body from the point between the eyebrows on down. It is easy to feel the stretching. We don't strain it. If there is some ecstatic conductivity in the spinal nerve, we can feel the stretching reach all the way to the perineum. It is amazing how it works. With jalandhara, we stretch the sushumna from the third eye to the root. This stretching greatly enhances the effect of yoni mudra kumbhaka, and promotes the rise of ecstatic conductivity in the spinal nerve. Later on, we will work more with jalandhara, using a dynamic version of it to stimulate huge amounts of prana up into the heart, throat and head. Jalandhara is a very important advanced yoga practice. Here in yoni mudra we are introducing the beginning of it – just letting the head go down easily while the breath is held in. Then we lift the head up while we are doing our exhalation and inhalation. We keep it comfortable.

The other component we will add is uddiyana. This also comes in several versions, which we will explore fully down the road. At this stage we are introducing a basic version for yoni mudra. When we are retaining the breath during yoni mudra, we gently lift our diaphragm a little and pull our belly in. This ties in with mulabandha coming up from the anal sphincter through the pelvis. Uddiyana does wonders as we are sitting in siddhasana too. Uddiyana, which means, "to fly up," is connected with the activity in the pelvis, and carries it all up much higher. Because we are full of air in yoni mudra kumbhaka, we will not be pulling up with the diaphragm very much. Just a little.

You will feel the pressure coming up through the body from uddiyana. Don't overdo it. If you have learned yoga postures (it's highly recommended you do this), you will no doubt have learned to do uddiyana while standing up with all your air expelled (see addition to lesson #71). This is a good way to get some familiarity with it. There is a lot that will be done with the diaphragm and abdominal muscles. We will get further into it later. For now, just pull up a little during your yoni mudra kumbhaka. Let it go as you are exhaling and inhaling between breath retentions.

So, there are a lot of things being done in yoni mudra. Most are physical habits that can be easily cultivated. In time, once we are through the clunky stage, all of these things will come together into one integrated reflex of the body that happens automatically when the breath is retained. Then, as ecstatic conductivity rises, these maneuvers will refine into subtle coordinated inner movements responding the natural flow of divine ecstasy within. All that we have been discussing here is an introduction to a new and natural style of bodily functioning. In its advanced form all these components of practice discussed above will manifest as intimately connected, automatic "micro-movements" in the body, occurring invisibly as the energy moves in us day and night. All of these physical procedures we are learning now relate directly to the biology of ecstatic experience rising in the body. Though we are very clunky right now with these things, you will be amazed at how subtle, smooth, and naturally connected they become. Daily yoni mudra kumbhaka, with the full array of bandhas and mudras added gradually transforms us into the ecstatic equivalent of a fine tuned Ferrari. It may not seem like it now, but that is what happens. Yoni mudra kumbhaka is advanced spiritual training for the biology.

We will take a very gradual approach to yoni mudra kumbhaka, starting slow and easy with three repetitions between pranayama and meditation, as discussed. Those who find the practice of yoni mudra kumbhaka good and smooth can ramp up by baby steps. Do not overdo it. Kumbhaka is the most powerful of all the direct kundalini stimulators. If three repetitions are good, then maybe in a month try four. After a few more months, you could consider trying five repetitions. Like that. Don't start doing five or ten right out of the gate. A very slow buildup is the way to go, and then only if you are smooth in all your practices and in daily activity.

We've talked about how to do yoni mudra kumbhaka, but not much about what yoni mudra kumbhaka does inside us. Put simply, it works to open every nook and cranny of our nervous system and draws kundalini (sexual energy) up at the same time. It produces a huge amount of purification in the body. It also cultivates the subtle habits of ecstatic biological functioning in us.

The multiple angles we take on the third eye produce a purging effect at the upper end of the sushumna and throughout the entire head. So, yoni mudra is a third eye cleanser for sure. The entire spinal nerve is stretched and permeated with prana coming up from the pelvic region. Also, kumbhaka, by creating an extra demand for life force in the body, pulls a large amount of sexual energy (kundalini) up from the vast storehouse of prana located in the pelvis. Siddhasana, mulabandha, and uddiyana promote this drawing up going on in the lower part of the body.

This is a broad overview of what happens. Many other things go on in the biology and nervous system as a result of yoni mudra kumbhaka. Way more than can be discussed in these few paragraphs. We will fill in the details in future lessons as experiences come up.

Finally, it should be mentioned that this is an optimized version of yoni mudra, aimed at promoting a broad range of openings in the nervous system. Formal yoni mudra involves using more fingers to seal the ears (thumbs) and mouth (ring and pinky fingers), and fewer of the bandhas and mudras given here. What we are learning here is a hybrid practice for the sake of efficiency. In a few extra minutes during our twice-daily sittings, we can add a big boost to all of our practices, and to our experience of the rise of pure bliss consciousness and divine ecstasy in our life. That is what this yoni mudra kumbhaka is for.

The guru is in you.

Addition – The introduction of kumbhaka here is for the retention of breath inside during performance of yoni mudra. This is called "internal kumbhaka." Since this lesson was posted, several inquiries have been received regarding "external kumbhaka," where the breath is expelled and held outside with the lungs empty. This is a practice taught in some traditions, but not in AYP, and it has not been discussed in the lessons. A Q&A on this is being added here for completeness.

Q: have you ever heard about negative effects from kumbhaka on exhale? I did experiment with it for while, but recently read a number of warnings that it could be destructive in a long run.

A: If you mean by "kumbhaka on exhale," holding the breath outside with the lungs empty, yes, I agree that that there can be some risk there. In the lessons we use it for short periods with uddiyana/nauli (to be fully covered in lesson #129), but not much beyond that. If it happens automatically in our practices, we let it if it is not extreme. Sometimes the breath will suspend outwardly automatically during meditation. All that is fine. The nervous system knows what it needs. The lessons do not prescribe deliberate external kumbhaka, holding the breath out for extended periods. The reason is because the lungs are not designed for that, and the forceful negative pressure in the lungs can do damage over time.

For the same reason we do not restrict inhalation during ujjayi (lesson #41) or brahmari (lesson #229) pranayamas in spinal breathing.

The lungs are designed to hold air in, and that is very natural, as everyone knows. Holding the air out forcefully is not so natural, though it will happen during brief times of uddiyana/nauli, and sometimes in automatic yoga. Neither of these put a strain on the lungs for an extended time. So that is the approach to doing external kumbhaka in the lessons – sparingly, and only in the situations just described.

Lesson 92 – The Star

Q: I have meditated for the past 10 years. I would say that I was never really good at it. I felt that way because I was easily distracted during meditation by thoughts. With that in mind, it was a hit or miss as to whether I meditated or not. In other words, not a daily practice. More like 3-4 times a week.

Prior to joining your group, I was told how to do yoni mudra. I wasn't really doing it right, but the first two times I saw this beautiful circle with a star in the middle. I did not know at that time that it was something that would happen after doing yoni mudra. A couple of days after seeing it, I received a flyer in the mail from the Self Realization Fellowship, and on the flyer was the exact thing I saw. I had not seen it again even with trying yoni mudra.

So, now fast forward. I joined your group. I really liked the fact that the thoughts that come are ok. Just keep going and go back to the mantra. I felt like maybe I was doing it right before and that my expectation was off. I've committed to doing the practice twice a day. I wanted to keep the "time line" in mind so that I didn't rush through this. So I added the advanced practices slowly. I haven't really had any rush of kundalini energy like some of the people, but I decided to keep practicing.

This morning I tried the yoni mudra for the first time since joining your group. As soon as I started, I saw a bunch of crazy lights. I just watched and kept doing it. Then came the circles with the star in the middle. There was a bright circle with a dark circle inside. In the middle was the star. The star would fade in and out. I didn't want it to go away. I went into my meditation and it did leave.

My question is, what's the star all about? Why do I want to see it so badly when I don't even know what it is all about? I know it is part of the process but how and why is not known. Will I see it when I meditate, or only during yoni mudra? Is there something I can do to retain the star during meditation? What made it come during yoni mudra? Am I supposed to do something with the star?

A: The simple procedure of meditation doesn't mind thoughts at all, or anything else. It is the art of gentle persuasion, letting the mantra refine to pure bliss consciousness. The mind goes to stillness easily when we give up the fight with thoughts and just favor the mantra naturally at deeper levels whenever we become aware we are off it. This is the way in.

On seeing the star, it is a natural outcome of purifying the sushumna (spinal nerve) and opening the third eye. It was mentioned in the lesson on yoni mudra kumbhaka that the attention will sooner or later be drawn out beyond the point between the eyebrows. This is an extension of the sushumna beyond the body. At the end of the sushumna are the infinite realms of bright white light. They are seen as a bright star in the beginning. The colors ringed around the star are the inside of the sushumna. You are looking out from the inside, so you are seeing the inside of the sushumna in your body, and the end of the sushumna off in the distance, which is the star. You are looking through the tunnel of the sushumna, seeing "the light at the end of the tunnel," as they say. Inside the tunnel, we are literally a rainbow of light, beginning with dark red at the bottom and ending with blue and violet at the top. You have heard the expression, "She has a heart of gold." Well, we all have hearts of gold. We just need some housecleaning to see it. That is the outer ring you are seeing.

Some of the most graphic and beautiful descriptions of the inside of the sushumna are presented by Norman Paulsen in his book, *Sacred Science*. Mr. Paulsen is one of the few remaining direct disciples of Paramahansa Yogananda, the famed yogi, founder of the Self Realization Fellowship, and author of *Autobiography of a Yogi*. In his book, Mr. Paulsen discusses a more intricate form of spinal breathing. There are a variety of approaches to spinal breathing, different styles. The approach to spinal breathing we use in these lessons is chosen for its simplicity and known effectiveness. Each person is free to choose, so different styles of practice are honored here.

The sacred diagram, *Sri Yantra*, is also a representation of the inner reality of humanity – concentric circles of divine feminine energy forming a tunnel leading to the final union of Shiva and Shakti in the center. When we do spinal breathing we are joining these two energies everywhere inside the sushumna, and in every part of the nervous system. This is one of the few instances in life where "tunnel vision" has some positive connotations to it.

What are we to do with this star when we see it, and a rising awareness of the sushumna tunnel that often goes with it? It is an important question you raise. Yes, we are naturally attracted to the star. It is "heaven." It is where we go when we die. Reports of the tunnel and white light are common among those who have had a near death experience. The tunnel is the way by which we have come into this earthly existence as well. Now you can see why spinal breathing is so important in our practice. We are clearing our highway to heaven. But it isn't time to leave yet! Therein lies the answer to the question: What do we do about the star? You will get different answers from different people on this question. There is a lot of hub-bub about it.

The answer in these lessons is, we don't do much with the star. We let the experience of it evolve naturally, just as we do with everything coming up as a result of our practices. As the star comes up we regard it as any other part of our inner workings and go back to the practice we are doing. It is, after all, just another feature of our spiritual anatomy, like nadis, chakras and the like. Everything in heaven and earth is contained within us. We don't have to go anywhere to be what we already are. If our ecstasy inside or outside practices draws us into the star, then this is just fine. Whatever happens there is part of our experience of divine expansion. If our ecstasy draws us elsewhere in our spiritual anatomy, that is fine too. If we are in practices, we easily favor the practice we are doing, like always. We don't get all hung up on this or that experience that may come up. If we are not in practices and we see something happening in our spiritual anatomy – let's enjoy! In these lessons we are yogis and yoginis first, and tourists second. It is fine to enjoy the scenery when we are outside practices. There will be plenty for us to see. While inside practices, we stick to the easy job of favoring the practice we are doing.

On this earth we are in the business of putting our nervous system in good spiritual working order. That is what we are here for. This can only be done by continuing to nudge the nervous system every day to higher levels of functioning. As soon as we become fixated on any particular aspect of our spiritual anatomy, we may be doing so at the expense of the overall enlightenment project. For this reason, we do well to consider all the inner mechanics and experiences to be going on "under the hood" as we zoom along on our road of advanced yoga practices to enlightenment.

Let's go back to our analogy of taking a trip to California. Let's suppose we are building ourselves a road to California. One that will enable us to have easy access to come and go as we please. As our road under construction gets close enough to Los Angeles, we will see the bright lights shining off in the distance. We might be tempted to stop working on the road and just run across country to the lights of LA. Doing that, we end up in LA, leaving an unfinished road outside town somewhere. Not that LA needed another road anyway, but it is just an analogy. Sooner or later we will have to go back and finish that road. LA is not completely LA until we can come and go as we please. Like that, heaven is not completely heaven until we can come and go as we please. For that, we need a fully purified nervous system.

Enlightenment is not about running off to heaven and leaving an unpurified nervous system behind that we will have to come back to and finish later in another life. It is about doing the work of completely purifying the nervous system. Then we have it all, become it all – heaven, earth, the cosmos, LA, everything. Then we become an expression of heaven on earth, and can do much for others who are expressions of heaven also, just needing a good housecleaning to realize it. So, it is not about going off into the star. It is about bringing the star in here, into the earth plane. That we do by purifying and opening the nervous system. As Jesus said, "You are the light of the world."

So, if you are seeing the star or having ecstasy reaching out beyond the point between the eyebrows, go there as part of your normal spinal breathing. It will add a lot to your practice. If you see the star or have ecstasy extending out beyond the point between the eyebrows during yoni mudra kumbhaka, just be there easily during kumbhaka as the instructions say. Don't try and hang on to it. A natural purification and connection is occurring. Just let it happen. Keep in mind that we are working to purify our nervous system here on earth. That is what we are doing in meditation, spinal breathing, kumbhaka, bandhas, mudras and all the rest. Enjoy the bliss of heaven when it kisses you. Bring it back into your body naturally in practices. Remember, the work we are doing is here in this earth form. What we accomplish here we will take with us wherever we go when we leave. This nervous system is the gateway. If we attend to that, everything else will take care of itself.

It has been said that the angels in heaven are a bit jealous of us mortal human beings. Why? Because on this plane of existence we have the nervous system readily available to purify, and the motivation (our mortality) to do something about it. It is much easier to do that work here on earth than in heaven. So the angels are a bit jealous. They are waiting for their turn to do what we can do here and now – advanced yoga practices. So, before we go running off to heaven, let's make the best of our opportunity here and now. Heaven will be there when it is our time to go. The more we can purify our nervous system here and now, the easier it will be for us later on.

There is a tendency in some approaches to get into some particular vision. To have that vision means everything. It doesn't have to be like that. The manifestation of truth won't be exactly the same for everyone. So, picking a specific vision to strive for could be a mistake. Maybe some will never see a tunnel or star. Maybe they just zoom through at some point and it is all pure white light. Or maybe some other kinds of colors, and then the white light. Maybe no white light, and just more and more ecstasy, until one day, boom! … white light is everywhere inside and outside the body. It can happen many different ways, depending on the unique purification process going on in each person. No one can tell how it should be for every person. For this reason we don't worry much about visions in these lessons. We do the practices every day that we know encourage the nervous system to purify and open naturally. The experiences will be whatever they will be. If we keep clearing the highway to heaven, there can be no doubt that we will arrive in the best shape, and have the everlasting ability to come and go as we please.

A vision is not the big payoff in yoga. Eternal freedom in enlightenment is!

The guru is in you.

Lesson 93 – Changing Times

Q: I feel like meditation is going good, and I just took up spinal pranayama which is proving to be challenging to get through the clunky startup as you call it. With all the other things you introduced, I feel like I am going underwater. So many wonderful practices, and me so inadequate to do them. I doubt my worthiness for all this, yet I have so much desire to pursue the path to the end. I wish I had started this twenty years ago. I am going crazy with impatience, yet I know if I push too hard it could make problems. What should I do?

A: You are doing just right taking it one step at a time. While your emotions may be raging for the divine, you are clear on what must be done in what order, what you can undertake now, and what you can undertake later. And you will. It is coming together just right. Just take it one day at a time. You will know what to do next.

You suffer from a most blessed disease – intense bhakti. We should all have this disease. If we all did, the world would be transformed in one generation. I know it may not stem your impatience to hear that, but that is how it is with bhakti, you know. When we become acutely aware of our separation from the divine, we crave yoga like mad. We become mad for God. It is a blessed condition to be in. It will get much better as your experiences of union advance, and they will as you continue with daily practices.

Bhakti will continue to increase in all of us as time rolls on. There are powerful forces at work that are putting the spiritual winds at our back. All we have to do is put out the sails in the form of practices, and the spiritual winds constantly fanning our nervous system will do the rest.

Let's step back for a minute and take a look at the big picture that we are all part of. We are living in very interesting times. Back in the 1960s, Bob Dylan sang, "The times, they are a-changing." It was certainly true then, and it is even more true now.

Depending on which astrological approach you consider, the earth has been, or will soon be, entering a "new age" of enlightenment. In Sanskrit, these ages are called "yugas." The new one may have started over a hundred years ago. Or it may be starting now. It has been a popular topic since those early Dylan days. But an emergence was occurring in the world of yoga long before then. The start of a new age is not an instantaneous event. It starts with a long gradual build-up, and it keeps accelerating as momentum grows. Quite a lot has happened already, and we are whisking along at an ever-increasing pace.

Around the turn of the last century, Vivekananda, a leading disciple of Ramakrishna, came to the West and planted the first seeds of yoga that found some fertile soil and sprouted. Twenty years later, Paramahansa Yogananda came and found even more receptivity than Vivekananda did. By the time Maharishi Mahesh Yogi came along in the 1960s, a whole generation of disaffected baby boomers was ready to jump into yoga in a big way, with a little help from the Beatles, of course. Since those days, hundreds of yogis have come to the West from India, and thousands of "next generation" Western yogis and yoginis have stepped up to the teaching podium. Actually, in the past couple of decades, things have gotten a bit muddled, a bit confused. So many different approaches to yoga have come up that it is hard to know which brand of yoga is the real one, if there is even such a thing as "the real yoga." Will the real yoga please stand up? There are many volunteers for this exalted position, of course. Some have even gone to court to stake their claim on your nervous system. There have always been those who would like to be in charge of your gateway to heaven. Well, never mind that.

So, in a century we have gone from having no yoga to having so many different kinds that we are looking at a proverbial yoga "Tower of Babel."

That's okay. It is a good thing. Obviously, it can't stay splintered in a thousand pieces like that forever. Sooner or later it will be distilled down to something (or several somethings) that the average ready-to-become-enlightened person can grab hold of. In the next few decades the name of the game is going to be, "consolidation," "integration," "optimization," "simplification."

Pick any of those, and you will have the idea. It will be the scientific method that will produce this distillation of the knowledge of yoga, so the widespread application of it will become practical.

When personal computers first came out, you needed to know an archaic language like "BASIC" or "DOS" to get anything done. Computing was an esoteric world for geeks. Then the mouse pointer and graphical user interface came along, and suddenly the doors to easy computing were flung open for everyone. It was a revolution.

This has been the story with many applications of knowledge over the centuries. It starts out with a few "geeks' who establish a beach head in applying a type of knowledge. Then, later on, some researchers figure out how to make it easy for everyone to apply the knowledge. It nearly always boils down to simplifying the user interface, the main controls, so anyone can apply the knowledge with good results. Useful technology is "user friendly." Remember the Wright Brothers? Remember Henry Ford? Remember Thomas Edison? They all simplified the interface between users and the application of powerful knowledge.

This is what is going to happen with yoga. It must happen. Millions of people are feeling the spiritual winds rising inside them in this new age, and the sails of practice must be pulled up. It is time for the full range of yoga knowledge to be made user friendly.

Nothing is new in yoga. All of the components of practice have been around for thousands of years. Natural principles don't change. The human nervous system has always had the same natural abilities. There have been enlightened times in the past when yoga has flourished. In darker times, the vision was less clear about the possibilities in us. There was heavy doubt, superstition and fear. But a few have always been playing around with applications of yogic knowledge – doing it in secret in the darker times, because they'd get strung up if they got too public with their endeavors. They have been the "geeks" of yoga, you know. The pioneers who created the esoteric traditions. We owe much to the great old-time yogis. They have given us the seeds of knowledge necessary to proceed full speed ahead into the new age. Now it is up to this generation, and the coming ones, to develop and utilize simplified interfaces with the human nervous system, optimizing the application of yogic knowledge so many will be able to take up yoga practices and have good success.

The new age is not just about the spiritual winds coming up behind us from the cosmos. The enlightenment game is not a spectator sport. We have to get in the game if we want to have the benefits. We have to put up the sails of practices to take the ride. As we do, this earth will continue to become a better place. As we bring the reality of pure bliss consciousness and divine ecstasy into the earth plane through our practices, everything will change. There will be light and love rising everywhere in abundance. It will not be an ideological occurrence. It will be a real energy transformation, palpable to all who live on the earth. With nervous systems everywhere becoming powerful radiators of pure bliss consciousness and divine ecstasy, no one will be left in the dark.

Lingering doubts will be swept away. The winds of bhakti will carry us ever forward. All we have to do is keep up the sails of our daily practices. Our nervous system will take care of the rest.

The guru is in you.

Lesson 94 – Some House Cleaning Tips

The goal in Advanced Yoga Practices is to provide the most important yoga methods in an easy to manage way so you can begin and continue a daily routine of spiritual practices without having to turn you life upside down. We have taken a "building block" approach, where you decide when to add on each new piece according to your time line and capacity. Each building block is a pretty easy practice by itself. When you have two, three, four, or ten pieces, it will still be easy if you have not gone too fast in adding on components of practice. Easy in practices and easy in daily activity is our objective, with pure bliss consciousness and divine ecstasy coming up ever so steadily to become a 24/7 experience (meaning 24 hours per day, 7 days per week).

What we are doing in all our practices is giving our nervous system the opportunity to clear out the old accumulated obstructions that block the ongoing experience of our inner truth, which is bliss, bliss, bliss!

It is a house cleaning that is going on in our nervous system. The experiences that come up during the house cleaning cover a wide range from the spectacular to the dull and dreary. No matter what the experiences are, the house cleaning goes on, as long as we are doing our daily practices.

It is important to be clear about the difference between practices and experiences. This is especially true since we have been stimulating kundalini, and maybe having some pretty ecstatic feelings and even some impressive visions coming up. So here are a few tips on what to do if some of these things happen in practices.

If you are doing spinal breathing and, as you come up to the third eye on inhalation, your ishta (your chosen ideal – Jesus, Krishna, Moses, Mohammed, Mother Divine, etc.) comes galloping up to you in a golden chariot, beckoning you to climb in and go for a ride, what do you do? You easily exhale and go back down the spinal nerve. In other words, you favor the practice you are doing. If the chariot with your ishta in it goes down the spinal nerve with you, great. If it doesn't, that is okay too. We don't push visions out. Neither do we hang on to them. We just favor the practice we are doing. If these visions are real, they will be with us for a long time both inside and outside practices. Your ishta will understand that you are doing practices, and will be happy to take you for a ride afterwards. It is the practices that have created the opportunity for such experiences in your expanding spiritual nervous system. Always keep that in mind. Don't let your experiences distract you from the practices that have facilitated them. If you remain steadfast in practices, your experiences will become greater and greater, eventually never leaving you. You will find yourself trooping around during the day with your ishta, and an entourage of angels too! Experiences do not beget greater experiences. Practices do.

If you are doing yoni mudra kumbhaka and you are filling up with divine light rushing in through your third eye, with more and more light coming, and you are wanting to do more and more yoni mudra kumbhaka because it is so good, what do you do? You stick with the number of repetitions of yoni mudra kumbhaka you are doing. Well, maybe add one, if it is that terrific. But keep in mind that it is easy to overdo when such wonderful experiences are occurring. Then, the next thing you know, you are frying inside for a few days because you did too much. The nervous can only handle so much at any given level of purification. If too much is put through the nerves before they are ready, the frying effect can happen. It is like being in a fire. It isn't hell, though it might feel like it. It is just too much energy too soon. That's all. Take the gradual approach to purification, and you will have a much more pleasant journey, and will not jeopardize your ability to do advanced yoga practices over the long haul. It is doing well-measured practices over the long haul that leads to enlightenment. Then all the light and bliss will be there without the fire. The fire comes from fast house cleaning – sometimes we stir up too much dust and it is too fast with so much coming out. There are no overnight wonders in this house cleaning business.

While meditation is usually a more gentle and blissful process, settling the nervous system down to deep silence and letting obstructions go in a global way, still, powerful experiences can come up in there. When we have thoughts, sensations, lights, ecstasy, restlessness, visions, negative emotions, whatever, we just easily come back to the mantra. We do not meditate for any particular experience other than the experience of favoring the mantra when we realize we are off it. It does not matter what we are off into. If the heavenly hosts come and fill our inner vision during our meditation, and we realize we are off the mantra, what do we do? You guessed it. We easily go back to the mantra. If we are true to the simple procedures of our practices, we can revel with the heavenly hosts whenever we want – while we are having a sandwich, in the shower, taking a walk, or anywhere ... except in our practices. If we are seeing them in practices and realize we are off the mantra, off the spinal breathing, or off the count in yoni mudra kumbhaka, then we do best to ease back to the particular practice we are doing.

A word that sometimes comes up when discussing practices is "expectations." We all have expectations. They are desires. Our desires are always wanting more, reaching for this or that thing. We can slip into the habit of expecting certain kinds of experiences. If we apply the technique of bhakti, we can transform the energy of our expectations, channeling them into motivation to do our daily practices. If we find expectations for visions, or whatever, coming up in practices, we treat them like any other thoughts or feelings that come up, and easily go back to the practice we are doing.

This is the way to get the house cleaning done most effectively. We aren't giving anything up by taking this approach. We are gaining everything.

The guru is in you.

Lesson 95 – Stabilizing Ecstasy

Q: I can't begin to express how much I am enjoying the practices. I have held at siddhasana for now because I feel so much bliss and at times incredible energy surges as if my whole body pulsates! My whole outlook is bliss. I see God the universal being at times everywhere. Today, while driving, I felt so good. I felt as if I should scream out the window and tell everyone I love them and to join the practices. I had to dance when I got home ... Now my question is do I hold where I am and just enjoy, or do I add on the other practices? I don't want to stimulate the kundalini too much so she gets angry with me. Right now I feel the bliss connection some days stronger, some days only lightly.

A: I'm very happy to hear things are going so well. Given your sensitivity (wonderful!), it would be a good idea to bide your time at the level you are at for a month or two. Maybe more. You have taken on a lot in a very short time. Give things a chance to even out. Make sure practices and daily activity continue smoothly. The big rushes of ecstasy have to do with purification. It is the fun part of house cleaning, but it is still house cleaning. In time, there will be less friction in the nervous system and the ecstasy will become refined, like a quiet divine smile forever radiating outward from inside you – very peaceful and very powerful.

You will know you are ready for the next step when the level you are at becomes steady without so many big rushes. Yoni mudra kumbhaka is very powerful, and you want to be sure you are stable before getting into it. When you do, start slow, maybe with only one or two repetitions per session, and see how it goes. Be very measured with it, as there can be a delayed reaction with kumbhaka. Feel your way along according to your own capacity.

As for telling others about the lessons, by all means do so if you feel this is good stuff. This unorthodox approach of open transmission of advanced yoga practices will grow only if many come on to it and find good success. Then who will be able to question the validity of it? It is really a test of how ready we all are for wide open spiritual science, where everyone can sit in their own driver's seat. Time will tell.

The guru is in you.

Lesson 96 – Spinal Breathing Startup Review

Q: My question is about what I should expect to experience during spinal breathing. I do not visualize well or easily, and it's very difficult for me to imagine anything moving up and down my spinal column, as I cannot yet feel anything happening. I sometimes talk to myself during this exercise ("...the light goes up to my third eye ... the light comes down from my third eye..."). Sometimes I try to do it silently.

If I am intent on imagining the breath moving up and down the spinal nerve, is this sufficient? I am concerned that in trying to concentrate I am becoming too tense. On the other hand, I become caught up in the challenge of trying to move the breath up and down my spine, and I usually find that I spend more time on pranayama than I meant to. And I do enjoy it! Can you tell from my description whether I am doing this technique correctly?

A: Yes, you are doing fine. Just continue imagining the breath going up and down inside that little spinal nerve. It takes a while to develop the mental habit. Be easy about it, like in meditation. If you wander off the spinal breathing, just easily come back to it. There is nothing more to expect than that you will continue that easy process. If other visions come and fill your attention, just favor the practice of simple spinal breathing – breath with the attention going up and down. No big effort at concentration is necessary, and no big visualizations are needed. You should be able to let go of the verbalizations pretty soon. It is best to be easy and relaxed with the process.

Review the lessons on spinal breathing (beginning at #41) in a month or two and you can pick up some of the refinements. By then you will be through the "clunky" stage and much smoother in your practice. In time, you will want to add more elements of practice. It is all in the lessons. You will know when you are ready. Just take it one step at a time, and be easy with it. Make sure you always follow pranayama with meditation.

Something good is happening.

The guru is in you.

Lesson 97 – Tantra – Help for Sex Maniacs and Ordinary Lovers

Q: I am sort of a sex maniac. I can't seem to get enough of it. My wife takes every opportunity to encourage me, so she must be one too. Needless to say, we have a very active sex life. In the past year we have gotten interested in Tantra and Yoga, but we have not been able to get our sex under control. We don't even know if we are supposed to get it under control. It is beginning to concern me that I am draining myself of vitality every day. I know it can't go on like that forever if I hope to achieve anything spiritually. You have given many practical methods for Yoga and we are very grateful, but we are still hooked on sex. What do you suggest?

A: If your desire is strong to bring your active sex life into the realm of yoga, much can be done using the methods of tantra. It will not necessarily mean curtailing your sex life. That can go on naturally as before. It will mean developing some discipline in the form of specific techniques you can use during sex, and these you can practice together. There are other techniques you can practice alone. Then you will find sex gradually becoming part of the larger picture of your overall yoga practices.

In most situations, it is the man who holds the keys to tantra in sexual relations, because it is he who experiences the greatest loss of prana, and it is he who usually determines the duration of the sex act. No matter how much a woman may long for tantric unions, it is the man who must first facilitate them. Then it can become heaven for both the man and woman.

Once a man becomes committed to manage the loss of prana, thereby lengthening the duration of sexual union, a new mode of lovemaking will evolve that is in the direction of yoga. Then sex can become a strong facilitator of the union of the masculine and feminine energies within us, along the same lines as mulabandha and siddhasana.

Tantric sex, while not at the heart of Advanced Yoga Practices, is an important skill to develop, especially if we are inclined to have sex often. It is an extension of the principles of siddhasana, really, where we are cultivating sexual energy upward into our nervous system as it is being gradually being purified using the full range of advanced yoga practices.

The sexual methods of tantra we will discuss are to support the overall goals of the advanced yoga practices we have been using in these lessons, without putting any sort of draconian limits on our freedom to make love whenever we like. Applying and gradually mastering the sexual methods of tantra frees us from the negative stigmas that sometimes get attached to sex. Sex becomes another aspect of our spiritual anatomy that we have the means to nudge toward the higher purpose of our enlightenment. Sexual relations become an aid to our spiritual evolution rather than remaining an obstacle. At the same time, we gradually come to enjoy sex in ways we may have never imagined. Good tantra is very liberating all the way around.

To honor requirements regarding the posting of sexual content in this group, we will continue the tantra discussion in a separate adults-only group that has been created for this purpose. It is the same format as this group, except it is for adults only. The tantra lessons are included in this book following the main lessons.

So, for those of you who are inclined to learn how human sexual relations can be utilized directly in support of your advanced yoga practices, the rest of the focused tantra discussion can be found in the separate lessons. These include questions and answers that pertain to tantric sexual methods and experiences. As you will see, the tantra lessons ultimately tie back into the main lessons quite naturally.

The main lessons will continue along the lines that have been indicated. As you know, there is much more to cover on Advanced Yoga Practices, and we will carry on here.

The guru is in you.

Lesson 98 – Yoga and Marriage

Q: Can a person get married and still practice meditation and attain the "goal?" How does marriage help/disturb the spiritual growth of a person?

A: Marriage is not necessarily incompatible with spiritual practice. Marriage can be an important part of spiritual practice, for it can help us grow into a life of loving service. The sexual aspect need not be a deterrent either. It all depends on how you approach it. The previous lesson on tantra begins the discussion on this subject.

I am married with grown children, and deeper into practices than ever, finding life filled with joy. The greatest challenge that marriage and raising a family places on spiritual practices is the need to provide for everyone and then make the time for practices too. It takes a strong commitment, a lot of bhakti. There are many rewards if one can manage to do it all.

Some may prefer to focus only on their spiritual life. This is not so simple either. Renunciates can become ingrown and narrow in their outlook, with little regard for others and stunted in their spiritual progress even while doing many yoga practices. Service to "a family" of some sort is necessary to keep the heart and spiritual progress growing. The family may be our neighbor who needs help, our spouse and children, our community, or all of humanity. A joining of some sort that connects us to others in service is important. If it is marriage, that is great. If it is not that, then something that puts us in a position of having some responsibility to help someone other than ourselves.

If we are helping others, we are helping ourselves. It is the oldest wisdom in the scriptures.

Ultimately, spiritual progress is less dependent on our external environment than on our internal environment. This is why meditation is first. It goes right to the source and immediately begins building the right internal environment – pure silent bliss consciousness. Then we should go and do something with this inner silent quality. We will be wise to take our pure bliss consciousness and give it to the world in some form of service. Then we are like a channel, and the pure bliss consciousness and divine ecstasy come up through us going out to others.

With a commitment to developing the internal environment, all external environments become natural fields of service, which is also practice. It is called karma yoga, the yoga of action in loving service. Karma yoga isn't something that can be forced into happening. It just happens as the spirit expands inside. All of yoga is connected like that. All of life is connected like that. We are One, expressing as many.

So, let's do advanced yoga practices and come out of our meditation room and consider how to help someone. We will be helping ourselves.

The guru is in you.

Lesson 99 – Practices – Front End and Back End

Q: I want to give you some feedback and seek some further guidance from you. The spinal breathing pranayama had an almost immediate calming effect, reducing the intensity and wildness of the emotional storms I was experiencing. I am currently, and so far, comfortable with the practices up to but excluding yoni mudra kumbhaka. Comfortable in the sense that whilst the practices are still somewhat clunky I have not been experiencing any surges and imbalances.

I did try yoni mudra kumbhaka for one day, and 3 days later after a "severe" emotional roller coaster ride. It felt as though my entire nervous system had been fried – I was utterly exhausted. So I have very quickly backed off from that for the time being. Questions:

Whilst I have had what I could describe as two peak experiences in my life (one of these before I had had ever meditated), I do not experience feelings of bliss or anything similar. For the most part, mediation is just "meditation." If I slip into any form of expectation, it then very quickly becomes an exercise in frustration. Suggestions or comments?

I am in general able to direct energy at will, including kundalini. Yet, my body seems unable to cope with the energy if I do so – kind of like having a racecar with no oil in the engine. If you start it, the engine just blows. Again, any suggestion or comments you may have would be most welcome.

A: I am very glad that the spinal breathing helped. It is a wonderful practice, not only for balancing, but also for gradually and safely awakening the Shiva/Shakti union in the sushumna and everywhere – experienced as the rise of ecstatic conductivity. And, of course, spinal breathing is a powerful enhancer of meditation as well, a primary reason we do it.

If you have taken on mulabandha, sambhavi and siddhasana in such a short time with no overloads, you are doing really fantastic. Yoni mudra kumbhaka is another big step. It turns up the volume on everything. Even just a few minutes of it goes a long way. When you feel like trying it again, just do one repetition and see what happens. There can be a delayed reaction with kumbhaka, as your experience confirms. You have to feel your way along with it very carefully. For now you are taking the pause that refreshes. There is no rush. You will know when you are ready to try again.

This business of "directing energy" wherever can be a two-edged sword. It can bring some ecstasy, or it can fry us inside. It is really premature to be doing it if it leads to the difficulties you describe. It is questionable if it should be done at all outside the structure of practices, though we all are curious to see what we can do inside.

Whether you are moving energy yourself or in structured practices (as in bandhas, mudras, siddhasana and kumbhaka), what is needed is much more "global purification" of the nervous system. This is done with meditation and spinal breathing. If meditation is rough (boring, frustrating, uncomfortable, etc.) at times it is a sign that much cleansing is happening – the very thing that is necessary to remove the source of the blockages you have been running into. The discomfort can be minimized by following the guidelines for practice. Check the early lessons on how to deal with the various things that can come up in meditation. Remember, expectations are regarded as any other thoughts that come up in meditation, and we easily go back to the mantra.

Always take enough time when coming out of meditation. If you don't, there can be some irritability or other discomfort during the day.

Meditation is where you will get the most done to allow you to eventually do more on the back end of practices (yoni mudra, etc.) So, consider doing more on the front end of practices to help you on the back end.

There is much you can do to enhance the depth, power and smoothness of your meditation. The length of meditation now is okay. Twenty minutes is optimal for most people. If you put asanas in front of pranayama, that will give you an extra step going inward, and help smooth things too. Then, if pranayama is smooth, you can inch it up in time to take you even deeper before you get into meditation. Try adding five minutes to pranayama. If it is smooth for a few weeks, then try another five minutes. Spinal breathing will not only help meditation, but "direct energy" in a more balanced way for inner awakening. Do your energy directing up and down the sushumna between third eye and root in spinal breathing and you will accomplish the most, with the least chance of problems.

If you can get to ten minutes asanas, twenty minutes pranayama and twenty minutes meditation, you will be doing global house cleaning by the truckload. If all that stays smooth, you will be pouring lots of oil into that racecar of yours – cleaning and lubricating your nervous system to enable more flow of prana. You will know it is working when you can do yoni mudra kumbhaka with no emotional upheavals, but ecstasy instead. You will experience more pleasure from the other practices as well. It could take a while to get to that stage, but you will be on the right track if you focus more on the front end practices. You seem to be a bit ahead of your nervous system with your energy flows. So you have to go back and take care of cleaning out the vehicle. There really isn't any way around it, unless you want to go the Gopi Krishna route of having too much energy running around inside, and spending years in difficulties, until finally the nervous system is burned clean inside and the smoke clears. That isn't a very good short cut. It can be much more fun than that.

The guru is in you.

Lesson 100 – What is Enlightenment?

Q: Before we do all the practices would it not do justice if we clearly define enlightenment? "What is enlightenment?" I guess many people practice the techniques for powers, problem solving, etc. Few of them practice for actual enlightenment ... would it make a difference?

A: Yes, I agree that it is important for everyone to know what the ultimate objective of Advanced Yoga Practices is. But does it make a difference? Let's explore that.

We have focused on the subject of the enlightenment process several times (including the fruition in unity/Oneness), and also on the subject of "powers." Here are a few of those lessons:

#35 – "Enlightenment Milestones"
#76 – "Siddhis – Are Powers Real?"
#85 – "Enlightenment Milestones Revisited"

In addition to these, there is an ongoing discussion on where we are in the enlightenment process throughout all the lessons. There are many sub-milestones that can be recognized. In general, I try and keep out of philosophical and theoretical speculations, and instead tie everything to practices and direct experiences we are having. The lessons attempt to keep it relevant by keeping the discussion as "experience-based" as possible. That has a practical value as we have experiences coming up. If we understand where our experience fits into the overall enlightenment process, we can have a much better handle on our practices and what to do – when to make small adjustments, when to forge ahead, and when to hold back. So, everyone gets to sit in their own driver's seat – a new approach, really. It seems to be working for many, which fills my heart with joy.

It should be emphasized that undertaking meditation and the other advanced yoga practices does not have to be with the end goal in mind. We'd all like to find some relief from the burdens of daily life – more inner peace, more bliss, and find more energy and creativity to carry on toward our goals, whatever they may be. Everyone has their own ideal they are aiming for, their own bhakti process, if you will. Their own idea of "enlightenment." So, while there is an enlightenment process, everyone has their own approach to it, their own ideal they hope to fulfill.

As we move forward with daily practices, our ideal will expand as our nervous system purifies. Over time, we reach higher and higher. That is how bhakti unfolds in our nervous system. Then, one day we are seeing everyone as an expression of our blissful self, and we have become a fountain of love. There may be a thousand levels of expanding experience on the way to that one, each as valid as the one before and after.

To tell you the truth, it really does not matter why people do advanced yoga practices. We each have our own reasons. Doing them will open our gateway to the infinite regardless of our original motivation for coming on to the path. Purifying and opening our nervous system to the truth will expand our point of view to what is true, no matter what point of view we started with. So, while it is good to hear about our final destination of enlightenment, it is even better to be a more fulfilled person today than we were yesterday. This is the real draw of advanced yoga practices, because they do work day by day with regular practice, and that is where the rubber meets the road.

So, what is enlightenment? It is a process, a journey. Most important, it is the ideal you choose that turns you on to doing daily practices.

The guru is in you.

Lesson 101 – What is Brahmacharya?

Q: What is brahmacharya?

A: Brahmacharya means, "walking in Brahma," or "walking in the creative force of God."

This is commonly translated to mean celibacy, but it does not mean only that. It really means preservation and cultivation of the creative life force, the sexual energy, which can be either in celibacy or in tantric sexual relations. These two modes of behavior produce the same outcome, for both involve preservation and cultivation of sexual energy upward into the divine processes rising in the nervous system through advanced yoga practices.

The approaches to brahmacharya are discussed in more detail in the tantra lessons, particularly in lesson #T9, "The relationship of brahmacharya, tantric sex and celibacy."

The guru is in you.

Lesson 102 – Importance of Smooth Long-Term Meditation Routine

Q: I've been struggling with the meditation and it has been about 6 weeks now. Could I just have a lot of "cleansing" to do before I add the breath work? I am not really reaching "bliss" yet at all. Still, I've been devoted to the two 20 minute intervals and find that I am subtly more calm but I still have many "episodes" during the day were I am not that calm…

Nonetheless, I am still very appreciative that you've initiated this group and enlightenment of many. Just 5 years ago, I felt so alone in this world ... that my spiritual beliefs were not shared by many because there were just too many that revered the Almighty Dollar over Spirit. I used to pray almost daily at that time to have more like-minded earth angels (or warriors as some like to call themselves) and happily I can say that I've started to have much more Spirit in my life and it increases every day.

A: It sounds like good things are happening, but a more comfortable ride would be better for you. It is uncommon for meditation to be rough on an ongoing basis. It could be a lot of obstructions coming out, which is good, but more smoothness in and after meditation is necessary if you are going to be motivated to stay with it for the long haul.

Roughness could come from forcing the mantra, coming out of meditation too fast, or maybe meditating too long for your constitution. Ask yourself the following:

Am I picking up the mantra easily, not forcing a particular pronunciation of it? Am I fighting with thoughts to go back to the mantra? We want to be gentle with the process, just easily favoring the mantra when we realize we are off it. It does not have to be a clear pronunciation. In fact, if it goes naturally to a very fuzzy pronunciation, that is just right. That is the mind taking us naturally to stillness.

Am I getting up too soon at the end of meditation? If we get up too soon, we can lock up obstructions coming out during meditation, and that can give rise to roughness in activity during the day. So we always take at least a few minutes of quiet with no mantra at the end of meditation. If meditation has been rough with a lot of thoughts and emotions coming out, then lie down for five or ten minutes, however long it takes for the roughness to settle down. That can make a big difference in our experiences during the day.

If smoothness in meditation still doesn't come, try five minutes of spinal breathing before meditation. If that does not bring some smoothness into meditation, then back off the breathing. Try five or ten minutes of yoga postures before meditation. That can help smooth meditation too.

If none of the above helps smooth things out, then consider trying fifteen minutes of meditation twice a day instead of twenty minutes.

These are just suggestions on different things to try. Experiment with it and see if you can find a smooth rhythm. The ideal routine will have asanas, pranayama and meditation in that order. The times can vary a bit, but typical would be 5,10 and 20 minutes in that order. You have to find your own balance and comfort zone, Once you do, then you can go on with your routine for many years, adding on additional advanced yoga practices along the way. Then much progress is assured. You are tasting inner silence now. That is wonderful. Now the thing is to grow steadily in That (pure bliss consciousness) over the long haul without falling off the track of practices due to discomfort from too much purification happening too fast. You are the one behind the wheel, so drive smart and smooth.

I wish you all success on your journey, "earth angel." You've got lots of company these days.

The guru is in you.

Lesson 103 – Destiny and Free Will

Q: I have been practising yoga and meditation for many years with slow and steady improvement on the "experiences." The only problem I presume is I keep trying out many techniques without sticking to one for long. Is it one's own karma that prevents progress in meditation? Should we give it up and allow things to happen or should we use our free will to make things happen? To me it's sometimes free will and sometimes destiny that takes over ... well, sort of confusing! Please comment.

A: I think your question on free will is covered in part in lesson #84, "The Art of Doing Nothing." If we allow ourselves to become part of evolution, we will be doing something. All of nature is doing something. To consciously not do something is still a doing. The trick is to be doing something that is very little that facilitates the natural opening of our nervous system to pure bliss consciousness and divine ecstasy. We want to hand the process over to our nervous system's natural abilities. To do that we have to nudge a bit here and there with efficient levers. That is what Advanced Yoga Practices is about.

Karma/samskaras/obstructions embedded in our nervous system are what stand between us and divine experience. Spiritual practices are for stimulating the nervous system to purify itself, removing the obstructions. Not doing that and leaving it to "destiny" prolongs the journey, leaving the house cleaning to be done later. There is free will in this. We all have the freedom to choose. We can do it now or do it later. That is the choice we have. If we do it later, we may have an easier time of it due to the efforts of others and the position of the stars. Most prefer to pitch in, rather than sitting around in the dark waiting for someone else to turn on the lights.

You might want to review lesson, #93, "Changing Times." It discusses how the rise of this "new age" relates to the spiritual choices we make. Bottom line: Destiny is in the stars. The rest is up to us.

As for trying many methods, the "digging the well" analogy applies. If we dig in one place long enough, we will eventually find water. If we dig here, there and over there, maybe it will take longer to find water. So, in general, sticking with a practice is better; assuming it is a tried and true one.

In these lessons we talk about a full range of tried and true practices, and put them together in a building block fashion to be undertaken by each person on their own reconnaissance according to their unique capacity and time line. For those already on another path, it is all offered as "food for thought." That is the approach.

The guru is in you.

Lesson 104 – Stubborn Energy Blockages

Q: I have a couple of questions I'd appreciate your feedback on. If someone is having some rough kundalini energy experiences, do you think it would help to go see a healer that works on the energetic level, like a Reiki master or something, or is this cheating or like taking a shortcut that won't really pay off in the long run? Assuming that one continues with the practices, of course. Just looking for a little outside assistance in removing blockages.

When I meditate I do get a fairly intense pain in my back, which could be posture related but it could also be a blockage (my suspicion). I have tried all sorts of support and leaning on things and props but I haven't found anything that works yet. I can meditate while lying on my back. I get enough rest that I can stay for half an hour and not fall asleep, but intuitively it feels like there is something special about the vertical position, something about the up/down relationship that feels important and that I'll miss out on if I do it in a horizontal position. What do you think?

Also, I'd like to know if mulabandha, sambhavi and siddhasana can be carried over from pranayama into meditation. Is that ok?

A: If there are rough kundalini experiences, chronic blockages, or anything like that, whatever means that can be found to relieve them are okay. We'd like our journey to be as comfortable as possible, or we may not wish to continue it. So if Reiki, massage, energy healing, chiropractic, Tai Chi, or any other means are available that can help relieve a stubborn energy blockage, by all means go for it. You may want to go back and review the lesson on kundalini remedies from a few weeks ago. Don't forget yoga asanas. These are particularly good for spinal blockages, assuming there is no medical problem. If you think there could be a medical problem, be sure to seek medical advice.

Of course, we can also manage our practices to mitigate discomfort if it is energy related. This is really the first place we look to make adjustments if our energy is running into an uncomfortable wall. The evolutionary energy comes from within, loosening and pushing obstructions out, and there is much we can do to accelerate or temper this process in practices. It is the whole game, really. Each of us is different in how we respond to spiritual practices. We'd like to be chipping away at those obstructions in our nervous system with gentle nudges each day, rather than with a sledgehammer. So gauge your practices to accommodate your experiences. What we do here is "experience-based."

If you are meditating more than twenty minutes, that is too much. Sometimes less than twenty minutes is necessary when lots of obstructions are coming loose.

As for posture in meditation, yes, vertical is better than lying down, but we are not fanatic about it here in the lessons. Meditation should be comfortable first, otherwise why bother with it? So, until the back situation eases up, lean back as much as you have to. But have the goal to work your way gradually up straight. Maybe use one pillow this week, two next week, three the week after. See if you can gradually inch your way up to a comfortable sitting position with back support. If the back pain is an energy blockage, it should clear up sooner or later.

Regarding what to let carry over from pranayama to meditation – only the things that do not divide the attention to do them. At this stage, that is only siddhasana, because it takes no extra attention to sit in it. Of course, it can be distracting in the beginning stages with the stimulation at the perineum, so leaving it out of meditation is recommended until it becomes a familiar and easy habit in pranayama. It is your call. Mulabandha and sambhavi require attention to maintain at this stage, so we don't try and do those in meditation. The idea is to keep our attention free to follow the simple procedure of meditation. This is very important.

As time goes on, various yogic things will sometimes occur spontaneously during meditation as the processes of yoga become more fluid in our nervous system. Some of these "automatic yogas" will be familiar to us, like spontaneous mulabandha and sambhavi. Others may be brand new, and we may see these show up miraculously in practices introduced later in the lessons here. There are some examples further on. We don't encourage automatic yogas, but we do not struggle against them either. When we become aware of an automatic yoga, we just easily go back and favor the practice we are doing. If we find ourselves standing on our head in the middle of meditation, what do we do? Yes, we sit back down and easily go back to the mantra.

Well, we probably won't find ourselves standing on our head spontaneously very often, but other unusual things can and do happen. It is all part of the connectedness of yoga. The nervous system knows what to do if we give it the opportunity to open up. The nervous system is the source of all yoga. We are just lending a helping hand here and there. Facilitating the automatic process of enlightenment, you know.

The guru is in you.

Lesson 105 – Hitting a Wall at Mulabandha

Q: I started the practices at the beginning and was doing well until I hit #55, "Mulabandha." I find it near impossible to "gently flex" the sphincter muscle. When I try, I become completely tense and experience a variety of aches and pains as a result. I keep trying, but can't wait to get out of pranayama – which up to this point I had been quite comfortable with. I'm also concerned with the sexual emphasis the lessons have taken. I'm looking for spiritual enlightenment and now I wonder if I'm doing the wrong practice.

A: If mulabandha is not good at this stage, it is a good time to back off to a comfortable level of practice and bide your time there for a while. It could be months or even much longer before you feel ready to go to the next step. That is okay. What you are doing is very advanced already. You will be purifying and opening at a good clip. It is your journey.

This approach to practices is unorthodox in that everyone can go at their own pace, so you must be measured in your approach and gauge your practices to your experience. Many of the practices described in the lessons have historically been reserved for the very few (esoteric), until now. So we all have a big responsibility in using this new approach. It is hoped that many more will be able to benefit from advanced yoga practices than in the past dark age.

It is not possible for anyone to zoom right through everything in a few months without hitting a wall at some point. It is a long journey we are on. Remember the lesson, "What is your time line?" The lessons are being put in place for the long haul, to provide an ongoing resource for aspirants at every level. The practices will become progressively more advanced as you read on, and some will seem outrageous. Naturally, at higher levels fewer will be ready, but there are folks at every level here now, so we go on. Over time, everyone will go as far as they are able and willing. The goal is to blaze the trail clearly from beginning to end for everyone's use.

As for the sexual aspect, it can't be separated. It is part and parcel of the middle of the journey. I have not been able to figure out a way to keep it out. So we are facing it head on. You will see how it fits in as you read on. Eventually sex is transcended to something much more. To ignore it is to hit the worst wall of all – pretending something is not there. Sex is there, and the energy will expand up at some point. If it does not, it only means there are obstructions to be cleared out. It is a fundamental reality in the transformation of the nervous system to higher functioning. If you are not ready to deal with it directly in practices, that is okay. Just bide your time. Meditation and spinal breathing will work to open and enliven the entire nervous system in more subtle ways, and you can avoid the direct stimulation of sexual energy if that is best for you. So leave mulabandha for now, and stay away from siddhasana too. Even sambhavi (at the third eye) is sexual when it connects, bringing ecstatic conductivity up the spinal nerve from the pelvic region. That is just how we are wired for enlightenment, you know. But you can do it all with meditation and spinal breathing. It just takes a little longer, and the sexual aspects are more behind the scenes. The experiences will ultimately be the same, and you will be ready for them. The nervous system will open naturally to its own truth, and you will be filled with light and bliss.

There is no particular place you are supposed to be on this broad spectrum of practices. Everyone is on the leading edge of their own journey to enlightenment. Wherever it works for you is where you are supposed to be. As purification occurs, you can move on at your own pace. Be careful to not overextend and expose yourself to ongoing difficulties. This is supposed to be fun. Choose your level of practices for a smooth, enjoyable ride.

The guru is in you.

Lesson 106 – Mantra and Breathing in Meditation

Q: As I attempt to develop a better habit of meditation, which though fairly new in the process, I am enjoying tremendously. Does it matter if I imagine/hear inside myself saying *"I"* on an inhale, *"AM"* on an exhale, or if I hear *"I AM" "I AM" "I AM"* on an inhale and then the same on an exhale, etc?

A: Some systems of meditation involve using mantra with breath. The approach in these lessons is to not do that. So, no, it doesn't matter if the mantra is with the breath or not. We just let the breath go in meditation and don't mind what it is doing. The reason is we want the mantra to be free to change naturally in speed of repetition and degree of clarity so the mind is free to go to stillness easily. We want meditation naturally leading the breath, not the other way around. If we favor the breath leading the mantra, we will drift into pranayama mode of cultivating the nerves on a less subtle level than the mind will go if given the opportunity in deep meditation. This is a fine point that is easy to miss. It will become clearer when we enhance the mantra, giving it more syllables.

Cultivating the nerves is very good and pleasurable, and we do that in pranayama. But meditation with breath leading is not as deep as meditation without breath leading. In deep meditation when the mind comes to stillness, the breath and metabolism will automatically suspend. We'd like to be free to pick up the mantra on very subtle/quiet levels in the mind without having it habitually tied to breath. If the mantra follows the breath, we don't favor or push the breath out. We just follow the procedure of easily favoring the mantra on whatever level of stillness we are at in the mind. Then we will be going to more stillness and purifying the entire nervous system from deep within with the rise of pure bliss consciousness.

So, pranayama is for cultivating the nerves with attention and breath, and meditation is for letting the mind go deep – awakening the silent seed of pure bliss consciousness deep within the nervous system. In this approach we do not cultivate and plant at the same time. There is further discussion on this in lesson #43, "Relationship of Pranayama to Meditation." You will find if you let the breath go in meditation, you will go much deeper into silence, especially if you have done spinal breathing pranayama before meditation.

The guru is in you.

Lesson 107 – Self-Pacing in Postures and Practices

Q: I have been "dabbling" (sometimes a lot, sometimes little) in ashtanga yoga for over five years, and my yoga has helped me with the breathing and mulabandha. Ashtanga is very enjoyable – even for an xc skier/tri-athlete who is not too flexible. Recently I was in a car accident that has strained my wrist. Do you have any suggestions on how I could modify sun salutations and asanas to most effectively continue my practice, as I had just started to get on a roll again before the car crash?

A: For sun salutation, asanas, and, in fact, all yoga practices, the first rule is to never force, and always use gentle persuasion. If there is some stiffness, injury, or discomfort, then we just go to our natural limit and test it a little. Never to the point of pain or strain. Just to the point of the limit of movement, and then be there for the time of our posture. This may be nowhere near the full posture, which is perfectly fine. We do what we can comfortably in the direction of the posture without strain, knowing we will be doing gradually more in subsequent sessions. If any degree of stretch becomes uncomfortable, we back off to a comfortable level. Or, if it can go a little further without strain, then we let it. This is what we have talked about many times as we go through Advanced Yoga Practices. It is the principle of "self-pacing." It is the fine art of progressing in yoga – never forcing, always using gentle persuasion. With this approach, the body and nervous system slowly but surely move to more flexibility, purification and greater experiences of inner peace and bliss.

There is the old saying, "By the yard, life is hard. By the inch, it's a cinch." It is easy to become advanced in yoga if we know how to handle self-pacing.

The guru is in you.

Lesson 108* – Kechari Mudra – A Giant Leap for Humankind

Kechari mudra is a subject of increasing discussion and debate these days. It is a good sign. It means it is coming out of the shadows of esoteric yoga and into the early morning sunshine of this rising new age of enlightenment.

What is kechari mudra? Let's put it in terms that we can easily relate to. A centimeter or two above the roof of our mouth is located one of the most ecstatically sensitive organs in our whole body. It can be reached relatively easily with our tongue. It is located on the back edge of our nasal septum, and when the nervous system is purified enough through advanced yoga practices, our tongue will roll back and go up into the cavity of our nasal pharynx to find the sensitive edge of our septum. When this happens, it is like a master switch is closed in our nervous system, and all of our advanced yoga practices and experiences begin to function on a much higher level. When kechari is entered naturally, we come on to the fast track of yoga. It is the major league of yoga, if you will.

Ramakrishna said, "When the divine goddess comes up, the tongue rolls back."

Many have experienced this natural phenomenon at times in their yoga practices. When the nervous system is ready, it just happens. The tongue wants to go back. But few are able to follow through, and this is just a matter of education. If strong bhakti is there and the tongue is rolling back, it is a short trip to make the connection in the pharynx to a higher level of spiritual experience.

Not many people on earth today have made this important transition in yoga. However, it is likely that the number of people entering kechari will increase dramatically in the coming years. As this happens, it will be a giant leap forward for humankind, for it will mark humanity's shift to a predominantly spiritual mode of functioning of the nervous system. This will bring with it the many benefits of rising enlightenment spreading out through our modern society. Kechari is that significant, that powerful, and that indicative of where the human race is heading. Only a few yogis and yoginis in kechari can have a huge effect on the spiritual energies in everyone. They radiate energy that quickens the rise of the enlightenment process in all. So, while kechari is an individual phenomenon on the road to human spiritual transformation, it has global implications, as do all of our advanced yoga practices. As Jesus said, "You are the light of the world."

But enough about the spiritual destiny of the human race. What about each of us, and our relationship with kechari?

Since kechari was first mentioned in the lessons some time ago, several have written about having the early symptoms of it, wondering what to do. "Should I stop the tongue from rolling back?" "Should I proceed? And, if so, how?" These are the questions that have been asked.

If the tongue is rolling back and we feel we are getting ahead of ourselves, there is no rush. If we have doubts or excessive kundalini experiences, it may be best to wait. It is the application of self-pacing, you know. Only you can know when the time is right. No one can tell you when it is time to go for kechari, or for any other advanced yoga practice. Your experiences and your bhakti will be your guides.

Even though we are talking about a journey of a couple of centimeters, kechari is a big undertaking. Not so much physically, though there is some physical challenge, but more so in the psyche and the emotions. Kechari is a big deal. It goes to the core of our spiritual identity. Are we ready to close a neurological switch that will transport us to a higher plane of existence? It is not that we are changed instantly and forever. It is not like that. The day after we enter higher kechari for the first time, we are still the same person. We may even stop doing kechari if we entered prematurely. No harm done. Kechari has its "clunky" stage, just as all advanced yoga practices do. It takes some determination to get through the awkward beginnings of kechari.

We are not instantly a different person the minute we start kechari. Only in time with daily practice are we changed, and this will be a substantial change. In a real way, we have become a different person before we enter kechari. The decision to do it is the crossover as much as the act is. In this sense, kechari is more than a physical act. Deciding to do kechari is recognition of the nervous system being ready for the next level. The nervous system tells us when it is ready. We have become kechari even before we enter it. Isn't this true with all advanced yoga practices we undertake? We feel ready. We begin the practice. If we are in tune with our nervous system, the practice will stick. If we are premature, there will be roughness and we will have to back off. This is okay. It is how we test and find our openings to move forward in yoga. Kechari is like that too. Only with kechari, we are doing a bit more to get into it, and the experience is pretty dramatic, so it requires strong motivation to do it – strong bhakti.

Kechari means, "To fly through inner space."

This sounds poetic and dramatic. Yet, kechari is much more that that. It is much more personal than that. Regular practice of kechari takes us into a permanent lovemaking of the polarities within us. The effects of kechari ultimately exceed those of tantric sexual relations as discussed in the tantra group. This is amazing because kechari involves no external sexual activity at all. Kechari is one of the great secrets of enlightened celibates. Not that celibacy and kechari have to go together. Anyone can do kechari and continue in normal sexual relations. But if one chooses a path of celibacy, then kechari, along with other advanced yoga practices, will provide more than enough cultivation of sexual energy upward in the nervous system. It is a natural internal process that comes up in us.

With kechari do we "fly though inner space?" The greatest part of the kechari experience is the rise of ecstatic bliss. The senses are naturally drawn in and it is like we are flying inside. Our inner dimensions are vast, and we soar through them in a constant reverie.

The connection we make near the top of the sushumna, ida and pingala in kechari is an ecstatic one that brings ecstatic conductivity up in the nervous system more than any other practice. Every other advanced yoga practice then becomes increasingly effective at doing the same thing – raising ecstatic conductivity. So kechari is an ecstatic connection that illuminates our entire nervous system. The sensitive edge of the nasal septum is an altar of bliss. The more time we spend there, the more bliss we experience. Kechari is the perfect companion for sambhavi. The two practices complement each other. Together, sambhavi and kechari draw divine ecstasy up, filling us with divine light.

Advanced yogis and yoginis use kechari continuously throughout their sitting practices, and often during the day when not engaged in conversation. In other words, kechari is home for the advanced yogi and yogini. We do not even know that they are in kechari. Only the subtle glow of divine light gives them away. Inside, they are in the constant play of divine lovemaking.

We will cover four stages of kechari here, all pertaining to the location of the tip of the tongue:

Stage 1 – To the point on the roof of the mouth where the hard and soft palates meet. This is the line of demarcation that must be crossed before stage 2 can be entertained.

Stage 2 – Behind the soft palate and up to the nasal septum. It is a short trip, but a momentous one. Initially this is done with help from a finger pushing back under the tongue, going to the left or right side of the soft palate where entry is easiest. This may require "breaking the hymen" of the membrane under the tongue. See below for more on this.

Stage 3 – Gradually working to the top of the nasal pharynx and septum. This takes us to the bony structure containing the pituitary gland.

Stage 4 – Entering the nasal passages from inside and moving upward beyond the top of the pharynx toward the point between the eyebrows. It is not as far for the tongue to go as it seems. Put you thumb on the hinge of your jaw and put your index finger at the tip of your tongue extended straight out. Then pivot the fixed length to your index finger up on your thumb to the point between your eyebrows. See? It is not so far for the tongue to go straight up from its root.

Many years may pass between stage 1 and stage 4. Kechari is a long-term evolution, not an overnight event, though it certainly has its dramatic moments of transition, especially between stages 1&2 and stages 3&4. Now let's look at the four stages in more detail.

Stage 1 puts us in contact with the bottom of the septum through the roof of our mouth. This has already been suggested as a goal to work toward in the lesson on yoni mudra kumbhaka (#91). Some ecstatic response can be felt at the point where the hard and soft palates meet if the nervous system is rising in purity. Stage one is not easy, as it takes some effort for most people to keep the tongue on the roof of the mouth and work it gradually back over time. A habit gradually develops. Once the tip of the tongue passes the point where the hard and soft palates meet, and the soft palate can be pushed up with the tongue, then stage 2 is close at hand.

Stage 2 is very dramatic. The tongue is pushed back with a finger to the left or right side of the soft palate. These are the shortest pathways leading behind the soft palate. One of these will be a shorter route than the other. At some point you will experiment and see for yourself. The long way in is up the middle. The soft palate has an elastic tendon running across the back edge. When the tip of the tongue gets behind it for the first time, the elastic tendon can slip quickly around the bottom of the tongue as though grabbing it. Then the tongue is suddenly in the nasal pharynx and touching the edge of the nasal septum for the first time.

The first reaction is surprise, and the tongue will probably come out quickly. It is easy to pull out. No finger help is needed. It is also easy to breathe through the nose with the tongue in the nasal pharynx. On the first entry, the eyes and nose may water, there could be sneezing, there could be sexual arousal, and strong emotions. All of these things are temporary reactions to the event of entering stage 2 kechari for the first time. Upon repeated entries, things settle down. In time, the finger will no longer be needed to get behind the soft palate. The elastic tendon across the edge of the soft palate stretches out and stage 2 kechari becomes quite comfortable. In fact, it is easier to stay in stage 2 kechari than to stay in stage 1 kechari. The tongue rests very easily in the nasal pharynx with no effort at all, making it simple to use during pranayama and meditation. The tongue is obviously designed to rest blissfully in the nasal pharynx.

There are two practical matters to consider once in stage 2 kechari. First is lubrication in the pharynx. Second is the accumulation of saliva in the mouth.

The pharynx can be a little fickle. Usually, it is naturally moist and well lubricated for the tongue. Occasionally it is dry and not so well lubricated. In the former situation, kechari can be practiced practically indefinitely. In the latter situation, only sparingly. When the pharynx is dry there can be a stinging sensation when the tongue is in there. So, this is not the time to do kechari. We just go to stage 1 when that happens. Interestingly, the pharynx will almost always be moist during practices. But there is no telling for sure. We just go in when we are welcome, which is most of the time. And when we are not welcome, we honor the situation and refrain. Like that.

When we are up in stage 2 kechari, saliva will accumulate in the mouth down below. Since we can't swallow what is in our mouth with our tongue going up into the nasal pharynx, and we don't want to drool, then we come out of kechari as necessary to swallow the saliva in our mouth. In the early adjustment period to stage 2 kechari there can be a lot of saliva, so we will have to swallow more often. In time, the saliva goes back to normal levels, and coming out of kechari to swallow will become infrequent.

So, in stage 2 kechari, we are just letting our tongue rest easily on the edge of the nasal pharynx, and that sets spiritual processes in motion everywhere in our body.

In the beginning of stage 2 kechari we will be curious. We are in a new place and want to find out what is in the pharynx. There is the sensitive septum, the "altar of bliss." We have no problem finding that, and realizing that the best way to do pranayama and meditation is with our tongue resting on the sensitive vertical edge of the septum. It is like having a powerful siddhasana working simultaneously on the other end of the spinal nerve, awakening our entire nervous system ecstatically from the top. When we are not enjoying bliss at the septum, we will no doubt explore, finding the prominent "trumpets" of the eustachian tubes on either side of the nasal passages. We also can't miss the entrances to the nasal passages on either side of the septum, and quickly find the extremely sensitive erectile tissues inside them. Too much. Better stay away from those for a while. So, we go up the septum on our journey to the top of the pharynx, to stage 3. For some this is a short journey. For others, it can take a long time. In going there we expose the full length of the edge of the septum to our tongue, and prepare ourselves to eventually enter the nasal passages and go higher.

A practice that can help as we go beyond stage 2 kechari is the so-called "milking of the tongue." It consists of gently pulling on the tongue with the fingers of both hands, alternating hands, as though milking a cow. A good time to do this is for a few minutes while standing in the shower each day. That way you can get the benefit of it without slobbering all over your clothes. Over time, the tongue can be lengthened by this method. This is not a very useful practice for getting into stage 2. Dealing with the frenum is most important for that, as discussed below. Milking the tongue is helpful for going beyond stage 2 kechari, especially in stage 4.

Stage 4 is another dramatic step. It could be years away from stage 2&3. Everyone will be different in approaching it. There is a trick to it. The nasal passages are tall and narrow and the tongue is narrow and wide, so the tongue can only go into the nasal passages by turning on its side. But which side? One way works better than the other. The tongue can naturally be turned with the top to the center by following the channel on top of the trumpet of each eustachian tube into its adjacent nasal passage. This naturally turns the top of the tongue to the center and allows it to slide up the side of the septum into the nasal passage. Turning the tongue inward to the center is the way up into the passages. Entering stage 4 is as dramatic as entering stage 2, because the tissues in the nasal passages are extremely sensitive, and connecting with them in the way described takes the nervous system to yet a higher level. Stage 4 provides extensive stimulation of the upper ends of the sushumna, ida and pingala, and this has huge effects throughout the nervous system, especially when combined with our pranayama and its associated bandhas and mudras.

Going to stage 4 is natural once stages 2&3 have been mastered and become second nature. Before then we are not much attracted due to the sensitivity in the nasal passages. Our opening nervous system and rising bhakti take us to stage 4 when we are ready.

Once the nasal passages have been entered, the tongue can be used to do "alternate passage" breathing during spinal breathing pranayama. This provides alternating stimulation in the nasal passages, which produces additional purifying effects in the sushumna, ida and pingala. Our pranayama becomes supercharged in stage 4 kechari.

The four stages of kechari foster major neurological openings in the head, and throughout the entire nervous system. Kechari is one of the most pleasurable and far-reaching of all the advanced yoga practices. Kechari represents a major transition in our advanced yoga practices to a much higher level.

Now let's talk about the membrane/tendon under the tongue called the "frenum." For most of us, the frenum will be the limiting factor in moving through the stages of kechari. There is debate on whether the frenum should be trimmed or not. Some say that we are deserving or not deserving of kechari according to what kind of frenum we have under our tongue, and that the only way into kechari is by stretching the frenum. If we can't stretch it far enough to get into kechari, it is "God's will."

In these lessons, we don't subscribe to that limited point of view. The view here is that, "God helps those who help themselves."

In these lessons we view the frenum as a tether to be trimmed back when the time is right. It keeps us out of kechari until we are ready. When we are ready, and each of us knows when that is, the frenum can be trimmed. It is like a "hymen." When a woman is ready for sexual intercourse, the hymen goes. Until then it serves to provide protection. This breaking of the hymen can be a stressful and painful event if it is forced. Sooner or later the frenum will be forced open too, because going into kechari is as natural as going into sexual intercourse. It is biologically preordained. It happens when the nervous system is mature enough. Advanced yoga practices bring us closer to the transition with each day of daily practices.

Kechari results from a second puberty in us – our spiritual puberty. As our nervous system becomes pure, our bhakti increases. More than anything else it is bhakti that sends us into kechari. When every fiber of our being wants God, then we will go there. The tongue will roll back and go up. Like that.

Once our bhakti is hurling our tongue back into kechari, breaking the hymen of the frenum does not have to be stressful and painful. It can be very easy and gentle. Above all, it can and should be gradual. It is done with very tiny snips. Tiny snips, each as small as a hair or a very thin string. A sterilized, sharp cuticle snipper (like a small wire cutter) can be used to do the job, bit by bit. When we lift our tongue up, we can see right away where the point of greatest stress on the frenum is. If we take a tiny snip there, not bigger than a hair, it probably won't even bleed. Maybe one drop. If more than one drop, we did too much. The tiny snip will heal in a day or two. The tissues of the mouth heal very quickly. Then maybe in a week or a month, whatever we are comfortable with, we will be ready to do it again. And then, in another week or more, do it again. If we are sensitive, a little ice can be used to numb the edge of the frenum, and we won't even feel a little pinch when we snip. Don't use ice to take a big snip though. That is too much, and brings in some risk of infection. We should not snip if we have any kind of infection in the body. With tiny snips, the frenum will be allowing the tongue to go further back in no time, and before we know it we will be using our finger to push our tongue behind our soft palate.

We can continue with the tiny snips once we are in stage 2 kechari, and this will help us move on to stage 3. Then we can continue with the tiny snips once we have gotten to the top of the nasal pharynx, and this will help us move on through stage 4. It will take years. There is no rush. We may go for many months, or even years, with no snipping at all, content to enjoy the level of kechari we have attained so far, and the steady spiritual growth that comes with it. Then we may become inspired to continue going up with the tongue, and do some more snipping.

As the snipping progresses past stage 2 kechari, it becomes very easy to do it. As the frenum gives way slowly, the edge it presents when stretched becomes like a callus. There is no pain snipping it, and no blood. It is not difficult to trim it back so the tongue can go further up into more advanced stages of kechari. It is a long journey in time, and a fulfilling one. It can take decades to complete stages 1 through 4. There is no rush. The nervous system knows what must happen. When it knows, we know through our bhakti.

Everyone's frenum is different. A few will enter kechari with no snipping necessary. Others will need a lot of snipping. The rest of us will fall somewhere in-between. Whatever the case many be, we will know what to do when our bhakti comes up. No one else can tell us what to do when. Everything in this lesson is offered as information so you will have a better idea on what your options are as your bhakti comes up.

Some will have medical concerns about snipping the frenum. Most doctors will not be for it. Is there risk? There is always some risk when we undertake new things. That is life. The practice of trimming the frenum for kechari has been around for thousands of years – at least as long as circumcision, body piercing and tattooing. Not that any of these other types of body alterations are in the same class as kechari. They are not. Kechari is one of the most advanced yoga practices on the planet. When we know we are ready for it, we will be willing to accept whatever risk may be associated with entering it. We each choose our own path according to the feelings rising in our heart.

This lesson is not to promote stage 2 kechari and beyond for everyone. It is to provide useful information for those who are experiencing kechari symptoms and finding themselves stretching naturally past stage 1. What you do with the information here is your choice. Remember to always pace yourself according to your capacity and experiences.

The guru is in you.

Addition – There is a fifth stage of kechari mudra which is presented in the *Hatha Yoga Pradipika*, and it is appropriate to mention it here, though its practical application is pretty far down the road for most yogis and yoginis. Not to worry, kechari stages 1-4 are more than enough to complete the journey. In fact, it is possible to complete the journey without going above the soft palate at all. Each of us will have a different manifestation of the many aspects of yoga in our nervous system. So, when we discuss kechari, we are speaking of possibilities and options. Whether or not you are moved toward kechari is a function of your own journey. If you are moved that way, it will be clear enough. And if you are not, that will also be obvious. No one should force their way into practices that are not beckoning from within.

Having said all that, let's look at **Kechari Stage 5**. What is it? It is going down the gullet (the esophagus) with the tongue. Obviously, to do this the tongue has to be all but free from the limiting influence of the frenum, the tendon under the tongue. By the time this has occurred, by daily tongue stretching-milking and/or snipping, kechari stages 1-4 will have already been achieved. This is why going down the gullet is called stage 5, even though it is in the opposite direction from the other stages.

Why would anyone want to swallow their tongue? What is the yogic benefit in doing this? For those who have made it into stage 2, 3 or 4, the benefits are self-evident. Advancing kechari gives a great boost to the rise of ecstatic conductivity in the nervous system.

In the case of kechari stage 5, something new is being added. It is associated with a late-stage step in the evolution of the divine union that occurs within us. The blending of inner silence and ecstatic energies in the nervous system (the union of Shiva and Shakti) goes on everywhere in the body. At the same time it gradually rises to find its focal point in the head. Kechari and sambhavi are important influences in this rising union. Of course, all the other elements of yoga practice are behind this also – meditation, spinal breathing, kumbhaka (breath retention), siddhasana, mulabandha, etc. So the union that is happening in every cell in the body gravitates upward, with its focal point arriving finally in the head. Once this has occurred to a sufficient degree, something else begins to happen – the focal point of the divine union in the head expands downward into the chest, and the heart melts.

The neuro-biology of this heart melting is quite complex, with many things going on at once. First, the union of ascending and descending pranas reaches a critical mass in the head. This causes the secretions from the brain (amrita/nectar) flowing down into the GI (gastrointestinal) tract to increase. This, in turn, creates a natural attraction of the neuro-biological energies in the head downward. This tends to draw the tongue downward into the throat, and eventually down the gullet. Once this occurs, the neurology in the throat and chest is stimulated to a higher level of functioning. The experience of the union of inner silence/Shiva and ecstasy/Shakti is ecstatic bliss, with the focal point of it in the head. When this joining expands from the head down into the heart area, the experience becomes one of outpouring divine love. This is why enlightened sages are an endless source of love and compassion. Their hearts are in a constant state of melting due to the divine union going on continuously inside. This corresponds with the highest stage of enlightenment, where all is seen and profoundly loved as an integral part of Self. At this level of functioning in the human nervous system, there is the divine power to aid healing and spiritual transformation in everyone near and far.

Kechari stage 5 has its greatest use once the neuro-biology in the head has been fully awakened via a full range of advanced yoga practices. "Fully awakened" means with the third eye fully activated and sambhavi fully engaged in the process of ecstatic conductivity. Much more will be covered on these prerequisites as the lessons unfold.

For now, we have touched on kechari stage 5 enough. When it calls to us, it will not be such a mystery, and we can move forward from there. Or maybe stage 5 won't call to us. Enlightenment can happen without it, just as it can happen without stages 2-4. All of this discussion on kechari is just to let you know the possibilities, so if it starts to happen, you will know what it is. Let your bhakti and common sense be your guides in approaching the various stages of kechari mudra, and, for that matter, all advanced yoga practices.

The following illustrations show kechari stages 1-5.

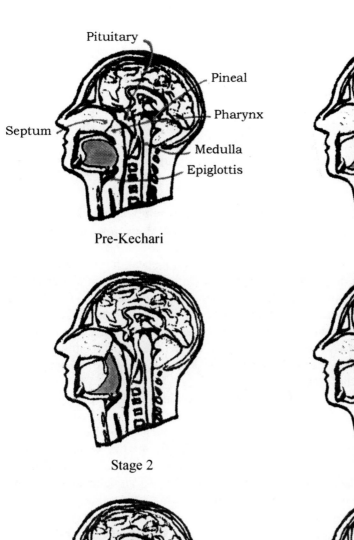

Pituitary

Pineal

Pharynx

Septum

Medulla

Epiglottis

Pre-Kechari

Stage 1

Stage 2

Stage 3

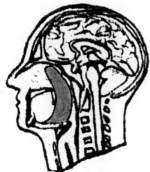

Stage 4 – left nostril

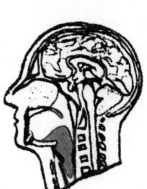

Stage 5

Lesson 109 – Bhakti, Meditation and Inner Silence

Q: Is it possible for kundalini to, let's say for lack of a better word, talk to you? Let's go back. After reading the bhakti lesson I have been working on redirecting desires towards spirit – sometimes not so well, but at other times I feel as if my steps and thoughts are where they should be. At one point I asked God to direct me through the divine kundalini energy to let me know what is spirit and what is just ego pretending to be spirit. At times I get guidance from the energy in the form of blissful feelings and surges if I am working in a spiritual way. So my question is can kundalini speak to us with her energy, or is this a direct answer from God/angel thoughts? Is this Bhakti? Are there any techniques that we can use to help purify old habits and desires and redirect them with bhakti?

A: Yes God can speak to us, and does all the time. It can come through kundalini or any other God-channel we choose. By choosing and focusing on a spiritual ideal, we can filter out the noise in us and receive guidance constantly. In time, we become one with the guidance, for the guru/God is in us, and is us. It is not so much in the mind. God does not speak to the intellect, so be careful about the mind games we can play with ourselves – we can build castles in the air in a hurry with the intellect. He/She speaks to us in the heart with feelings and intuitions. This is also how we speak to God, with our heart, with our feelings. If we are intense in our bhakti to our ideal, our needs will be communicated automatically and we will know what to do next. It is like that, a very intimate process that emerges as a oneness inside us on the inner levels of feeling.

We experience a knowingness deep inside before we know. If that is how it happens you can be sure it is divine guidance, and not some trick of the mind.

The best way to cultivate bhakti is to purify the heart, which is done through all the advanced yoga practices we have discussed to date – especially meditation. A purified heart is a blissfully silent heart. Meditation brings up the "silent witness" in us, which is the deep heart awareness that enables us to choose what direction our emotions will go in. Before the witness, we were dragged every which way by our thoughts and emotions, because we were identified with them as our self. With the silent witness we experience our self beyond all that, so thoughts and emotions become like objects we can redirect before they manifest outwardly. We can pull an ongoing "inside job" on our thoughts and emotions and avoid problems that come up when everything flying around inside us shoots out. In essence, working from the level of the silent witness, we are able to develop the habit of redirecting thoughts and emotions deep in the mind before they reach the surface. This was mentioned in the first lesson on bhakti (#67).

This inner process of bhakti is more about feeling than about thinking. Deep inside us there is a fine line between feeling and thinking. The line is where mind and heart meet, and that is the point of stillness. Functioning at that blissfully silent balance point between heart and mind is the destination of yoga, living in union with God. Meditation and the other advanced yoga practices are for cultivating that.

There are more practices coming (mantra enhancements, samyama and physical techniques) that will expand our silent presence in the heart, and these will make our witness (pure bliss consciousness) and bhakti much stronger.

If you want to do more now, favor an attitude of service, and be mindful about surrendering desires/emotions to that. All emotions can be redirected in that way. It is a path of surrender, and is something we can do anytime, anywhere. Very good for the heart. But don't get too carried away with it. We don't want to do it at the expense of sitting practices. The best bhakti is the bhakti that puts us in practices every day.

The guru is in you.

Lesson 110 – Romantic Love

Q: What would be effective yoga practices to stop feeling romantic love for someone?

A: If it is an infatuation, it should pass. If it is an obsession, then daily practices discussed so far (particularly meditation) will gradually help you to transform it to something more evolutionary. If it is a sexual addiction that is holding you back, then, if you haven't already, see the techniques given in the tantra lessons.

If it is pure love for someone, I would not recommend stopping it. Better to let it expand to divine dimensions through sitting practices, bhakti and loving service.

If the other you love is harming you, then keep in mind that real love is wise and strong and can say, "No."

If your love is unrequited, then let it redirect through bhakti, expand, and flow out to those in need around you. Expanding love knows no boundaries and expects nothing in return.

There is nothing wrong with romantic love if it is expanded to divine romance. Enlightenment is a never-ending divine romance inside, overflowing with love everywhere.

The guru is in you.

Lesson 112 – Bhakti – Up Close and Personal

Q: My question is about bhakti. It is described as love for the divine, which could be love for people, nature and all the manifestations. Sometimes it is viewed as a certain practice, such as chanting, or sitting and singing spiritual songs. Bhakti is so highly touted; I am wondering how to really practice it. To "love God" is abstract. You can love God's qualities, such as unconditional love, guidance, light, and therefore yearn to be in God's presence and think about God, being preoccupied by God. This word "bhakti" is just a word though – what is it?

A: A very good question. Love of God (bhakti) can be very abstract. Nebulous even. There are so many external forms of bhakti, as many as there are ishtas (chosen ideals) and attributes that we can imagine. Unlimited! In the lessons we don't get into that very much. It is the province of the religious traditions. For those who love to worship in their tradition, that is very good. For those who are not inclined that way, it is not the end of the world. Yoga can progress very well with or without formal modes of worship. Yoga works either way.

The kind of bhakti we talk about in the lessons is the "up close and personal" kind. It is a non-sectarian approach. Here, bhakti is about you, your nervous system, your desires, your practices, and your experiences. When we talk about bhakti as "love of God" here, what we mean is, what is our highest desire? What is the highest ideal we aspire to for ourselves? Maybe so far it is only a question we want to answer, like, "Is there more than this?" If we ask that question in our heart with sincerity and give our emotions to it, we will have some good bhakti going. Real bhakti is very personal. It is about our innermost desire to become something more in our life. It is about wanting to know the truth and using our emotions to move toward it. It can be as simple as the bare wanting – hungry with wanting to know. This is bhakti. Or it can be very involved as a relationship with our chosen ideal, our ishta. This is bhakti too. In whatever way it is occurring, the process is the same – the emotions are harnessed toward an ideal, which moves energy through our nervous system, purifying and opening it.

When longing is strongly expressed deep in our heart, things happen. Answers start coming. Practices come to us. Then we begin to open and want to go higher. Then there will be more opening, more answers, more practices. Like that. Bhakti is like magic as it spirals up. It corresponds with the opening of our nervous system. We have called the nervous system the gateway to the infinite. That goes both ways. We can see out into the infinite through our nervous system as it becomes purified. And God can come in through our nervous system. God comes in as bhakti in our heart. God, the guru and bhakti inside us are all the same thing. It is the infinite, responding to our inner cry, coming in through the gateway of our nervous system.

You may wish to review the following lessons for further detail on the approach we take to bhakti here:

#12 – "The Essential Ingredient – Desire"
#67 – "Bhakti – The Science of Devotion"
#68 – "The Relationship of Traumatic Experiences and Bhakti"
#88 – "The Magic of Bhakti"
#109 – "Bhakti, Meditation and Inner Silence"

The dynamics of bhakti are woven through many other lessons as well. Spiritual desire comes up naturally as our nervous system opens, and our practices are married to our expanding desire. It is a personal process for each one of us, yet it is quite easy to recognize in its different stages. Not abstract or nebulous at all.

Directed desire is the essential ingredient in all spiritual practices. Not in the actual performance of the practices though. The procedure for each practice we follow according to its particular form, whether it be meditation, pranayama, bandhas, mudras, asanas, etc. It is the bhakti that gets us to our meditation room. Then we easily favor the particular advanced yoga practice we are doing. The practices are designed to open our nervous system steadily each day, month and year. So we do them precisely according to the procedures that have been discussed in the lessons. Then we have a constantly purifying and opening nervous system, growing desire for truth and enlightenment, and we are always hankering to go to the next level of practices. And so it goes, up and up.

The guru is in you.

Lesson 113 – Bliss, Ecstasy and Divine Love

Q: Can you explain the difference between bliss and ecstasy?

A: Let's look these two words up in the dictionary:

- Bliss means, "complete happiness, heaven, paradise."

- Ecstasy means, "overwhelming rapturous delight."

They seem a bit similar, but not the same. In terms of how we interpret these two words in Advanced Yoga Practices, the difference is in where these two experiences originate. This is the key to understanding how we use them in the lessons, and how they relate to specific practices we are doing. There is also a tie-in with the inner divine romance we have been discussing recently, and also our steps along the path to enlightenment.

We are putting names on experiences we have during and after our practices. So, the words are experience-based here, like everything else we discuss in the lessons. They are words we use to describe what is happening inside us. The experiences comes first, then the words. Not the other way around.

Bliss is associated with the "pure bliss consciousness" we experience in meditation and gradually more and more in our daily life as we continue to meditate. It comes up is as a pleasant, peaceful silence, a sort of unending inner smile, if you will. It is happiness that comes out of nowhere inside us as we take the mind and body to stillness over and over again in meditation. Is inner silence we come in touch with during meditation "complete happiness, heaven, paradise?" As its presence grows in us it comes pretty close. It is unshakable, always positive no matter what is going on around us, and it has the feel of eternity in it as well. Most important, it is our awareness standing alone, independent of body, breath, mind, emotions, senses and all external events. It is the proverbial "rock" that will not wash away in the storms of life. Once our sense of self has become that inner silence, where have we gone? Everywhere, and nowhere. Pure bliss consciousness is a mystery. Yet, it is what we are in our essential nature. We experience it as bliss, a complete unending happiness. Our consciousness is the source of bliss. Our consciousness is bliss. No one has to take my word for it. As we meditate each day, we gradually come to know what pure bliss consciousness is. As the *Psalm* says, "Be still, and know I am God."

Ecstasy, on the other hand, is an undoing. I mean, we get lost in a reverie of pleasure. "Overwhelming rapturous delight" is a good a description for it. Where does ecstasy come from? While bliss emanates from our consciousness, ecstasy arises in our body. Ecstasy is the result of prana ravishing us in delicious ways. You will recall that prana, the life force, is one of the first manifestations coming out of pure bliss consciousness. When prana moves in evolutionary ways in the nervous system it produces vibrations that we experience as overwhelming pleasure. Ecstasy is the goddess moving in us. Ecstasy emanates from an awakened kundalini, which we know comes from our sexual energy, our great storehouse of prana.

Now comes the tie-in, the relationship between bliss and ecstasy, which sometimes causes us to jumble meanings together into phrases like "blissful ecstasy," or "ecstatic bliss." What is going on here? Is Yogani confused when he uses these phrases? You bet. Who isn't when lovemaking is going on?

The truth is that bliss and ecstasy want to merge in us. Metaphorically, pure bliss consciousness is Shiva, present everywhere in us as inner silence. At least if we have been meditating he is. If we have awakened kundalini Shakti with spinal breathing and other advanced yoga practices, she is on the hunt for Shiva in our nervous system. We know she is because we can feel her moving through us as ecstasy (or fire), cleaning house as she goes. At some point we have inner silence stabilized inside us, and ecstasy moving around inside us as well. What happens?

Activation of the experiences of bliss and ecstasy through advanced yoga practices corresponds to the first two stages of enlightenment, which have been discussed in previous lessons – the rise of inner silence and the rise of ecstasy, best done in that order. The third stage of enlightenment comes following the union of bliss and ecstasy in divine romance inside. While this is going on, we tend to get the descriptions jumbled, because both pure bliss consciousness and divine ecstasy are present at the same time, joining inside us!

What comes out of this union of the masculine and feminine polar energies inside? We have described the third stage of enlightenment as "unity," where we see all as an expression of the One that we have become. That One is pure bliss consciousness coexisting within all the (ecstatic) processes of nature. When it gets to this stage, we become a channel for an unending flow of divine love. We act for the good of all, expecting nothing in return, because we perceive all as an expression of our own self. In this stage, personal need is expanded to encompass universal need. This is enlightenment, divine love naturally manifesting through us, born of the union of pure bliss consciousness and divine ecstasy inside us.

Advanced yoga practices are for facilitating this evolutionary process of transformation in our nervous system. Everyone is born with the ability to make this glorious journey.

The guru is in you.

Lesson 114* – Kechari – Throat Jamming in Stage 1

Q: I am one of those whose tongue has been rolling back. Your recent lesson on kechari is wonderful, a real eye-opener. My question regards some difficulty I am having as the tongue goes back on the roof of the mouth. In the beginning I was having a gag reflex in my throat, which seems to be getting less. Sometimes when my tongue is back during meditation, my breathing gets blocked temporarily. Are these normal experiences?

A: These are transitional experiences that can happen in stage 1 kechari. The reason for them is something I call, "throat jamming." It is a temporary phenomenon that can occur between stages 1 and 2.

Because the tongue cannot go up beyond the roof of the mouth in stage 1, the further back it goes, the more the base of the tongue will tend to be pressed down into the throat. This can create a "jamming" effect deep in the throat that can lead to some gag reflex and/or some closing of the epiglottis over the entrance to the windpipe (trachea). The epiglottis is a trap door-like flap connected to the root of the tongue that closes the windpipe when we swallow, and also when we hold our breath in the normal way.

Everyone has a slightly different physical anatomy, so some may experience these transitional experiences during stage 1, and others may not. In any case, the experiences should be temporary. As the frenum under the tongue stretches out, or is trimmed, the tongue will eventually go up behind the soft palate into stage 2 kechari. When this happens, the throat jamming should naturally end, because the tongue goes up into the nasal pharynx and will no longer be pressing down into the throat as much. I say "as much" because with the frenum still pulling down on the tongue, there could still be some throat jamming in stage 2 kechari, though much less, and less likely to create any distracting experiences in the throat. As the tongue goes higher up, the frenum will continue to be stretched, or trimmed, and the tendency for jamming will go away.

As mentioned, for anatomical reasons, only some people may experience the throat jamming symptoms mentioned above, while others will not have them at all. Whatever the case may be, the phenomenon is a transitional one as kechari evolves upward in us.

The experiences of ecstatic bliss we find in stage 2 kechari far outweigh the inconveniences we may encounter on the way there.

Take your time with kechari. Approach it in your own way. Your bhakti will take you up when the time is right.

The guru is in you.

Addition – Another question on going from kechari stage 1 to stage 2:

Q: I have a question/suggestion on your very helpful kechari mudra lesson. When you describe the four stages of the journey of the tongue, it might be helpful to include some familiar landmarks. For example, you don't mention the uvula or the tonsils. I'm wondering where they lie on the path?

Also, the critical first step is to reach "the point on the roof of the mouth where the hard and soft palates meet," but I'm not sure I fully understand where that point is, exactly. Can it be described in terms of teeth, uvula, tonsils, etc?

A: More can always be said about the kechari journey. Could we ever say enough? It is such a profound practice. On the uvula and tonsils, I did not mention them so far because they are very quickly bypassed as the tongue slips from stage 1 to stage 2, up into the nasal pharynx. There really isn't much to do with them.

There are those who place a lot of emphasis on the uvula – nectar coming down through there and all that, but I don't see much significance in it. Once the "secret spot" is reached on the back edge of the septum above the soft palate (see lesson #T34), then there is a whole new level of stimulation far beyond anything that can be done with the soft palate or uvula. The soft palate is a doorway, little more.

Significant stimulation can be achieved below the soft palate too, at the point where the hard and soft palates meet on the roof of the mouth (stage 1). It is easy to find if you go back along the roof of the mouth. The roof is hard, yes? Then you get to a place where it is soft. That is right below the septum and nasal pharynx. It is about half way between the front teeth and uvula. The nerves from the septum (secret spot) reach down to that place where the hard and soft palates meet on the roof of the mouth, so significant stimulation can be achieved once the tip of the tongue reaches that place. Of course, it will also depend on there being some ecstatic conductivity in the nervous system cultivated through a daily routine of yoga practices.

Lesson 115 – Mantra, Language and Meaning

Q: English is not my first language. I am wondering if I should translate the mantra *I AM* to my own language and use that for meditation.

A: It is a good question. Others have asked it too. Even those of us who have English as our first language should take note of the following suggestions.

No, don't translate the mantra. As has been said before, the mantra is not about language or meaning. If we had been given it orally, there would be no spelling, no language, and no meaning. Just a sound vibration to use in meditation in that specific way that allows the mind to go naturally to stillness.

Since we are doing all this in writing, we have to spell the mantra. With or without spelling, it is just a sound that is found to have certain good qualities deep in the nervous system. This was reviewed in lesson #59, "Some mantra particulars." It is found in the English/Christian tradition as "I AM." It is also found in other traditions and languages in similar forms, and sometimes identical. The natural vibrational qualities in our nervous system are universal, and not determined by language.

If the *I AM* spelling is distracting, then think of the same sound spelled another way like – *AYAM*. Same pronunciation, no English meaning. If we try and attach a meaning to it, we will not be doing our meditation a favor. Let there be one sound in our life that does not have a worldly connection. Let it be the mantra. The mantra should mean only one thing – It is our ticket to ride to the infinite. Let us use it for that, and for that alone when we are meditating.

If meanings and language come up in meditation, we just regard them as any other thoughts coming up, and easily go back to the mantra at whatever level of quietness or fuzziness it is. Then we continue our inner march to stillness, inner silence, pure bliss consciousness.

The mind settles down to stillness best when using the vibration alone. Meanings tend to pull us to the surface of the mind, so we easily let them go and favor the finer levels of the vibration of the mantra. Meanings and language are for the outer word. Vibrations naturally becoming finer and finer are for the inner world of pure bliss consciousness. The mantra is for that. It is not a word of meaning. It is a vibrational vehicle that refines and disappears as we ride to the infinite every day.

In time, with the easy daily practice of meditation, our inner world of silent pure bliss consciousness becomes always present in our outer world, and vise versa. The gateway of our nervous system opens wide. We experience the truth of yoga, the joining of the infinite with our everyday life. We come to find we are That.

This glorious outcome has nothing to do with language or any outer meaning of the mantra. We leave all that behind when we meditate.

The guru is in you.

Lesson 116 – Meditation – First Enhancement of Mantra

As we continue to use the mantra, *I AM*, in that particular way that allows the mind to go to stillness, we are clearing out obstructions deep in our nervous system. Over time, our experience will become smoother and deeper as the purification progresses. We will experience more inner silence.

With rising inner silence, at some point in time we will be ready to take broader strokes deep in the nervous system without getting bogged down too much on the surface of the mind. We will be ready for an enhancement of our mantra.

Think of it as shifting gears in a car. With a manual transmission, we go along in first gear, and then at some point we are ready to shift to the next gear, which enables us to go faster with ease because we have gotten up to an adequate speed with the first gear. If we shift into the second gear too soon, what happens? We bog down and don't get much out of it, because there is not enough speed yet. Shifting too soon is a strain, and does not help us go faster.

Taking on a mantra enhancement is like that. If we have smoothness and good depth in meditation with *I AM*, we can think about moving to the first enhancement. It could be in a few months after starting, or it could be in a few years. Everyone is different. It is one of those situations where self-pacing is important. There is no rush to step up too soon. We can make the entire journey using the *I AM* mantra for our meditation if we wish. Nothing is missing. It is only a matter of how fast we want to go. If and when it is time to shift, we will know. Then we can do it and the transition will be reasonably smooth with minimal clunkiness, like making a good shift of gears in a car.

The enhancement adds syllables and sound vibrations to our mantra. This will make a "bigger footprint" in the nervous system as we meditate. Meditation will be slower going into silence and slower coming back out of silence. This creates the effect of making pure bliss consciousness stick more in our nervous system and in our awareness. That is the benefit of the enhancement. It speeds up the cultivation of inner silence to be more prevalent and steadier in us. It is a "higher gear."

The first enhancement is an expanded mantra. It is:

… SHREE SHREE I AM I AM …

We use it exactly the same way as we have used *I AM*, following the same easy procedure of meditation we learned early in the lessons. Once we have made the change, this will be our mantra from then on.

We will notice a difference right away. Our mind will go to stillness slower, and come out of stillness slower. Interestingly, this slowing down of the attention moving in and out speeds up the infusion of pure bliss consciousness into our nervous system.

Think of the mantra as something we are systematically penetrating the fabric of our subconscious with. A mantra with few syllables goes through more quickly, clearing out obstructions easily a little bit at a time. Then it gets to the point when we can use a "wider" mantra and cover a bigger area as we go in and out through the subconscious, clearing out more obstructions with each pass through. A mantra with more syllables does this, but only after we have prepared the ground with the first level of mantra – *I AM*.

If you have just begun meditating recently, give yourself time to develop a good habit using the *I AM* mantra, and to develop smoothness and good depth of inner silence before jumping ahead to the first enhancement. Several months at least. It could take a year or two before meditation with *I AM* clears the nervous system enough. Maybe longer. We each have our own unique journey to take (and time line) as we open our nervous system to the infinite. The mantra enhancement will be here when we are ready, so let's take our time ... and enjoy!

The guru is in you.

Lesson 117 – Finding a Mantra with no Meaning?

Q: Since all mantras have meanings attached to them, even Sanskrit ones, how do I find a mantra with no meaning?

A: Meaning or absence of meaning is in the way we use the sound. In the procedure of meditation the sound of the mantra is favored over thoughts that come up, including meanings, so the mantra has no meaning in that application of sound inside.

Take the sound, "AM." Not only is it a word in English, but it appears in hundreds of other words – ham, lamb, sham, bam, cram, and so on, not to mention the innumerable meanings in other languages. Do we think of all these words and meanings when we think the sound, "AM?" No. It is a matter of context, a matter of what the situation is when we use the sound.

The mantra has a unique context of use. It is used in a specific way for going inward to stillness of mind. In this method of use, we let go of meaning. We don't have to worry about pushing meaning out or anything like that. The method of meditation will take care of it for us. It is very simple. When we use the mantra we follow a particular mode of thinking, a procedure, which we develop into a habit that we use whenever we sit to meditate. Part of that procedure is easily favoring the sound of the mantra over any thoughts that come up. Once the habit is in place, meanings don't come up when we sit to meditate. It is just the mantra. That is what we mean by the mantra having no meaning. Whatever particular sound we use as mantra in meditation has no meaning by virtue of the way it is being used.

For details on the procedure of meditation, see the series of lessons beginning with #13.

The guru is in you.

Lesson 118 – Strong Pulse in Meditation

Q: Is it possible that energy is getting stuck in my solar plexus? To give you background, I have faithfully done the practices twice a day for about two months. During breathing, I include sambhavi and siddhasana. I do not include mulabandha, because I found I was not able to take a deep breath without releasing the lock, and that was distracting. I will focus on sambhavi until it is automatic and then try again. I'm doing 15 minutes of pranayama. During meditation I stay in siddhasana and meditate for 20 minutes.

Lately I have noticed during meditation a very strong pulse in my solar plexus that distracts me from the mantra. It can be quite a strong series of jolts. I do go easily back to the mantra but with nearly every breath I am distracted by the deep pulse. The pulse is strongest after I begin to exhale. (It is noticeable when I inhale and sometimes during pranayama) If I hold after exhaling – which I did just to see what happened – it subsides a bit. It does seem to grow stronger throughout the meditation and I often feel it up to my ears. It does not go below my navel at all. I guess I wouldn't mind if I could remain focused on the mantra, but it does distract. The occurrence of the pulse did not follow any new practice; I have been doing pretty much the same things throughout. Most days I also do some yoga before pranayama. The yoga does not have any affect on the pulse. I'm not sure if you have any suggestions. I seem to be at a point where I could relate to your discussions of bliss were it not for this issue. I appreciate any thoughts you might have and thank you for your time and consideration.

A: Sometimes pulse can happen like that in practices for a few days or weeks. It can happen almost anywhere in the body. Usually it will settle down as the nervous system adjusts. The solar plexus can be the blockage, or it could be something elsewhere in the nadis (subtle nerves). I presume the pulse is not prevalent in daily activity. If it becomes so and doesn't clear up, make sure to cover the medical angle. Not to be alarmist, but we don't want to be blind to potential health issues.

You might review the lesson on physical sensations that can come up in meditation – #15. There is a specific technique in there to deal with distracting physical sensations during meditation, which would include a distracting pulse.

After using the method in lesson #15, if it continues to distract you, you might consider backing down a bit on your pranayama (and siddhasana and sambhavi, if necessary) for a week or so and see if that helps. Then slowly come back when the symptom subsides. Self-pacing, you know. (You did not mention yoni mudra kumbhaka – it goes without saying that backing down on that is also in order if symptoms become excessive.)

Also, you could do some uddiyana (and learn to do nauli) as part of asanas before pranayama and meditation. Those can help clear the solar plexus. We will be doing nauli (special churning of the abdominal muscles) in the lessons pretty soon, and then another physical technique (chin pump) higher up that will bring energy up through the solar plexus and chest. So, we will be working on it from a few more angles.

On mulabandha, there is no need to keep it locked throughout pranayama. It will naturally go through its own pattern of pulsations as our inner spiritual biology comes up. Yes, it is distracting when the mulabandha comes alive. But the distraction gradually turns to ecstatic bliss as the inner process in us come up.

The first order of business is to get comfortable in your routine, and that could mean backing off temporarily on the things mentioned, until you get through this bump in the road. It is up to you.

Real yogis and yoginis are hungry to stay on the "leading edge" of their journey, and I admire you for it. Your bhakti is terrific. But we want to avoid having it become the "bleeding edge." It should be fun. In time it becomes much more than fun. It becomes infinite joy!

The guru is in you.

Lesson 119 – Some Other Approaches to Mulabandha

Q: I am still having some difficulty with mulabandha also. It is very difficult to keep the muscle flexed. Sometimes I'm not sure if it is unless I flex it strongly. Are there any intervening exercises I can do? If I just don't do it – I can't see how I will ever advance to the stage where I am able – yet it takes all my effort to do it during pranayama and I don't know if that is good.

A: It might be a bit easier if you do the gentle flexing on the rising inhalation during spinal breathing and release it on the descending exhalation. Then the breath will be a cue for flexing. This is actually called asvini mudra, the alternating flexing and releasing. If that does not work, then try a short flex at the bottom and a short flex at the top during spinal breathing, again, the breath is the cue. This last approach might be the easiest, as it is a short flex and done. Once you get comfortable with that, then maybe do two at the top and bottom of each cycle, and later move on to the rising flex and no flex going down. Later, you can let it become more spontaneous as it was originally given. Another thing you can do is flexing exercises for ten or more repetitions a few times during the day. It is just a matter of developing coordination and familiarly. Then it becomes second nature. The sphincter is part of an organ of spiritual ecstasy. We find them all over the body in yoga, sometimes in the least expected places.

Where we'd like to end up with mulabandha/asvini is with spontaneous subtle movements as ecstatic energy moves naturally inside us. It will evolve gradually to that as our inner ecstatic conductivity comes up. All the other bandhas and mudras will participate in simultaneous coordination, so it will be like one spontaneous whole body mudra going on subtly everywhere inside us. When it gets to that stage we have found our new natural spiritual biology. One slip of the eyes upward and we are in ecstatic bliss everywhere inside. Our nervous system is permanently transformed to a higher mode of functioning.

There is no one way to awaken mulabandha/asvini. There is no exact formula. Experiment and see what works for you. It is supposed to feel good. You may find an option that I have not mentioned that works for you and does not distract excessively from other practices. Of course, add siddhasana in with any of these mulabandha/asvini combinations and there will likely be distraction for the short term. That goes with the territory. It is a transition period filled with delight, and it gets more delightful all the time. Eventually it calms down to an unending divine smile radiating from within.

The guru is in you.

Lesson 120 – "Getting Enlightenment"

Q: The main aim of my remaining life is to make all possible efforts to get liberation from the cycle of birth and death in this life time only. I know that I have many weaknesses yet to overcome but still I wish to make all possible efforts to get rid of them and make this soul merged with the supreme soul during this lifetime. Is it possible or not? For this if I have to undergo more vigorous practices for a longer time I wish to do that also, that is, spinal breathing and meditation for a longer time or any other practices. Kindly guide.

A: Yes, I understand that you don't want to waste a minute to get enlightenment. Yes, absolutely! I have felt the same way since taking up practices in this life many years ago. You should continue with practices to your capacity using self-pacing, being careful not to overdo. If there is strain, then it is too much. We all have to go at our own pace, or progress gets stymied. I will do my best to see that everything you need will be here in the lessons. Everything but a purified nervous system. That you have to do yourself, swept along by your bhakti, your love of Truth and God, which is God alive in you.

Keep in mind that "getting enlightenment" is an ego strategy, and not likely to be completed in this life if it continues like that on the basis of "getting." This does not remove the necessity for practices to achieve progress. But getting enlightenment is a letting go. A paradox. Not letting go of practices necessarily, but letting go of something. Letting go of our need to "get it." How can we let go of the thing we need so desperately? How can we let go of the very thing we have been cultivating – intense desire for God?

It is a strange thing. Somewhere along the line we stop trying to "get" enlightenment and find ourselves "giving" ourselves to it. We may be doing everything the same – practices, bhakti, service and all that. Maybe even more practices – yes, definitely more practices. The nervous system wants to do them as it opens. But something changes. Maybe it is in the rise of kundalini, and we no longer feel in charge. It is easy to give in to a powerful divine process happening automatically inside, even while continuing aggressive practices. As the ego is dissolving to become pure bliss consciousness it still craves enlightenment and struggles to do more to "get it!" Then, magically, our need to "get" turns into a need to "give." This is an important turning point that has its foundation in practices and rising bhakti. It is a maturing that occurs in our nervous system as it becomes purified.

I think the most effective strategy is for day-by-day. It is a higher path to take. Never mind enlightenment somewhere down the road. Is it good today? Is today better than yesterday, last week and last year? That is something real and concrete. Enlightenment may be next year, or a hundred lifetimes from now. Who knows? How we feel today, and what we can do to feel better tomorrow – that is not so nebulous. It is real, while enlightenment, salvation, or whatever, is out in the imagination somewhere.

The future isn't real. Today is real. It is misery to want a thing in the future, keeping it out there, out of reach. The future never comes. It is maya (illusion). On the other hand, it is bliss to want what we are having today that this good, and tasting it being more already tomorrow. That is why I have said, "Do something nice for someone today." That is more enlightenment than we can find anywhere in our imagination of the future. If there is enlightenment, it is to be found today. It is a fine point. As long as we do practices for the future, enlightenment will remain in the future. If we do practices for happiness today and tomorrow, then enlightenment is suddenly much closer. Then we can relax a little and breathe. The relaxing and breathing is the enlightenment itself coming up.

Will we ever experience enlightenment in the future? No. We never will. We can only experience it in the present. That means today.

What does this mean in relation to our practices? Remember that meditation is going inward when we sit, and then going out into daily activity to engage the blissful silence we have gained. If we meditate all day we will have lots of silence. If we don't engage our silence in meaningful activity, we will not get full enlightenment. Maybe only the first stage – unending inner silence. That's not bad, but not the whole thing. Enlightenment is the union of inner and outer. If we are all inner and no outer, we will not be in yoga. We must move to all inner and all outer – two fullnesses. Then we are becoming it.

I have been doing all this writing here for months. Why? Well, it is a good thing that needs to be done for sure. Many agree with that. From my perspective, it is going out with my inner silence into many lives, and that is helping me expand tremendously inside. The more I give away, the more I am filling up with ecstatic bliss. I am a very selfish person doing all this transmission of knowledge. Yet, my self is becoming more and more in everyone. Your joy is my joy. You can do the same thing in your life. Do your sitting practices, however much and whatever kind you find is good for you, and then go do something good for someone. That is rising enlightenment.

If we don't share it, we don't get it. It can happen today. Don't worry about enlightenment in the future. Claim enlightenment today by doing practices and then giving away your silence and your bliss to others. Whatever good feelings practices bring to you, give them away in daily activity. That is enlightenment coming up right now. All we have to do is say, "Yes" to the flow of divine love going out, and it will surge out through us like an endless river of ecstatic bliss.

Then we will be laughing like joyous innocent children all the time. That is what we are when all the obstructions and holding on are gone.

Getting enlightenment is giving it away. Getting enlightenment is letting it go.

The guru is in you.

Lesson 121 – Pratyahara – Expansion of the Senses Inward

Q: During spinal breathing and meditation different sounds are heard. One is a low frequency fluttering sound that I assume is the AUM (*OM*). However, I do not always hear that frequency. Sometimes there are multiple frequencies heard. Are these pitches associated with the different chakras and does that indicate that they are active or perhaps cleansing? Should the attention become fixed on these sounds or should they be dismissed?

A: Someone asked a similar question and it was reviewed in lesson #53 – "Light and Sound in Pranayama." In a nutshell, yes, it is purification, and we just easily favor our practice over experiences that come up. And yes, the chakras are involved, but there is no need to manage the details of it. It's "under the hood," you know, to use the analogy from past lessons.

The truth is that all our inner senses come alive throughout our nervous system (nadis and chakras) as we progress on the path, so we have to be mindful not to get distracted from the practices that are opening our nervous system up to the divine experiences. In yoga the change in sensory experience is called "pratyahara" which is often interpreted to mean losing or giving up attachment to sensory experiences. This is sometimes taken to mean killing involvement in the senses, or controlling them. Something anti-sensual, like that. This has led to bizarre practices in some cases, running away from natural experiences of the world. This is a limited interpretation of pratyahara. What pratyahara really means is "expansion inward of the senses," meaning we sense more and more divine qualities inside that are initially more charming than physical sensuality, so we are naturally drawn to them. We do not reject physical sensuality. We just begin to operate on a broader spectrum of sensuality as our nervous system opens inside. In time, even our physical senses are heightened as inner sensuality opens up, and our sensuality is seen to be a broad continuum. All the while, we keep up our daily practices, which are the underlying cause of the transformation. The rise of pure silent bliss consciousness, a fundamental constituent in this process, keeps us beyond the grip of ego attachment to the widening sensory experience.

Some traditions use inner sensory experiences for practice. There is nothing wrong with this if it is a tradition we have chosen, and it works for us. But as you said, sometimes the experiences are there, and sometimes they are not, depending on the course of purification in various parts of the nervous system. What we do in Advanced Yoga Practices are global practices that will be purifying all of our nervous system, no matter what else may be going on inside. That is why we use meditation and spinal breathing first. These will do the global housecleaning, and we are not dependent on any particular experience coming up in any particular part of our spiritual anatomy.

Sooner or later, everything will open up. When experiences come up, great. We enjoy them. In time we will have them twenty-four hours a day, seven days a week. When they come up in practices, we just stay with the practice we are doing. When they come up while we are in daily activity, we can enjoy them however we like. Our perception of our inner and outer world will change very much for the better. This is the fruit of practice, not the practice itself.

Once meditation and spinal breathing are well established, we can add on practices for stimulating from both ends of the spinal nerve to awaken it to ecstatic conductivity, which spreads out through our entire nervous system automatically. These practices have been given already in previous lessons.

In upcoming lessons we will look at additional practices for moving prana more from both ends of the spinal nerve toward our center, our heart.

The guru is in you.

Lesson 122 – Witnessing

Q: I've been going through a process for a long time now where I just don't identify with the body. I don't identify with the emotions or feelings. Something else is feeling them, not I. Sometimes I am aware of an emotion trying to come up, but I just don't know what to do with it so I ignore it and it goes away. My grandmother died two weeks ago and it didn't bother me at all. I must have been the only one in the funeral smiling or trying not to smile most of the time. My cat whom is everything to me, my best friend, my companion, my love, I think is going to die or is dying slowly, and I am just not bothered by this. I am concerned and a bit worried, yes, but I am not bothered. It changes things externally, but not internally. I can fall down the stairs and just laugh not caring. I could get fired from work without a care in the world. I am just not attached to anything. More recently, I feel like I lost identity with my name. It almost hurts me to sign an email or a posting with my name. Is this normal and apart of Pratyahara? Are there stages to this, so I would be prepared for what's next to come?

A: Thank you very much for writing and sharing. The answer depends on what your state really is, and that has to do with how you got there. If you have been meditating and have this feeling of separation in silent witness, that is one thing. If you have separated from your life and the world as a psychological defense mechanism because of some trauma in the past, that is something else. The former is due to purification in the nervous system. The latter is a pigeon-holing of awareness in avoidance of subconscious obstructions involving a lot of pain. One is an opening up. The other is a kind of closing down. They can appear similar, but are not. Under certain circumstances, it is even possible that some of both could be happening at the same time.

If it is purification in the nervous system giving rise to the emergence of inner silence, then the thing to do is engage in spiritual practices and in life. Ultimately, our enlightenment is not about us. It is about everyone else. The first stage of enlightenment is the rise of an ongoing inner silence – a temporary separation. The second and third stages are about joining with the divine rising dynamically in us and in others (this is where ecstasy and pratyahara come in, not much before). Going beyond stage one (inner silence/witnessing) is not an inert do nothing process. It involves the rise of devotion, and engaging our pure bliss consciousness in the further processes of enlightenment, which include practices and involvement in the world. It is a natural evolution, part of which is in our deciding to participate.

Suggestion: When emotions come up, instead of ignoring them, consider the process of bhakti as described in lesson #67, "Bhakti – The Science of Devotion," and subsequent lessons discussing the finer points of witnessing and bhakti, especially, #109, "Bhakti, Meditation and Inner Silence." These might give you some tips on how to make better use of your witnessing state to move on to next steps. The relationship of witnessing and emotion is a key dynamic in this.

Pure bliss consciousness, the silent witness, is not touched by the phenomenal world, but it is not uncaring. Just the opposite. Inner silence is an endless well of love and compassion, and moves us naturally to engage in the ecstatic processes in the body, and in loving service to others. We can even get angry and cry in the witnessing state – the nervous system will continue to purify itself. Even though the silent witness is the ultimate unmoved spectator, the enlightenment game is not a spectator sport. This is one of the paradoxes of spiritual life. Until pure bliss consciousness becomes fully present in our nervous system, joining continuously with the ecstatic processes of creation (the divine inner lovemaking), there can be no completion of enlightenment. If we want to move to higher stages of enlightenment, we must actively participate.

So, my suggestion is to see if you can find a desire in yourself to grow beyond where you are. Any desire will do, because you can transform emotion easily into bhakti in the witnessing state, if you choose to. If you can, cultivate it. Then you will find it easy to do something – some daily practices, some service, doing something for someone else. If you find it difficult to "engage," then maybe the situation is psychologically more complicated than a natural process of purification coming up in the nervous system stimulated by spiritual practices. Or, sometimes there can be some tenderness during the witnessing stage (or any stage) where we just have to bide our time for a while – a sort of healing into a new state of being. Once we get comfortable where we are, then we will become more interested in moving on to the next step.

Whatever the underlying cause of your witnessing is, it will not hurt to be in daily practices – meditation and pranayama especially. Sooner or later, these will naturally bring you to the next step.

I wish you all success as you travel along your chosen path.

The guru is in you.

Lesson 124 – Keeping it Simple

Q: I have a guru who sends me healing energy. I'm confused by what I am to do with it. I've studied various techniques and I get confused as to breathing in or breathing out, or looking up or looking down. I'm a beginner to pranayama and I do not know how to use this energy that I'm being blessed with.

It feels like my spine is energized and I would like to use this energy to benefit my spiritual progression, my life. I am pretty sure that I am already benefiting from it since this began. Now, I struggle to find out what to do. I have, at different moments, gotten up and tried to meditate with it. It subsides. Then I just lay there sometimes but I feel like I'm useless through this whole process. I'm grateful for your teachings such that I have not yet found an outlet for these types of questions and answers. I'm sure you have already answered this somehow but please guide me to a technique or lesson I could use. I don't know if I'm working against this healing energy.

There comes a point in meditation that I feel I cannot move through like a barrier keeping me from the possible limitless. I also felt fear of losing my control, my self. Fear arose in me of letting go of something but I didn't know what I was supposed to do. Do I just go with it? Will it subside with further meditative practice and what could help? What in your library refers to kriya techniques that would work with this?

A: You certainly have a lot going on. My suggestion is to simplify your approach to making your spiritual journey, and take things one step at a time. If you want to use these lessons as a primary source of guidance, then go back to the beginning and review the lessons and Q&As on meditation, and find a stable routine in meditation first. Don't bother with pranayama or anything else until you have settled into meditation for at least a few months. The key to increasing practices is to operate from a stable platform of practice. That has to come first. In the Advanced Yoga Practices lessons, that means meditation first, and nothing else until you have that going reasonably smooth.

If you are having emotions or mental concerns during meditation, treat them as any other thoughts coming up, and easily go back to the mantra as instructed in the lessons. There is nothing to fear in letting go into yourself. What you will find inside is your own "Self" – all peace, love and bliss ... and freedom from fear. There will be some ups and downs in practice. That is normal. Just follow the procedures of meditation and everything will be fine. You will feel your inner silence coming up. It is a homecoming.

As for the inner energies, whether they come from an outside source or an inside process in your nervous system, they can be treated just the same. Just let them go during meditation, favoring the procedure of meditation. When purification/healing is going on inside, we don't have to supervise it. It will happen automatically. Just let it happen without undue concern or need to "do something" with it.

Later on, in a few months, when you are feeling stable in your meditation routine, try some light spinal breathing before meditation, as the lessons guide. When that time comes, see about expanding your stability in meditation to include some spinal breathing. Always keep a stable platform of daily practices. Very important.

The lessons are a specific step by step build-up of advanced yoga practices. If you follow them closely, you will be on a logical course. If you try and do too many things at once, you will be on a confusing course. If you follow multiple teachings, it can also be confusing. So, choose a course and stay with it. If you decide to follow a guru or teaching organization, that is fine. Then consider these lessons to be only food for thought. One teaching should be first – all the rest are food for thought only.

The guru is in you.

Lesson 125 – Kundalini Heat

Q: I've been studying kundalini for some time now, and have been feeling a great deal of internal heat due to the kriyas and meditations. However, recently I read that the part of the head (sushumna) that was once soft as a child, needs to soften again in order for the heat to be released, otherwise the kundalini experience can be painful. The way this is supposedly done is through Reiki Tummo? Can you shed any light on this for me? I have curtailed my meditations and my sadhana for a few days now, which I so did not want to do.

A: I am not very familiar with Reiki methods so am not able to comment much on Reiki Tummo, other than to say it appears to be a more aggressive method aimed at raising kundalini, beyond healing-style Reiki. So perhaps it is a cousin of other yoga systems aimed at raising kundalini first – which brings us to your situation.

As you know, in the lessons we go through practices for "global purification" of the nervous system before we go much for stimulating kundalini directly. These include deep meditation and spinal breathing. With these as a foundation, the risk of kundalini difficulties is greatly reduced. Of course, we'd all like to compress the time scale of reaching enlightenment, so we press ahead, and sometimes are tempted to skip the prerequisite global purification methods. Some traditions even skip them!

If you are running into too much heat, it can be obstructions in the nadis and chakras, and premature awakening of kundalini into those areas of your nervous system. Using only the kundalini methods can be a long, slow and uncomfortable grind to get through. Make sure you review lesson #69 on kundalini symptoms and remedies.

Besides inner obstructions there is another reason for heat, and you should consider this one carefully, because many kundalini traditions miss it. That is the matter of balancing the rising and descending pranas (Shiva and Shakti) in the spinal nerve. Traditional kundalini yoga uses mudras and bandhas for this, but these are often not enough. Spinal breathing can do wonders for balancing the rising and descending pranas, and in some cases can end uncomfortable symptoms immediately. Metaphorically speaking, Shakti is seeking her mate, Shiva, everywhere in our body. She purifies (housecleans) as she continues her hunt for Shiva. If he does not show up, she will get more and more frantic and raise all sorts of trouble inside us. If we gently bring Shiva down into Shakti's realm of the nervous system in spinal breathing, the two will be able to join in all the places where Shakti is looking – in every nerve and cell inside us. This is the metaphorical explanation of how spinal breathing works to stimulate and balance the pranas in the nervous system.

Also, with inner silence, the witness, all of this dynamic activity inside the nervous system will be much more manageable. Don't forget that the witness is not touched by any of this stuff going on, yet is in charge of it all via the bhakti connection. Pure bliss consciousness is our platform of "Self" that enables us to choose the divine desire to enter kundalini experience. Being established in Self/witness also enables us to manage much better whatever we might run into as we go though the dynamics of raising kundalini. Inner silence, by definition, is deep permanent global purification in the nervous system. This is why meditation is the first advanced yoga practice, and remains the core practice throughout the lessons. With inner silence, everything else can be like a cakewalk. Without inner silence, everything else can be like jumping off a cliff into an inferno. That's how it is.

Whatever your other practices are, if you make sure you are doing meditation and spinal breathing on the front end, you should find some relief on the heat. Once the balance between ascending and descending pranas is achieved through spinal breathing on an ongoing basis, we have the ability to do much more kundalini-wise with much less chance of difficulty. Our progress will be more and our discomfort will be much less. In fact, doing right practices can turn the journey into an endless joyride of ecstatic bliss. And we don't even have to feel guilty about it, because that is the way our nervous system is designed to operate. It is an ecstatic bliss machine. Everyone has one of these. Oh my gosh, let's not waste a minute getting them all in good working order.

As for the fontanel on top of the head, it is not my understanding that this is a kind of pressure relief valve for kundalini going up. The popular model of kundalini going up and out the top of the head is an over-simplification of the process. Rather, there is a joining on every level in the body of the two polarities that exist within us. On the physical level it occurs in the chest where ascending and descending pranas meet. From there it goes up the spine into the brain, then back down the front and again back up the spine, and so on in an endless cycle. It is part of our new spiritual biology. With adequate global purification and balancing of the inner polarities, all of this occurs with little heat and a lot of ecstatic bliss. So it is an inner closed cycle of union, rather than kundalini blowing out the top by herself. Blowing kundalini out the top could happen, but that is taking the process in the wrong direction, and is not very healthy. Better to cultivate the inner lovemaking and the rest will happen quite naturally, and quite pleasurably.

What does go out the top is a flood of radiant healing energy as a by-product of the inner joining of polarities. This comes later and is not experienced as heat – ecstatic bliss is what it is. Shiva and Shakti energies joined into something new, corresponding with the third stage of enlightenment – Unity – divine love flowing through the nervous system and out to everyone. In the Christian tradition it is called "Christ."

Whether the fontanel opens physically or not I don't think is a primary issue. Maybe it will happen, maybe it won't. If it does, it will be a natural outcome of the process of enlightenment, not something we have to worry about too much at this stage. The fontanel is over the pituitary gland, which is said by some to be the seat of higher consciousness. In the center of the head is the pineal gland, which is our receptor of divine light. Above the pineal is the corona radiata which turns up into a cup shape (which can be clearly felt and observed with the inner sight) as energy goes up. It is the sahasrar, the thousand-petaled lotus.

So we have the point between the eyebrows where a lot of ecstatic energy is stimulated in and out with spinal breathing and the other advanced yoga practices, the fontanel with energy going in and out mainly due to the illumination of the pituitary, and the sahasrar, above the pineal and spine, putting out a huge fountain-shaped aura. Things get pretty busy up there. Then, inside the brain, there are the dynamics between the pituitary and pineal (third eye activation) through the ventricles, down into the medulla oblongata, and connected all the way down the spinal nerve to the perineum/root. So many ecstatic energy dynamics are going on in the head.

Some day, spiritual neuro-biologists will sort it all out for us. In the meantime, we have to keep going with advanced yoga practices that will purify and open our nervous system, so the neuro-biologists will have someone to dissect. Only kidding!

These are exciting times for sure. I wish you much success on your journey.

The guru is in you.

Lesson 126 – Relationship of Pratyahara, Intellect and Bhakti

Q: Philo of Alexandria wrote about this matter of withdrawing from the senses in Egypt in the first century. His comments strike me as being mostly of historical interest, as showing that not only Indian but also Egyptian practitioners were interested in this. His remarks are confusing to me, but he seems to suggest that one should begin with an exquisite attention to the senses, then withdraw from them afterward so as to reside entirely in the intellectual nature. The mind was thought by these mystics to be divine in origin, and therefore the point of contact between the mystic and whatever there is in the universe that is divine.

A: Yes, the mind is the main connection with the divine, as we all can experience when we meditate. So, things haven't changed since ancient times on that score. However, the way the mind connects us to the divine is not through the intellect. It is through its ability to come to stillness. This is the great secret of the mind's divine connection. As it says in Psalm 46 of the Old Testament of the *Bible*, "Be still, and know I am God."

As you know, I take a different approach from the popular definition of pratyahara being, "withdrawal from the senses." I think it is an over-simplification that can be taken to be a kind of mortification of sensory experience, and I am not for that. In reality, we become less interested in stuffing the physical senses with pleasures as our sensuality expands into the divine realms, which are even more pleasurable. Eventually, the physical senses catch up as our inner divine experience comes back out into every day life. I don't think this process has much to do with the intellect, other than it is through the intellect that we choose to make the journey of yoga practices.

A great Indian sage, Ramana Maharishi, said that the intellect has only one useful purpose, and that is to continually ask the question, "Who am I?" Oddly enough, though Ramana was considered a very high jnani (one enlightened via the intellect), his perpetual question, "Who am I?" is a pure form of bhakti. If one is only interested in answering that question, life becomes pure bhakti/desire for truth. So, if the intellect is used in the right way, it merges with the heart's deepest longing for divine truth. That is how the intellect can help us make spiritual progress.

If the intellect is not brought beyond reason to the stage of simple divine inquiry ("Who am I? Is there more than this?"), then it is little more than a machine that is prone to build too many castles in the air. The intellect can be very seductive that way. From our inner silence the intellect can be channeled usefully. When it is, it merges with bhakti.

The guru is in you.

Lesson 127 – Siddhasana or Padmasana?

Q: I had been doing meditation in padmasana (lotus pose) for a long time. After reading your message I realized that it doesn't bring any pressure to perineum. Do I need to switch to siddhasana? I tried it but it looks like it would take quite some time for me to get accustomed to it. Let me know how should I proceed. In padmasana, one limitation which I find is after sitting for 45 minutes or so, my legs become slightly numb and it distracts me a little bit.

A: Padmasana is a very good seat with its own benefits, though not many can sit in it comfortably for long. Siddhasana in the simplified form given in the lessons is an easier seat to stay in, once achieved. Its effects can also be achieved using a prosthetic object at the perineum. See lessons #33 and #75 for details.

Which is best? It depends on your preference and approach to achieving your goals in yoga. If you are not inclined to directly stimulate sexual energy to raise kundalini, then siddhasana is not something to rush into. On the other hand, if you are inclined bring up sexual energy by direct means, then siddhasana is very desirable, more desirable than padmasana.

It is a matter of where we fall on the "tantra scale" at a point in time. Siddhasana is left of center on this scale, while padmasana is right of center. Left is working more with sensuality in practices, and right is working less with sensuality. As you know, we go far left in the tantra lessons. Siddhasana is in that direction. How inclined we are to go into siddhasana is a function of our bhakti, which is related to how much purification we have in our nervous system. It is interesting that more purification encourages us to be more involved in directly cultivating sexual energy upward in spiritual practices.

In yoga it is not possible to avoid dealing with sexual energy indefinitely, because sooner or later the nervous system becomes activated by the rise of kundalini, and inner ecstasy explodes inside. There is nothing more sensual than that. All of the advanced yoga practices are designed to promote ecstasy's natural rise in the nervous system. Even meditation is ultimately for that, coming from deep inner silence to union in ecstatic bliss everywhere in the body and beyond. That is why we call Advanced Yoga Practices, "easy lessons for ecstatic living."

Yet, everyone has their own inclination in yoga practice, and honoring each person's tendencies is much more important than giving everyone the same "cookie cutter" approach to enlightenment. A technology is good only if it is flexible enough so anyone can use it. That is why we keep all the practices as simple and direct as possible, and talk a lot about self-pacing. Each must travel their own way, at their own speed. The tool kit is here to be used, or not used, as you see fit. It we don't need a tool now, maybe we will need it later. Like that.

Given your interest, perhaps what you should consider doing is developing siddhasana. Work your way into it gradually, and see if it works for you energy-wise. If it doesn't, you can go back to padmasana. It won't hurt to know both seats. I went though a similar testing phase many years ago, and ended up in siddhasana for the long haul. I have stayed a bit left of center because, experientially, it has made sense to do so. Whatever it is for you will be fully respected.

The guru is in you.

Lesson 128 – Siddhasana and Pressure in the Head

Q: Thank you very much for that illuminating discourse on the "left" siddhasana and "right" padmasana; my experiences with these two asanas are fully in tune with what you have described. I notice that while sitting in siddhasana for more than a half hour, there is an intense pressure that builds up in the head (kind of like the same pressure one feels in the head while doing mulabandha). Is there something I can do to lessen the intensity of this pressure? I am wondering if one can use a prosthetic aid at the perineum while sitting in padmasana itself; this seems to me that it would confer the benefits of both siddhasana and padmasana together?

A: I'm happy you found the last lesson helpful. To balance the pressure in the head, make sure you are doing spinal breathing. Also do sambhavi along with your mulabandha and siddhasana. Ultimately you will have kechari too, which plays a big role in the new biology in the head. All of these will help the rising energies find balanced spiritual functioning.

There will be certain adjustments in the head as the spiritual biology comes up. I call them "growing pains," and sometimes we just have to heal our way through them. I had occasional soreness in the brain stem (medulla oblongata), and coming forward through the third eye off and on for years. It is all ancient history now (it became ecstatic bliss), and it will be for you too. If it gets uncomfortable, just back off the mudras, bandhas and kumbhaka and give it a rest. It should heal up in a day or two. It is a lot like athletic conditioning, taking ourselves gradually to new levels of capability we did not have before. Use self-pacing and don't overdo it. If discomfort in the head is chronic and unaffected by changes in practices, seek medical advice.

Soon we will get into dynamic jalandhara, which will put everything from the heart to the head in high gear. So hang on to your hat.

On the combined padmasana/siddhasana prosthetic aid approach, I have not tried that for any length of time. Since this is science (seeking the best applications of knowledge), and you thought of it, why not give it a try and see how it goes for you? Obviously, you will want to gauge it so as not to overdo the energy flows.

I wish you all success.

The guru is in you.

Lesson 129 – Nauli – Raising Kundalini with Your Abdominal Muscles

In the lesson on yoni mudra kumbhaka (#91), we introduced a maneuver called uddiyana, which is lifting the abdomen using the diaphragm. (It is also now covered in the addition to lesson #71 on asanas.) Uddiyana is called the "abdominal lift." You will recall that uddiyana means, "to fly up." Uddiyana is a bit tricky while we are doing breath retention inside, because the diaphragm does not go up as far when our lungs are full of air. So it was suggested that we also practice uddiyana outside yoni mudra kumbhaka. We do this by standing with our feet spread shoulder-width apart with knees a bit bent, and leaning forward enough to rest our hands on our knees. In this position, we look like a shortstop in baseball, leaning forward with his hands on his spread knees, intently waiting for the batter to hit the ball. Maybe sometimes in cricket they stand this way too?

In yoga (not baseball!), once we are in this "shortstop" position, we expel all the air from our lungs, and then lift our diaphragm. If we do this with a bare midriff, we will see our abdomen go in as the diaphragm is going up into the chest cavity. Most schools of yoga teach this standing uddiyana as part of a regular routine of postures, and this is a good time to practice it, during asanas before our pranayama and meditation. Uddiyana has good health benefits. It also draws energy up from our pelvic region, which is why it is part of yoni mudra kumbhaka, along with the other mudras and bandhas we do, all aimed at awakening and moving kundalini energy upward through the nervous system.

With uddiyana we use the abdomen in a fairly static way, not doing anything dynamic with the abdominal muscles. We just pull the abdomen in by lifting the diaphragm up. We can make uddiyana dynamic by going up and down with the diaphragm. We'd like to jazz things up even more, and put more stimulation on the kundalini energy in our pelvic region. By doing so, we will also be setting the stage for an integrated network of whole-body micro-movements that occur as ecstatic conductivity rises and matures in our nervous system. Part of this integration will be an automatic linkup between the movements in the abdomen and the movements in the pelvic region, eventually giving us ecstatic micro-movements from the root all the way up into the chest.

Of course, none of this starts out as "micro-movements." We have to begin with "macro-movements," which is what the mudras and bandhas are when we first learn them. If we are learning to play the violin, we have to master the long simple monotone strokes before we can indulge in the short complex multi-tone ones. Like that, the mudras and bandhas usually begin as pronounced and visible, and then naturally refine over time to be subtle invisible automatic manipulations deep within our increasingly ecstatic nervous system. Then it is the movement of ecstatic kundalini energy in our nervous system that performs the micro-movements all over our body, and we become a witness to an unending glorious display of luminous neuro-biology going on inside us.

The dynamic technique that takes us beyond uddiyana is called "nauli," which means, "to churn," or "to twirl." We begin in the standing "shortstop" position described above. Then we do uddiyana, expelling all our air, and pull our diaphragm up, which pulls our abdomen in. So there we are in uddiyana. Now we will do some other things to develop nauli. Let's take it step by step. It will be a good idea to do this with a bare midriff, so we can see how our abdominal muscles are moving as we are learning nauli.

Once in uddiyana, the first thing we do is contract our abdominal muscles by pressing down on our knees equally through both our arms. It is like doing a sit-up while we are standing up. Only no sit-up movement happens because our arms and hands are bracing our upper body on our knees. We are in uddiyana while we are doing this, so our abdomen is still pulled in by our raised diaphragm. Now something new is happening. Even though we are pulling our abdomen in with our diaphragm, we will notice our abdominal muscles bulging out in a line, up and down the center of our belly. This adds a great deal more suction on the pelvic region. Try flexing your abdominal muscles a few times while in uddiyana and see how they appear along the center line of your belly.

Summary: Stand like a shortstop, hands on knees. Expel all your air. Lift your diaphragm. Notice your abdomen being pulled in. Then pull your upper body (braced with hands on your knees) down toward your knees with your abdominal muscles in a sit-up fashion. See the line of abdominal muscles bulging in a line down the center of your belly.

See how easy it is? Feel the extra suction pulling up on your pelvic region? Great! Now you've got it. Now flex those abdominal muscles a few times. Get a rhythm going, doing a flex every few seconds. Find a rhythm that feels good for you. As you do this a few more times, you may find that flexing the abdominal muscle fits with whatever level of mulabandha/asvini you have become familiar with. Let them go together if you want. In time, they will become integrated together on a subtle neurological level and you will not be able to do one without being inclined to do the other. That kind of natural integration will happen with all the mudras and bandhas in the body. But more on that later.

So here you are, flexing away. Maybe you are feeling some nice energy coming up into your belly, and maybe beyond into your chest, and even all the way up into your head. The abdominals are very powerful for raising kundalini like that.

But, you know, this is not nauli yet. We haven't started "twirling" those muscles yet. The key to twirling is separating the flexing of our left abdominal muscle from the flexing of our right one, and then coordinating the two flexings into a twirling motion. We have two long abdominal muscles in there. One goes up and down the right side of our belly, and the other one goes up and down the left side. How do we separate them? It isn't very difficult to learn how, thanks to our shortstop position.

So, set up in the shortstop position for uddiyana and nauli, just as before. This time, instead of contracting down with the abdominals with equal pressure through both arms on to both knees, just contract down through one arm on to one knee. Take your pick on which one. Once in uddiyana, just contract with your abdomen down on to one knee though one arm. What happens? Did you see one side of your abdominal muscles flex out, and the other side stay in? If so, you've got it right. Now switch to the other side. Flex your abdomen with all the pressure going to the other knee through the other arm. Did the other side of your abdominal muscles flex out? Good. Now try going back and forth, with the same rhythm you used when you were doing both sides at the same time. Only this time, it will be left side, right side, left side, right side and so on.

Now you are drawing up on the pelvic region on alternating sides. This will be more stimulating on the kundalini energy. Are you ready to go for the whole thing? Let's see if we can twirl those muscles.

Assuming you have the abdominal muscles going smoothly back and forth from left to right, there is just one more step to have full nauli going. Instead of going in and out with the muscles from left to right one at a time, try doing a "sweep" across from left to right. This means that while your left abdominal is flexed out, you come up with the right one before the left one is releasing, so both are flexed in the middle for an instant. Then as you go more to the right side flex, the left will release. The effect is that you see one continuous movement of your abdominal muscles going across your belly from left to right – a sweep. Then as your right muscle releases going back in, the left one is coming back up. Then across you go again from left side flexed to right side flexed. And around and around you go, twirling left to right, left to right, again and again. You can sense and regulate the twirling by feeling the shift in pressure going through your arms from left knee to right knee as the flexing of your abdominal muscles shifts from the left side to the right side, and then back.

It is training to develop a habit that we are doing in this early stage of nauli. It will be "clunky" in the beginning, no doubt. But don't give up. You will get the hang of it. First learn it going one way. We started twirling the muscles out from left to right. Once you have that going well, then get it going the other way, from right to left. Once you are able to twirl either way, you will be on your way to being a nauli expert.

With some practice you will be able to twirl your abdominal muscles like a jump rope, with delicious effects on the energy in your pelvic region. Kundalini will not be able resist coming up with all that stimulation caressing her.

We don't do this macro-movement nauli during our sitting practices. We do it before we sit to do pranayama and meditation. It can be part of our asanas, included when we do uddiyana in our routine. Or, if we are not in the habit of doing asanas, we can do nauli by itself before we sit for practices. Doing nauli before our sitting practices awakens our nervous system in ways that are very supportive of pranayama, yoni mudra kumbhaka and meditation.

Try and do at least twenty rotations of nauli in each direction before every session of pranayama and meditation. If you are running out of breath while doing nauli, don't strain. Just pause, take a deep breath or two, exhale again and continue. As you become familiar with nauli, you will also be able to do it less formally in situations that do not involve the shortstop position. For example, once you have the habit of separate control of the two abdominal muscles, it will become easy to do while lying on your back relaxing, and, eventually, while sitting up. In time, nauli will refine to the point where you will be able to do it subtly with no visible motion just about anywhere, with wonderful ecstatic effects. This kind of nauli goes very nicely with subtle movements of mulabandha/asvini, while in kechari. These ecstatic exercises can be done in public without anyone knowing you are doing them, except for the glow, of course.

We will be using a subtle version of nauli when we move on to dynamic jalandhara (the "chin pump"), which involves the upper body to a much greater extent in the stimulation of kundalini energy between the heart to the head.

Nauli is a powerful practice with far reaching effects. We did not include the normal precautions at the beginning of this lesson because nauli is not usually a practice that can throw us immediately into trouble with kundalini energy. It goes without saying that if you have any health problems that could be aggravated by nauli, then you should refrain from doing it. Also, if nauli is practiced over a period of time without the benefit the global purification practices of meditation and spinal breathing, it could lead to energy imbalances in the body. It is beneficial to have good overall purification practices established before taking on any practices that target particular areas of the body for kundalini stimulation. This is why we started in the beginning of the lessons with meditation and spinal breathing, and continue to call them the core advanced yoga practices – the prerequisites for everything else we undertake.

If you want, you can do nauli before learning other advanced yoga practices beyond meditation and spinal breathing. Those two would be the recommended minimum prerequisites for nauli.

Always make sure you are smooth with your practices before taking on new ones. It is very important to maintain a stable platform of practices that you can sustain over the long run. When you know you are ready, you can methodically add on new practices as your bhakti calls you to more.

The guru is in you.

Lesson 130 – Vibrations at the Root

Q: I have been practising asanas (postures) for a long time. When I finish my asanas and do the shavasana (corpse pose) I sometimes feel a strange vibration or more of a palpitation in the region below my genitals. Most of the times I am able to stop it by will, other times I can't. I also feel this vibration sometimes at work. Then it gets very annoying. It almost becomes uncontrollable and I just can't seem to stop it. Is this some kind of cleansing process or is there something wrong with me? I just do regular asanas, which I had learnt during a hatha yoga course. I also do asvini mudra and nauli. Would appreciate your comments.

A: Yes, it is purification/cleansing. This is an early kundalini symptom. There is nothing wrong with you. Good things are happening. But maybe a bit in the wrong order.

A few aches, pains and vibrations can happen during purification of the nervous system. It is common in the perineum/root area as kundalini begins to stir. The symptoms should pass. If they do not, then the standard formula is to back off practices a bit until they do. It is called self-pacing in the lessons.

Mulabandha/asvini (anal sphincter contraction) and nauli are strong for stimulating energy in the area you mention, and are the likely culprits, so easing off these will probably bring some relief. It is not surprising you have this experience doing these particular hatha practices without prerequisite "global" practices.

Doing global practices of deep meditation and spinal breathing before going to raise kundalini is the best way to keep purification in balance and avoid unpleasant kundalini symptoms.

Perhaps it is time for you to consider getting into deep meditation. Then add spinal breathing once you have gotten a good routine of meditation going. The lessons go through it all, step by step. I think you will have no more difficulty with a bottleneck at the root if you do. As a matter of fact, you will be catching the difficulty early, before it happens further up in the body. The lessons go through all the reasons for doing global purification practices first, and more targeted (hatha-style) practices once global practices are well established. It is very important to do things in the right order, as it can save a lot of difficulties and bogging down with kundalini energy, and bring lots of ecstasy and rapid progress instead.

Asanas/postures are good for most people at any level, and make a great warm-up for pranayama and meditation too. Once you start with practices like mulabandha/asvini and nauli, then prerequisite practices of meditation and spinal breathing are needed to absorb and balance the energies that are stimulated at the root and then naturally move up through the nervous system.

The guru is in you.

Lesson 131 – Coordinating Sambhavi and Spinal Breathing

Q: I am facing a problem in doing sambhavi and spinal breathing simultaneously. I think when I concentrate on spinal breathing my eyes do not stay between the eye brows. My eyes go wherever the attention goes. If I do sambhavi separately, I don't have any problem. But when I start spinal breathing since the attention is in that, the eyes tend to traverse the spinal column. Can I imagine the picture of spinal column between the eyebrows to resolve this? If I concentrate on the physical position of the "sushumna" my eyes won't stay between the eyebrows. Could you suggest a way to synchronize these two practises?

A: It is a good question, and an important one. I think many have this same challenge to one degree or another. Coordination between sambhavi and spinal breathing is something that evolves over time. It is forming a habit in the beginning, and then it becomes very easy later on due to the rise of inner sensory experiences that draw the physical eyes and attention naturally to their optimal functions for rising ecstasy.

We have lived all our life with our attention going through our physical eyes. To expand our horizons to the inner spiritual life it is necessary that we develop the additional ability to have the physical eyes going one place and the attention going other places. Imagining the spinal column at the point between the eyebrows does not accomplish this, though it is a clever idea.

To fulfill its function in spinal breathing, the attention must traverse the physical length of the spinal nerve (sushumna) from the root at the perineum to the point between the eyebrows, again and again. Done with long slow cycles of breathing, and other aspects of spinal breathing practice, this is what induces the balanced movement of prana in the spinal nerve, and the cultivation of the entire nervous system. At the same time, the physical eyes are stimulating in a physical way the neurological and biological processes that begin in the brain and reach down through the spinal nerve to the root. So, while the attention is going with the breath in the spinal nerve, the eyes are physically stimulating the brain, which also is affecting the spinal nerve all the way down. Also, there is the furrowing of the brow (pulling the eyebrows slightly together) which is involved in the physical stimulation in the brain. This is the other half of sambhavi. The only time sambhavi involves attention, besides for the physical positioning, is when the attention comes up and goes to (or through) the point between the eyebrows. But even this is not engaging the attention through the eyes. The eyes just happen to be there too, but we are not looking through the eyes. We are looking through the spinal nerve, which is the same as the third eye at that location.

In spinal breathing, and at the times we fix our inner gaze through the point between the eyebrows (like in yoni mudra), we are not giving our attention to the physical eyes. We are engaged in inner seeing. The physical eyes are not used for inner seeing at all. The eyes, along with the brow, perform a physical function, squeezing the inside of the brain in a certain way, and that is all.

This separation of attention and the physical eyes is very important for the development of inner spiritual experiences.

When Jesus said, "If your eye becomes single, your body will be filled with light," he was talking about two things: The physical centering of the eyes, and the attention in the spinal nerve functioning through the third eye. These, done in concert, fill the body with light once ecstatic conductivity comes up in the spinal nerve and spreads out through the rest of the nervous system.

So, how do we achieve this separation of attention and the physical eyes? Sensory feedback is an important factor in it. The ecstatic sensations inside the body are the best sensory feedback. But what if we don't have the inner ecstatic conductivity yet? Then how do we separate the attention from the eyes? We still can use sensory feedback to develop the habit, and developing the habit will help bring up the inner ecstatic conductivity.

Pick an object on the other side of the room and gaze at it. Don't examine it, or even "see" it. Just put your eyes on it and leave them there. As you are doing that let your attention go to your perineum. It isn't hard to do, is it? Now, keeping your eyes on that object, let your attention go up the center of your spine and then forward from the center of your head to the point between your eyebrows. Don't worry about your breathing. Just do the gaze on the object and move the attention. When your eyes wander off the object, and you notice, just easily put them back on it. Use the object there in front of you as a visual feedback. Go up and down the spine a few times with your attention without taking your eyes off the object. Practice this for a while, until you can go up and down your spine with your attention without moving your eyes off that object very much. If the eyes or attention go off, then easily bring them back to the task at hand. It is a habit you are developing, much like learning to pat the top of your head with one hand while rubbing your belly in a circle with the other hand.

Keep doing the exercise until you can move your attention up and down the spine while keeping your unseeing gaze on the object. The object is your sensory feedback that enables you to keep your eyes in one place while your attention is going somewhere else.

Once you have good success doing that, then try it in actual spinal breathing. The furrowing of the brow produces a sensation at the point between the eyebrows that can also be used as a sensory feedback for the eyes. See if you can use that to bring the eyes centered and up while your attention is going up and down the spine. It is not a visual sensory feedback, so it may not be as easy in the beginning to use as the object across the room was. But try it. If it is too big a jump from using the object, then there is always the tip of your nose, or looking upward with your eyes partly open so you will have some visual feedback for sambhavi during spinal breathing. These are not ideal, but if you need visual feedback, then use it until you are ready to go up to the sensation at the slightly furrowed brow.

What we need in sambhavi is something the eyes can get sensory feedback from, something we can gently bring the eyes back to when we realize they have wandered elsewhere. As mentioned, later on it will be ecstatic pleasure inside our body that will cause us to raise and center our eyes. For now, we are using other sensory feedback that will enable us to train the eyes and separate them from the attention going up and down the spine.

If the attention keeps coming back into the eyes while we are doing all this, it is not such a difficult thing. We know how to deal with the wandering attention from our training in meditation. When we are doing spinal breathing the attention can end up anywhere – In the eyes, off in thoughts or emotions, at the grocery store, or even half way across the galaxy. Anywhere. When this happens in meditation, what do we do? We just easily come back to the mantra. In spinal breathing it is just the same. When our attention goes to the eyes or anywhere else, and we notice, we just easily go back to our spinal breathing. If we get lost on where we were in the spine, it doesn't matter. It doesn't have to be exact. We just pick up with the breath. If the breath is coming in, we go up the spine. If the breath is going out, we go down the spine. And so we continue. When the attention goes off somewhere again, we just pick up spinal breathing again. It will happen many times. It is normal. The eyes will wander many times too. It is normal. We never strain or struggle for perfection. There is no such thing. The practice works best when we are easy about it, favoring the procedure we are doing when we realize we have gone off it.

So, sensory feedback for the eyes, and easily favoring attention moving up and down in the spine are the keys to developing the two separate functions. It will evolve slowly. Rome was not built in a day. Eventually we will be doing lots of things at the same time during spinal breathing. They are habits we develop one by one that become automatic.

Somewhere along the line we will feel some pleasure coming up our spine from the root. Then we will notice it is affected by sambhavi. We will also notice that spinal breathing spreads it up and down and all through us. Then these practices will have very nice sensory feedback inside. We will be rewarded with ecstasy for doing them. We will become conditioned to respond to ecstasy very easily, and then all the elements of practice become a breeze. We all have this built-in ability. So, we start at the beginning with whatever sensory feedback we have, knowing that a whole new world awaits us inside. Before we know it, our body will be filled with light and we will be bathed all day and all night in the ecstatic bliss of God.

The guru is in you.

Lesson 132 – What is Sin?

Q: What is sin? Is it a condition we have no chance to overcome without intervention on our behalf by someone who is ordained? Are we sinners, or are we divine? I am confused.

A: Jesus said, "As you sow, so shall you reap." In the East, this same process is stated with one word, "karma," which means action and its consequences, including latent impressions (called samskaras) accumulated deep inside us over multiple lifetimes.

With yoga practices, we stimulate the nervous system's natural abilities to dissolve the many latent impressions of karma stored deep inside. We experience these impressions as limitations and tendencies in our thoughts, feelings and actions. These impressions are obstructions to our experience of the truth within us. As we clean them out, we come to know the divine truth within and we are set free from the binding influences of our past actions. Then we are naturally inclined to conduct ourselves in ways that do not build up obstructions that will limit us in the future – acting more and more as a channel of divine love. So, yoga has a direct impact on this whole process of sowing, reaping, and the latent impressions of karma.

None of this directly answers your questions about sin. I wanted to lay out the practical aspects of yoga's role first. Action, results of action, and the means for dissolving the binding results of action. That is how yoga fits in.

What is sin? If you look it up in the dictionary, you will see it focuses on the negative aspects of "As you sow, so shall you reap," and "karma." Sin is defined as, "An offense against religious or moral law, an offense against God."

Sowing and reaping is one thing, a process of nature, really. It just happens as we act in ways that are either in the direction of or away from purifying our nervous system and expressing divine love. What we put in is what we get out. If we do yoga practices and favor opening over closing, we give ourselves a big advantage in this process.

Sin is a step outside the natural process of "as you sow..." and karma. It is an "offense." An offense to who? Sin is colored with human judgement. If you do thus-and-so, you commit sin. You are doing bad. You are offending God. Who decides this? Most often, it is we who decide it through our guilt and shame over our actions. Maybe we have been conditioned by others since childhood to feel that way about ourselves. In our still-limited state of awareness we tend to act in ways that bind us, and in our conscience (the divine morality in us) we feel remorse. If we do not judge ourselves, others will certainly be there to do it for us. In doing so, they place themselves in the position of intermediary between us and our salvation. And there you have it, the psychological structure that holds most of the world's organized religions together.

The concept of sin is a human coloring of natural law. Sin is a spin on a process of nature. It rises out of our guilt and/or someone else's judgment. Overindulgence in the concept of sin can lead to a sense of hopelessness, and an unhealthy dependence on others for our salvation, when, in truth, there is only one place we will ever find it – within ourselves.

Expecting someone else, ordained or not, to relieve us of our sins is a formula for failure. Real religion is not a business transaction where we give this and get that. It does not happen like that.

Surrendering to a high ideal is something else. It is a private matter in our heart, not subject to anyone else's scrutiny or judgement. As long as we are letting go for a higher ideal deep in our heart, our bhakti will have great purifying power, and draw us to spiritual practices.

If we have been trained to see ourselves as hopeless sinners, it will be wise to reconsider it carefully. For if we do not believe in our own divinity, it will be difficult to find the desire necessary to make the journey home. Our identity as sinners is a label we put on ourselves, while our identity as divine beings is a demonstrable human condition we can claim as our own.

Saints and saviors over thousands of years have demonstrated again and again the ability we all have for human spiritual transformation.

Sitting to meditate for the first time can shatter the illusory grip of sin. It won't free us completely from all obstructions in us on the first day, but it is the beginning of a road we can travel that will reveal increasing divine light as we purify and open our nervous system further each day.

The guru is in you.

Note: Someone wrote in with this wonderful quote attributed to Paramahansa Yogananda – "A saint is a sinner who never gave up."

Lesson 133 – Nectar

Q: Sometimes I feel a very sweet taste at the end of my throat. It's not exactly sweet but what can be called as "madhur" (an Indian word ... not sure of the English equivalent). It happens on its own and goes off after an hour or so. I have not been able to relate it with anything. Neither to anything I do or eat. I really enjoy it when it happens and the more I gulp the more I can get the taste. Hope you can throw some light.

A: Your description sounds like nectar, called "amrita," coming down from the brain through the nasal pharynx. It is stimulated by spiritual practices, especially pranayama, kumbhaka and kechari, though it could come from any practices, sometimes even only with bhakti.

The biology of kundalini involves sexual essences going up the spine, and also through the digestive system and other channels. Then, in the brain, there is a process that brings the nectar down into the digestive system via the front passage mentioned, where it is reprocessed and sent up again. So, it is a circular process, up the middle and down the front, like that. This biology is the basis of rising inner experiences. It is part of human spiritual transformation. Advanced yoga practices are designed to promote this.

Nectar can be sweet with a fragrance like flowers. It is most noticed in early stages of kundalini awakening. Then later it is less noticeable. Don't get too fixated on it. Continue your practices, whatever they may be. The experience is part of the larger process, not an end in itself.

Good things are happening.

The guru is in you.

Lesson 134 – Yoga and Western Psychology

Q: I have recently joined your group and I am in strong disagreement of promoting meditation and other practices alone. When people begin to focus on themselves, sensations in their bodies, etc., they are in a very vulnerable position and at the same time they have the opportunity to uncover a great truth. In a situation where they do not have support they will end up in the same position or worse because they have not been able to understand their feelings, heal their pain, and express other emotions that might come along. You suggest that irritability is a result of an imbalance in a practice (note: as in coming out of meditation too fast) and I strongly disagree. I believe that and emotions that arise in meditation have a reason and the only way to work toward a greater awareness in this situation is to focus on that emotion, express it and understand it. Once a person has gone through this healing process they will achieve a greater awareness. If people pass it off as something else they will be going through the same cycle, and maybe for the rest of their lives. In this situation support plays a big role because the helper can guide the person into working through the situation.

A: The part you may have missed about meditation is that when correctly done, the obstructions being released in a particular session are gone. Gone. So there is nothing left to process or analyze, only the inner silence and light coming through from inside where there was blockage before. So let's be clear about those mechanics. That is effective yoga, a neurological cleansing where the effects of past actions are released, not on the basis of meaning, but neurologically dissolved from the inside by the pure bliss consciousness inherent within us, which we access in meditation. It is not a matter of belief or analysis. It is a mechanical process. It will work for anyone who does the procedure, even for someone who is a skeptic.

It sounds like you are involved in Western psychology, where thoughts and feelings coming to surface awareness are analyzed on the level of meaning – psychoanalysis. This has some value, but is far removed from yogic methods that go much deeper where analytical processes do not exist in the mind. Western psychology is like analyzing the waves coming up on the surface of the ocean, while yoga (deep meditation especially) is like cleaning the ocean from the bottom up, at levels where analysis is not possible. Only the procedure of cleaning is there. Obstructions are energy. Thinking is energy. Yoga deals with these at their root by going beyond the energy to pure bliss consciousness. Meaning is a less fundamental form of neurological energy, found near the surface of the mind. Meaning is the tail on the dog of thought energy, so to speak, and we all know that using the tail to wag the dog is not very effective. We can still use it if it helps us feel better in some way. If we are flexible, we will meditate daily also, which will be like having our cake and eating it too. It is not wise to try and do both methods at the same time, in the same sitting, as neither will be served.

Anyway, yoga is not only about cleaning up the psychology. That is a by-product. Yoga is about enlightenment, a direct pathway to the level of attainment of Jesus, Krishna, Buddha, Lao Tsu, Rumi, etc.

Compared to yogic methods, Western psychology is still embryonic in that respect. Keep in mind that psychoanalysis has been around for a little over a century, while yoga has been around for something like fifty centuries. Not that "time in the business" alone qualifies something as being more advanced, but it is a pretty good indicator. The experiences of modern practitioners support the conclusions of the long history of yoga. The proof of the pudding is in the eating.

From the standpoint of yoga, revealing "great truth" is not primarily about intellectual understanding or the resolution of emotional difficulties. It is about becoming the truth itself. This is done through systematic purification on every level in the vehicle of experience, the human nervous system. It is the divinity of the human being we are opening up here, using time-tested methods.

Logic suggests that Western psychology can learn a lot from studying the methods of yoga in an open-minded way. The great psychologist, Carl Jung, realized this late in his career.

The guru is in you.

Lesson 135* – Kundalini Currents in Legs and Arms

Q: I have been practicing asanas and pranayama for about six years. I started this practice to get rid of my asthma condition, and now I succeeded to 90%. Normally I do not do meditation except some self-affirmations and relaxation after my pranayama, as the sound *OM* has not much interested me. Now I found you and am practicing the meditation as per your instructions for the past 50 days.

When I started the meditation it was good, and in few days a sort of pleasant cool breeze (cool current) started flowing in my back during and after the meditation. During my prayers during the day and afternoon, I feel the same sensation in my back spreading to my upper back. I do pranayama and meditation in siddhasana.

My question is, for the ten days during the day around 10 AM until 2.30 to 3:00 PM I am having the cool current sensation flowing only in both my legs, and hands from the shoulders to the fingertips. Sometimes it is very strong, but pleasant. Please let me know what this condition is. As for my understanding, I thought the energy flows to the upper parts of the body, not down. Please let me know what it is. Is it ok for the energy to be flowing down instead of upward? Kindly advise.

A: It is kundalini energy, and it can go in any direction. It can be very evident in the legs and arms. You have heard the expression, "lotus feet?" Kundalini goes wherever the nervous system goes. This means to every cell in the body. It begins in the spinal nerve (sushumna) and radiates from there, sometimes instantaneously with the rise of ecstatic conductivity in the spinal nerve, and other times with some delay in time as kundalini energy works its way out from the spinal nerve. Also, energetically, the subtle nervous system reaches far beyond the body via the aura, and kundalini goes there also. That is how others can feel our rising ecstatic bliss. Good vibrations, you know.

Many years ago the same experience you describe rose in me. It was so pleasurably intense in my legs and feet that the only way I could calm it down was by walking barefoot all over the neighborhood. It was like having orgasms in my feet. I had the same thing in the arms and hands too. Being physically active helps smooth it out. You may want to check out the lesson on kundalini symptoms and remedies (#69) if you feel the need to smooth it out.

The symptoms have much to do with friction between kundalini energy and deep obstructions coming out. In time it evens out to be much smoother unending ecstatic feelings everywhere in the body. Ecstatic living!

If I have to take a guess, I'd say your pranayama has been opening your nervous system up over the past few years, and now meditation is taking advantage of that cultivated situation. You are very wise to be taking up meditation to complement your pranayama. The relationship of these two practices, and the importance of doing both, is discussed throughout the lessons, beginning with first instructions in spinal breathing. You may wish to bring your pranayama up to the spinal breathing level, if you have not already. This speeds up the effects of pranayama, while at the same time providing much more balance of energies in the nervous system, so there is more progress with less chance of excessive energy flows. Good things are happening.

The guru is in you.

Addition – Here is a Q&A that addresses the well-known hand mudra (jnana or chin mudra) where thumbs and index fingers are joined, in this case as a result of internal energy movements:

Q: In the lessons, one thing that has been conspicuous by its absence is the function of hands. So I have been putting them wherever I feel comfortable, i.e., either on the sides or folded on my feet. For the last few days I have observed that at some point in meditation my index finger and thumb of at least one hand (sometimes both) are moving with a jerk and are getting joined at the tips. I understand this could be a part of the automatic yoga positions you have mentioned. But I learnt that this position of hands is called jnana mudra. I wanted to know if it would be helpful to continue this voluntarily? Are there any other mudras that could supplement the practices?

This seems to have started with the practice of Amaroli I have taken up recently.

A: The top priority in the lessons since the beginning has been to focus on practices that bring the most return for attention and time put in. This is why the lessons start with deep meditation and then go to spinal breathing, mudras, bandhas, siddhasana, etc. Using this sort of prioritized approach puts some of the customary things in yoga in a secondary role. Even yamas and niyamas, including codes of conduct, diet, and certain bodily cleansing methods (shatkarmas), have been left behind for now. This is because we know that with meditation and spinal breathing, they will rise up by their own accord through the connectedness of yoga. They become "automatic" tendencies, and then we can incorporate them without being premature and gaining little spiritual benefit.

The hand mudra you mention (called jnana or chin mudra) is in this secondary category also, even though it is one of the most visible yoga "gestures." Because of that visibility it is highly ritualized, which is another reason why it has not been discussed in the lessons so far. Outward show of ritual is almost always either of no effect or an outright drag on progress in yoga, due to standards of external social conformity. Individual enterprise is essential for success in yoga, and this is a cornerstone of the AYP lessons, as you know.

Does this mean that jnana mudra is bad, and all such secondary and potentially distracting practices should be shunned? Not at all.

You have come on the hand mudra in just the right way – when your energy experiences have brought it up. That is perfect. As we do our core practices, and energy begins to move inside, eventually we discover the reality of things like jnana mudra. Then we find that if we touch the thumbs and index fingers of our two hands together to form circles, it is like closing an energy switch in our hands. It allows the kundalini energy to circulate more efficiently through our arms during practices. It can also help calm movements caused by the energy in our arms, and accentuate ecstatic feelings throughout the body. While doing jnana mudra, we can let our hands rest on our knees with palms up or down, or leave them in our lap, or wherever they are comfortable. Jnana mudra is an effect more than a cause, because without the kundalini energy flowing first, the mudra adds practically nothing to our spiritual progress. But once the energy is moving, and noticeable, we may be inclined to close that circuit in our hands. Or maybe not. Pranayama and meditation are just as effective with hands joined in the lap as with the hands in jnana mudra on the knees or anywhere else. So, it is personal preference more than anything that determines what is done with the hands, as long as we are not getting unduly caught up in the hands and distracting ourselves. In that case, we treat the distraction like any other in practices, and easily favor the practice we are doing.

Our spiritual progress will not be swayed significantly by using or not using jnana mudra. So it is up to you. My suggestion is, just let it happen naturally.

As for other mudras/bandhas, we have covered the main ones to use in practices already – mulabandha/asvini, sambhavi, uddiyana/nauli, jalandhara (static and dynamic), kechari, and yoni. There are a couple that show up in asanas that have not been mentioned much in the lessons so far – maha mudra and yoga mudra. Both of these involve leaning forward with the head and torso toward the floor or outstretched leg to stretch and loosen the sushumna. Both can happen as an automatic yoga in pranayama or meditation too. Lesson # 183 covers a situation like that. If we do these two mudras in our asana routine, it will help when we go into pranayama and meditation, because the sushumna will be loosened up beforehand. It can also reduce the chance of wayward movements occurring in sitting practices, which can be a distraction (lesson #183 again). All the asanas are for this, but those two are singled out, and do carry the name "mudra."

That's great about the noticeable rise in the interconnectedness of yoga since starting amaroli (see lesson #T32). Yes, it will do things like that. The nervous system can't resist opening when being stimulated yogically from so many directions.

Lesson 136 – Vigyan Bhairav Tantra – The 112 Techniques

Q: Pranam! Can I seek guidance based on practice as per dharnas of *Vighan Bhairav*?

A: I am familiar with the *Vigyan Bhairav Tantra* scripture mainly through the writings of Osho/Rajneesh in his volume, *The Book of Secrets*. It is a lengthly commentary on the 112 "Centering Practices" from *Zen Flesh, Zen Bones: A Collection of Zen and Pre-Zen Writings*, compiled and transcribed by Paul Reps and Nyogen Senzaki, first published in Japan in 1957.

The lessons of Advanced Yoga Practices cover the principles of *Vigyan Bhairav* in a concentrated and practical way, with a series of effective practices that can be taken up in a building block fashion as one becomes ready.

Besides *Vigyan Bhairav* (and other tantra yoga sources), these lessons integrate principles and streamlined practices from bhakti yoga, mantra yoga, kriya yoga, hatha yoga, kundalini yoga and tantra yoga, not to mention some good old-fashioned Christian common sense. AYP is an open and integrated system of practices, scientifically derived for ease of use, effectiveness and completeness. For further discussion on the sexual wisdom of *Vigyan Bhairav*, and how it is incorporated in the lessons, see tantra lesson #T21.

The guru is in you.

Lesson 137 – Getting Both Feet into Paradise

Q: I am ready to start meditation again so I can feel what I did in the past. It started when I was in school. I always strived for something, but until now I didn't know what. I started meditation back then. I always tried to meditate in shavasana (corpse pose) because it is mentioned that the asana is a position in which you can lay without straining your body for hours.

It is around five years back when one day I felt the light. I can't explain what it was ... but next day my whole family told me that in night I was up in the air and that is at least three feet above my bed, and my body is glowing. From that day I have been searching about what happened to me. I continued doing meditation and after this it happened various times that I feel like I am weightless and I feel a strange sensation in my third eye area. After that, because of studies, job and marriage, I left meditation and it is now around three years later, but still sometimes I have a smell of flowers, and sometimes I can't guess the smell but it is very pleasant. Sometimes I hear ringing bells inside and sometimes I here a sound of hreem, which is like hreeeeeeeeeeeemmm. Please help me out or at least tell me how to proceed as I am not meditating now and want to start it again.

A: Thank you for writing and sharing. You can go to the beginning of lessons go step by step through instructions on meditation, pranayama and then into combining with physical practices (bandhas, mudras, asanas, kumbhaka). There is also discussion on the "Why?" that comes up in us, and using that to increase bhakti – desire for the divine. There is not much on philosophy or theory in the lessons. The focus is on practices and on dealing with the different kinds of experiences that come as a result.

Your experiences of inner light, weightlessness, sweet fragrances, inner sounds, etc., are all symptoms of some good purification in your nervous system. Of course the greatest "symptom" to have is unending divine joy.

You will have good success once you begin practices again. Keep in mind that symptoms of purification are not the practices themselves, and that further progress is a function of practices, not focusing excessively on any particular experience, even the miraculous. This comes right from Patanjali's *Yoga Sutras*, and is good practical advice for anyone on the path of yoga having any sort of experiences.

Shavasana (corpse pose) is a wonderful posture, which is usually done at the end of an asana routine, and it can also be done at the end of sitting practices of pranayama, meditation, etc. It is not traditionally done during meditation, and there are a variety of reasons for this. Recommendations on easy ways to sit during meditation are given in the lessons (#33 and #75). You will see how the seat evolves as practices advance. If your desire to meditate is strong, you will find the time to make a daily routine of practice. It only takes 20-30 minutes twice a day starting out. Managing the time is covered in the lessons also.

If you decide to go back to your previous practices, or have a teacher or guru who will be assisting you, then just regard the lessons as "food for thought."

It seems you have had one foot nearly in paradise already. Maybe now is the time to get both feet in. I wish you all success as you travel your chosen path.

The guru is in you.

Lesson 138 – Would You Like to get Reconditioned?

Q: (On lesson #35, "Enlightenment Milestones") Re – your triad of silence, bliss and harmony, in your discussion of milestones are they close or similar to the description of brahman as existence-consciousness-bliss (sat-chit-ananda)? Is the body-mind purification process another name for reconditioning or unconditioning?

A: Sat-chit-ananda (existence-consciousness-bliss) is what we contact in deep meditation and it is what rises in us as silence, also called the "witness state," and stabilization of this transcendent reality as our sense of self 24/7 is the first stage of enlightenment. (24/7 means 24 hours per day, 7 days per week) The phrase "pure bliss consciousness," used often in the lessons, is synonymous with sat-chit-ananda, inner silence and witness. Bliss is a key word in this. The immutable inner witness is a blissful one, and so are we when we become it, and there is much more to come after that.

Ecstasy is the key word in the second stage of enlightenment, caused by the movement of prana (kundalini) in the nervous system. With refinement of inner sensory experiences, devotion (bhakti) rises, and we accelerate in our neuro-biological transformation toward permanent divine experience. Technically, the movement of prana/kundalini is movement of sat-chit-ananda, because all is that. But we make a distinction between the bliss (of pure consciousness) and the ecstasy (of the body) for the sake of the coming union of these two aspects of our nature in the third state, unity, which is where the word "harmony" comes in, and the rise of outflowing, unconditional divine love. Then we are a channel of the divine on earth, and loving every minute of it.

Lessons #85 and #113 revisit the stages of enlightenment from different perspectives, and it is looked at from different levels of experience in many other lessons as well.

None of this would even be mentioned, except for the experiences that come up with practices. There is a need then for a framework of understanding (and milestones), so it is discussed for that reason. Otherwise, who needs all this mumbo jumbo? With the experiences, the mental framework and metaphors (Shiva, Shakti, etc.) describing what is happening inside are helpful to inspire continuation of practices.

"Reconditioning" or "unconditioning" is a bit vague for me on what is happening. I like "purification" and "cleansing" better. Once cleansed, the nervous system becomes a clear two-way gateway to the infinite within us. It is semantics really. Whatever words work for you are okay, as long as you understand your experiences clearly on your own terms and don't misinterpret what is happening. Misinterpretation (and fear, when experiences get way out there) can lead to a loss of motivation to practice, so having an understanding of what is happening is important. Always, the main thing is that we are motivated to be doing our practices and getting reconditioned!

The guru is in you.

Lesson 139 – Dynamic Jalandhara – The Chin Pump

With meditation and spinal breathing we are doing global house cleaning in the nervous system, stimulating and balancing the divine energies in us at the same time. On top of these two wonderful global practices, we added a series of mudras, bandhas and asanas to directly target certain areas of the body, top and bottom. With kumbhaka (breath retention) in yoni mudra, we greatly increased stimulation of kundalini and the flow of prana in the spinal nerve, and beyond. Then we added nauli, and began targeted practice to bring kundalini up even more from the pelvic region, through the abdomen, and towards the heart.

Now, with all of that under our belt, we are ready to target the energy flows between the heart and the head. This is the territory of dynamic jalandhara. We learned static jalandhara bandha with yoni mudra kumbhaka. It is letting the chin go down to its comfortable limit toward the hollow of the throat. Now we will use it in a more dynamic way. The effect will be to stimulate the movement of prana between the heart and the head. I call it the "chin pump," because prana gets pumped up and down between the heart and head with this practice like you would not believe. It is a real clean out and energy stimulation practice for the upper body and head.

We will also be adding a new kumbhaka session with the chin pump. More on the logistics of that later. For now, what we will do is set up the same way we do for yoni mudra kumbhaka, except we will not be using the fingers on the eyes or nose. We want the head to be free to move around.

The same guidelines given for yoni mudra kumbhaka apply here regarding having the prerequisite practices in place and stable, and no health issues that could be aggravated by breath retention. You should be stable in all aspects of yoni mudra kumbhaka before you try the chin pump. An added precaution for the chin pump is that you should not have any neck or head conditions that could be aggravated by moving the head around.

So, we are sitting in siddhasana. We do our standard inhalation from the root up the spinal nerve to the point between the eyebrows, and we hold our breath closing the windpipe in our throat in the regular way we hold our breath using the epiglottis. Then we have ourselves in mulabandha, uddiyana, sambhavi and kechari, and looking out with attention through the third eye, all the same as in yoni mudra kumbhaka. With the chin pump, our hands are resting easily on our knees or thighs.

Now, with lungs full, we begin to rotate our head slowly to the left, then back, then right, and then we let it "fall" down toward the chest in a faster swooping motion, sweeping across the bottom from right to left, and coming back up the left side of the circle, slowing down, and then around and dropping down again, and again, and so on. So we are making a slow circle with our head, except for the faster falling/swooping down toward the chest going from right to left. We keep doing this circular head motion when we are ready to let our kumbhaka out at the comfortable limit and are going back down the spine with our breath. We keep the head going as we fill up again, going up the spinal nerve with the breath. Then, when we are full again, we reverse the direction of rotation of our head, so we are falling/swooping from left to right as we go down towards the chest. We continue like this for the breath retention and until we exhale and inhale again. Then, when we are full, we switch the direction of the head again. And so on, rotating left on a complete kumbhaka retention, and right on the next kumbhaka retention, and so on, switching the direction of head rotation each time we are full with air again. This is the chin pump.

Now let's talk more about some more particulars. When we are first learning, we limit this practice to four breaths. Later on, as we get comfortable with it, we can switch to the clock and do it for five minutes, and eventually ten minutes, using self-pacing to get there. The chin pump is done right after spinal breathing, right before meditation. When we add the chin pump, we move our yoni mudra kumbhaka to the end of our practice, after meditation and before rest. There is no change in yoni mudra kumbhaka practice. It only shifts to a different position in our routine. So we have kumbhaka with the chin pump before meditation, and kumbhaka with yoni mudra after meditation. There is great power in this combination.

The chin pump will feel clunky at first. You knew that would be the case, right? It takes some getting used to. It is worth the effort to make the adjustment. We don't force anything about it. We never go beyond the comfortable range of motion of our neck. And we go slow, being mindful not to strain. With practice, the range of our head motion will gradually increase. In time, our chin may come close to or even touch our upper chest when we swoop down. But don't rush it. We may never get that far down, and that is perfectly fine. As with all yoga, we never exceed our comfortable limit. Always start with a smaller motion of the head and let it increase naturally and gradually during a session to its comfortable limit. The chin pump will work optimally for you right there. You may notice some noise or sensation in your chest as you do the chin pump. This is normal. It can sound like a thumping, or feel like crunching, behind the breastbone. Your neck may crunch a bit too, which is also normal. But discomfort is not normal, so if you have any, back off right away. Do not overdo the chin pump. It will take some time to build up to it. Be very careful and be sure to use self-pacing, staying well within your comfortable range of motion. Remember that we continue to use all of the other indicated mudras and bandhas during our chin pump kumbhaka. And, of course, we are in siddhasana for our whole routine, as long as we are comfortable staying in it.

What might we experience as a result of dynamic jalandhara – the chin pump? If you have some active kundalini in your body, some prana moving in the nervous system, the chin pump will do two things. First, it will bring prana down into the heart area strongly where it is combined with prana rising up through the abdomen from the pelvic region. These are two different kinds of prana, characterized by the energetic polarities in the body. Second, the chin pump will bring the combined pranas from the heart back up to the head in large quantities. If kundalini is active in the body, the head will feel like it is being pumped full with vital essences and light. Every cavity in the head will light up. Even the sinuses can have these sensations. It can be a bit strange, but the strangeness passes soon. If kundalini is not very active in the body yet, the chin pump will facilitate its arousal, along with all the other means being applied. Everything is connected. It is only a matter of time with so many aspects of the nervous system being stimulated.

In the beginning, there can be some side effects from the chin pump. They shouldn't last long. Some dizziness can happen. Maybe a slight headache. Maybe energy currents not experienced before in the upper body and head. It is a powerful practice, and we are making a bid to break through to a higher level of functioning in our nervous system, so there can be a few bumps in the road. For this reason, you may wish to begin your chin pump practice for the first time on a weekend when obligations will be less. Be methodical and don't overdo. If any symptoms become uncomfortable, back off practice immediately, and give yourself time to recover. Then you can come back later and try again, slowly. Honor your limits and use self-pacing. Self-pacing is very important with the chin pump. We are moving a lot of energy with this practice, up through channels where the energy has not been in such quantities before. And we are dealing with delicate components of our anatomy, our neck and head. If we want enlightenment, we have to nudge open the doors so the spiritual energies stirring inside us can find their natural neuro-biological functioning. The chin pump is a powerful way to open the doors between the heart and the head.

As we continue with the chin pump daily over time, we will notice a strengthening in our chest, neck and head. It is a spiritual strengthening, as prana flows through us in commanding new ways. Our heart becomes full with a powerful and palpable love. Our spiritual vision will strengthen. The third eye is a direct recipient of the increased energy flow, as is the crown. It feels very good to have the energy moving in healthy ways in the higher regions of the body. There is also a physical strengthening that occurs with the chin pump. So there are many benefits, and it is a practice well worth learning and refining over time. Just start slow and build up very gradually.

When we finish our dynamic jalandhara session, we will feel energized and we may wish to take an extra minute or two to settle into meditation. It is more of a pranic energizing than a physical one, though both can be there after doing kumbhaka with the head going around for some minutes like that. So take a couple of minutes to settle down as you go into meditation. Maybe delay starting the mantra for a couple of minutes if you feel the need. Make sure you start the mantra effortlessly as originally instructed, and follow the easy procedure of meditation as always. We will be going from high pranic energization to deep silence. Mixing these two is very powerful, and it will be a different kind of experience in meditation. It is the pranic energy cultivation of chin pump marrying the silence of deep meditation. A new kind of luminous fullness will be born in our nervous system, and it will follow us out into our daily activity. So we will be both silent bliss and ecstatic radiance happening at the same time.

Translation: Ecstatic Bliss!

The guru is in you.

Lesson 140* – Chin pump – Coordinating Head Rotation and Breathing

Q: This (chin pump) is just wonderful. I tried it a couple of times to the best of my understanding and it is indeed very powerful. Thank you for sharing such precious teachings.

However, before I can incorporate this effectively in my daily sadhana, I need some clarification. I want to make sure I understand the technique properly. When I go from right to left and left to right, is it done in one round of breath or they are separate rounds? As the head movement is in progress, one should also breathe?

You have mentioned when we are first learning, we limit this practice to four breaths. Please can you clarify this point? Does it mean we do four rounds of head movement in each direction or take four breaths in each chin pump for a specific direction either right to left or left to right?

A: One full breath (kumbhaka/retention, exhale, inhale) is with head going in one direction. Then at the end of a new inhalation, switch and go the other way with the head for the next breath cycle beginning with kumbhaka/retention again. Then switch head direction again when full of air again on the next breath cycle.

The head never stops, only switches direction upon starting each new kumbhaka (breath retention).

Four breaths means four kumbhakas (retentions) with four series of head rotations, switching direction at the beginning of each of the four kumbhakas. We always switch direction with the head at the beginning of a new kumbhaka. When it gets smooth and comfortable with four breaths, then you can go from counting breaths to using the clock, and do five minutes. The number of breaths does not matter when we are on the clock. Just do as many comfortable kumbhakas as happen naturally until time is up. When five minutes gets comfortable, then try ten minutes. Don't rush to that level. Just go there when your practice is smooth and you can step up easily. If you go too far, then back off and bide your time at a comfortable level of practice until you feel ready to try and step up again.

The chin pump is very powerful, with far reaching effects. More lessons on it are coming soon.

The guru is in you.

Addition – Here is a short interchange on chin pump with an advanced practitioner:

Q1: This chin pump practice may take getting used to, as it is not easy to coordinate the pranayama breath with the rotations. I also want to try some half rotations and explore it a little as I did get a bit of neck soreness and stiffness the next day after attempting it. I will persist however and explore because it is absolutely consistent with neck movements and positions (automatic yoga) that I have already benefited from.

A1: Definitely don't overdo on the chin pump. Doing partial rotations, or whatever works for you within your capacity, is the right way to go. Sometimes automatic movements can get a little over-enthusiastic, and we should limit them to stay within the boundaries of what is safe practice for us. This is a matter of balancing our bhakti and automatic movements with good old-fashioned common sense. This is good self-pacing.

Q2: The chin pump (within my limit) feels great now, and I am also doing stage 3 kechari during both pranayama and meditation.

A2: It all sounds very good. Enjoy!

Lesson 143 – Chin Pump – Effects in the Lower Body

We have discussed the chin pump (dynamic jalandhara) as being a "targeted" advanced yoga practice. Its main focus is in opening the channels for prana going in both directions between the chest cavity and the head. But it is much more than that.

All yoga practices are linked. Sometimes we can see (or feel) the connections, and other times the connections are not so obvious. It is a matter of how much purification we have cultivated in our nervous system. The more the purification, the more perceivable the connections will be.

Back in lesson #91 on yoni mudra kumbhaka, we introduced the static version of jalandhara, which is letting the chin go down to its comfortable limit and rest there during kumbhaka (breath retention). We mentioned that jalandhara stretches the spinal nerve for its full length from the point between the eyebrows all the way down to the root at the perineum.

The chin pump takes this stretching effect on the spinal nerve quite a bit further. The rotations of the head affect the spinal nerve all the way down to the root also, in a much more stimulating way. The effect is a subtle twirling of the spinal nerve from top to bottom. With ecstatic conductivity rising in the spinal nerve, this twirling is also ecstatic, and plays an important role in the union of pure bliss consciousness (Shiva) and divine ecstasy (Shakti) in the heart, and throughout the whole body.

The chin pump evolves over time to find natural coordination with all of the mudras and bandhas in the body. In the end, there is only one subtle "whole-body" mudra that is made up of all the parts we are learning one at a time now. All the pieces start out "clunky" and end up subtle, smooth and intimately connected as unending ecstatic bliss is born and radiates out from the body. The chin pump is part of this refinement. Later on in practices, when the head stops, the spiritual twirling will keep right on going inside, centered around the spinal nerve and sending divine energy out in all directions. Don't worry, by then you won't even notice and no one will be able to tell by looking at you, except for the glowing smile on your face, and the pleasure of being around you. A mere intention on your part will be enough to set the spiritual currents in motion. Then you will be twirling the ecstatic energies without moving your head at all.

If you are inclined to let the inner spiritual twirling manifest outside, you can go visit the Sufi whirling dervishes and dance the night away. Many spiritual rituals and dances are geared to our inner spiritual whirling. It is natural for some to openly celebrate the inner light. Others may prefer to sit quietly and dance in ecstatic reverie within. No matter what the culture, religion or personal preference is, it is the same dance. It is the dance of the divine inside us.

As you become acclimated to doing the chin pump, you will notice many things happening. The energy flows between the heart and the head we already discussed earlier. You will also notice the stretching and twirling of the spinal nerve going into the lower body. As your head is on the up-swing during rotation, you may find a tendency for your knees to lift slightly, and then go down again as the head falls toward your chest after it goes around the back side of its rotation. Then, later on, you may find the knees going slightly up and down at different times during the chin pump. A kind of coordination between the rotation of the head and the small movements of the knees will develop.

What is this? It is the beginning of the micro-movements of subtle nauli, as mentioned in lesson #129. And what is nauli for? Twirling kundalini energy upwards. There is that word, "twirling," again. In time, the chin pump and nauli naturally team up on the level of internal micro-movements to foster this twirling of the spinal nerve. It becomes visible as our chin pump advances and the legs, hands and abdominal muscles naturally find their way into the practice. Do not try and put all this together at this beginning stage. Just be aware of it. It is not mainly a physical act. It is the body's response to the movement of ecstatic energy in the spinal nerve. Ecstatic conductivity is the basis all natural connectivity between practices.

The rise of these subtle movements during the chin pump also puts a new spin on siddhasana, making it subtly dynamic, and even more delicious. You can figure that mulabandha, sambhavi and kechari eventually get into the act as well. These are all techniques that stimulate different aspects of our nervous system. The nervous system is a single entity, and, sooner or later, all practices merge into a single multi-dimensional act that is the expression of the nervous system. At that point, we are no longer the instigator. God is. That is what yoga is, becoming what we are – the gateway to infinite bliss, ecstasy, love and joy.

The guru is in you.

Lesson 144 – Chin pump Lite (Without Kumbhaka)

Q: I have a problem holding my breath and it is very claustrophobic for me to do kumbhaka. I dunno, maybe I smothered to death in a coal mine in my last life or something. Can I do the chin pump without holding my breath? And yoni mudra too? I am OK in spinal breathing as long as I don't go too slow.

A: Yes, with the chin pump you can. If kumbhaka is difficult for you, even in the easy way it was instructed to be done, then don't do it.

This question has come a few times from different angles recently, and it is time to address it. Sometimes kumbhaka is not only uncomfortable, but can stimulate excessive kundalini. In either case, the instruction is to back off and return to a comfortable platform of practices that we can be stable with until we are ready to step back up.

If we are comfortable in spinal breathing, and bandhas, mudras and siddhasana we use during spinal breathing, we can do the chin pump easily in the last few minutes of our spinal breathing session. If we are doing spinal breathing for, say, ten minutes, then for the last three to five minutes we can do the chin pump along with our spinal breathing. It is the same procedure as when we are using kumbhaka, only we do not stop to hold our breath. The head rotation changes at the same point in the breathing cycle as when using kumbhaka, at the top of the breath after we have inhaled. You could call this approach without kumbhaka, "chin pump lite."

This is a good time to mention that spinal breathing, and all pranayama methods, are forms of kumbhaka in the sense that "restraint of breath" (what pranayama means) places a slight challenge on the oxygen supply in the body. This is what draws prana up into the nervous system from its huge storehouse in the pelvic region. So whether we are doing spinal breathing or kumbhaka, we are doing restraint of breath. It is only a matter of degree. The more restraint, the more kundalini flows up. That is why it is okay to do the chin pump with spinal breathing. There will be good effects, just not as much prana moving as when using kumbhaka. That is okay. We move what we can move without causing excessive flows. Whatever level we operate at, we will always be purifying our nervous system to more. That is the whole game – maintaining forward progress without falling off into messy energy flows that will force us to stop our practices.

Of course, the daily practice of global deep meditation is very important in this purification process. With the silence of pure bliss consciousness, it is purifying gently underneath everything going on in the nervous system, and this helps all other practices work much smoother and faster.

In future lessons we will be exploring another form of pranayama called "bastrika." With that one we will be saturating the body with oxygen in one way and challenging the oxygen supply in the body it in another way, both at the same time, with powerful purifying effects.

As always we use self-pacing in our practices, including in spinal breathing and kumbhaka. If we find the chin pump (or chin pump lite) producing excessive kundalini energy flows, we back off to a comfortable level of practice.

As for yoni mudra, this is a different story. Kumbhaka is central to yoni mudra, because we are using gentle air pressure coming up from the lungs to cleanse the sinuses and stimulate the third eye. So, without kumbhaka, yoni mudra is reduced to the fingers pushing the eyes toward the point between the eyebrows. That is ok, but it is probably better to just let go of yoni mudra if we are not comfortable doing kumbhaka, and stick with a good spinal breathing session with chin pump near the end, if it is comfortable to do. If we are doing good sambhavi during spinal breathing, then this is as good as doing the finger thing with the eyes. So, if kumbhaka doesn't want to be there, just forget yoni mudra and do the other practices, as discussed.

There is a small time advantage in doing chin pump lite. That is the overlapping of spinal breathing and chin pump in time. For busy people this might have some attraction. If you can do pranayama (with chin pump lite at the end) and meditation in 30 minutes, instead of 35 or 40 minutes with kumbhaka, it can help preserve our practice that day when the schedule is full. Trimming practices is not the first recommendation here, but as has been discussed in earlier lessons, brief practice is better than no practice. So, when time is short, we find ways to prioritize and optimize our practice. It so happens that chin pump lite done during the last few minutes of spinal breathing is in that direction.

Obviously, as we progress and become steady in our practices, whatever level that may be at, we look for our next opening to move up. Purification and growth of the inner divine presence are always happening at every level of practice.

In time, as your nervous system purifies as old karmas are dissolved from within, you will have less difficulty with holding your breath. In fact, you will find that the breath tends to suspend on its own more and more during easy practice of pranayama and meditation, with no intention or strain at all. It is as though we are nourished at times entirely by the prana flowing up through us from within. Then kumbhaka is no big deal. It just happens, sometimes for surprisingly long periods. At that stage it is no longer restraint of breath. It is natural suspension of breath. Then we can breathe air from outside, or breathe prana from inside. Either way is okay. No fuss, no strain.

The divine light rises and flows in us, and we surrender into the loving arms of God.

The guru is in you.

Lesson 145 – Overdoing it with Asanas

Q1: After dabbling for years, I have begun practicing yoga and meditation in earnest (for about a year now). During a recent yoga class, we practiced about 85 minutes of asanas, and then took a short break before resuming with pranayama. During the break, I found myself overwhelmed with emotion, shaking, unable to speak or make eye contact. When we resumed with pranayama, tears began streaming down my face. It has been several days, and I am still (uncustomarily) emotional. It is painful to the point of wanting to discontinue yoga, but I know that I must continue, that I am on the brink of a breakthrough. It feels as if my chest has been ripped open, that my heart has been exposed. The opposite of the bliss that I have been seeking. I am sad about the death of my father, but this heartache seems to be directly caused by my practice of yoga. Thank you for any insight you can offer.

A1: Thank you for writing and sharing. Sorry to hear you are having some difficulty. It sounds like you might have overdone it with practices – 85 minutes is a lot of asana time, especially if you have not built up to it gradually over time as a steady daily diet.

If you didn't overdo, then maybe you did not rest long enough at the end of your routine and something went out of balance from getting up too soon instead of getting released during practices and rest.

It could also be the mix of your practices. Physical hatha methods are notoriously hazardous when done to excess as stand alone practice. Much better to mix them in moderation with global purification practices of deep meditation and spinal breathing. That is the approach in the lessons. A flexible guideline is 10 minutes asanas, 10 minutes pranayama, and 20 minutes meditation, twice a day. That is not including add-ons like kumbhaka and other practices we will be discussing later. The times can be adjusted up or down to fit the individual via self-pacing.

Anyway, none of that is going to make you feel better right now. It is just advice for the future. For now, be very nice to yourself. Back off your practices as necessary until your heart heals. But don't give up. Some light spinal breathing and deep meditation might help. Take some long walks. You will heal, and maybe in the future consider moderation and balance of practices. Yoga is powerful stuff, and works well when done in correct proportions. Too much in the wrong combination can lead to trouble – too much purification too fast. It is just a matter of education, and prudent self-pacing according to experiences.

I wish you healing and continuing progress on your chosen path.

Q2: Thank you for your thoughtful response. I admit that I am not a moderate person, and I probably am overdoing the asanas. That particular class was filled with many more advanced people, including professional yoga teachers. My desire for progress exceeds my abilities/experience. I will practice non-violence toward myself, and will focus on meditation and spinal breathing.

I have found your postings to be insightful and useful in my daily life. Thank you for sharing them with me and others.

A2: The desire is good. It (bhakti) fuels practice. Of course, the tendency to overdo is the caution. As you go through the lessons, you will see a lot of situations in the Q&As where it is very similar to what you have been through. Self-pacing has a lot of nuances to it. With ongoing bhakti/desire and wise self-pacing you can't miss. I wish you all success.

The guru is in you.

Lesson 146 – Shaktipat – Direct Transmissions of Spiritual Energy

Q: Is it necessary at some point to receive shaktipat before one can experience samadhi? Even the great Paramahansa Yogananda received shaktipat from Sri Yukteswar before he could achieve samadhi. If this is necessary how does one go about obtaining shaktipat?

A: Shaktipat is direct transmission of spiritual energy from guru to disciple. Transmissions of spiritual energy can also occur in the form of darshan (blessing from a master), satsang (keeping spiritual company), through our chosen ideal by the intensity of our own internal bhakti, and even from reading inspired spiritual writings. It is all spiritual energy flowing in us by various influences, and it can happen in a lot of ways. It is our bhakti that determines the degree of flow more then anything. When the bhakti is intense, the energy will flow from somewhere, from everywhere. So, shaktipat really has its origin in the aspirant, not in anyone else.

There is another stimulator of spiritual energy in all of us these days, and that is the stars. The stars are giving us their darshan every minute of every day. This is because a new age of enlightenment is rising, and we are all increasingly being stimulated to open from within. In the past dark age, spiritual awakening stimulated by other people was more important than it is today. In those days, a sage was like a candle in a vast sea of darkness. That candle was a rarity, and only a few had any hope of being lit by it. It was a time of spiritual poverty, and the flame was kept alive by being passed between a very few. Thanks to them, and changing times, it is much different now.

In present times, we are all on the verge of enlightenment. It may not seem like it. There are still many obstacles to be dissolved inside, but it is much easier to do it now than it has been for thousands of years, or even only a few decades ago. The sun of God is rising. Hatred is making its last chaotic stand in the world, and it will not win. When the light comes, the darkness disappears.

It is important to see shaktipat and the traditional guru-disciple relationship in the light of these changing times. We are no longer wholly dependent on individual sages and teachers for our enlightenment. We are all becoming spiritually self-sufficient. We are all becoming capable of generating our own spiritual transformation.

The best way to become enlightened is by doing daily yoga practices. It is the surest and safest way, because it is we who determine how much energy will flow from within by our prudent self-pacing as we use powerful spiritual practices that were not available to most even a few decades ago.

There is another important spiritual influence working in the world today. It is now greater than the power of all the gurus on the planet. As more and more people come along on the way to enlightenment through their own efforts, the divine radiance of spiritual energy from so many opening nervous systems is increasing, and this is quickening everyone's opening. As more people do daily practices, the influence increases exponentially. So, doing your practices is not only good for you. It is good for the world. There is great strength in numbers, and this is how the world is being transformed spiritually. It is the ultimate shaktipat/darshan/satsang for everyone.

Is individual shaktipat still necessary to reach enlightenment? Maybe at some point we will get an individual infusion like that from somewhere, or maybe not. We don't have to go wandering around looking for it. Be wary of anyone who offers you a shaktipat shortcut. It does not work like that.

All we have to do is sit in our meditation room every day, and then go out and give our love away. Samadhi (unbounded pure bliss consciousness) comes in meditation. Full enlightenment comes by giving our samadhi to the world. The spiritual energy of transformation we need will come from inside and outside as we purify our nervous system by our own efforts. If our intense desire for enlightenment is there, everything we need to achieve it will be there too.

The guru is in you.

Lesson 147 – Sequencing of Asanas, Pranayama and Meditation

Q: I combine some other strengthening exercises like push ups, squats, etc. along with yoga. Some of these exercises consume lots of energy. So, when I follow this with pranayama and meditation, I feel the "freshness" of the meditation is reduced due to the other activities. So, is it all right if I first do the meditation and then do the yoga/exercises and then pranayama? I would like your suggestion to resolve this problem. Thanks a lot for the continued guidance.

A: Thank you for writing and sharing. As you have figured out, exercise is best done after meditation, not right before. With meditation, we are systematically bringing the mind and body to stillness. This stillness is a primary source of all spiritual progress.

Asanas and pranayama are part of this process of going to stillness. With easy bending and stretching we begin to loosen and quiet the nerves, and prepare the spinal nerve for pranayama. With pranayama, we further quiet our entire nervous system and cultivate it in a way that prepares it for deep meditation. That is the traditional sequence for best results in a routine of practices – asanas, pranayama and meditation. And it really does work.

I suggest you consider doing the easy bending and stretching portion of your asanas at the beginning. Then do pranayama, and then meditation, so you can get the full benefit of the above-mentioned sequence. After meditation and adequate rest coming out, then it is a good time to do more vigorous physical exercise. See lesson #80 for more on physical exercise and yoga.

So, first we do those things in the best order to take us in to pure bliss consciousness, and then we come out refreshed and ready to be active in the world. Vigorous activity after meditation is not a problem once we have taken time to come completely out. Activity helps stabilize the bliss and ecstasy in our nervous system. That is how we transform to become the walking enlightened, instead of the walking whatever we were before.

The guru is in you.

Lesson 148 – Why Practices Twice a Day?

Q: What is the importance of doing practices two times daily?

A: When we do practices, we coax our nervous system into a different style of functioning – sustaining deep silence (pure bliss consciousness). And in later stages when kundalini is active – ecstatic bliss. To stabilize all this we go out and are active in the world every day. There is fading of the higher functioning during activity as we work it into daily living. The fading happens over 5-10 hours. Then we can do practices again and re-establish the higher style of functioning again, to be faded in activity again. This cycle can be done twice a day by doing practices morning and early evening. It provides for the most purification and growth possible during waking hours for people with active lives.

Doing practices once a day is much slower – it is only one daily cycle of cultivating and fading, instead of two. And it is too much fading before reinforcement of the higher style of functioning happens again the next day. Twice-daily practice is a matter of effectiveness and efficiency.

With twice-daily practice over time, the fading of ecstatic bliss in activity becomes less and less, and the higher style of functioning of the nervous system becomes steady and unshakable 24 hours a day. This is the fruit of the process – enlightenment in daily activity, and all night too. It is the ongoing cycle of practices and activity that produces this result.

During retreats, where responsibilities are suspended, more than two routines of practices per day can be undertaken, alternating with meals, light activity, and satsangs (spiritual gatherings). Three or four cycles of practice can be done in this kind of environment. Maybe more for diehard yogis and yoginis. It is a matter of self-pacing for comfort and effectiveness. Then one can go very deep over a period of days, weeks, or months in retreat. This introduces another cycle between retreats that lasts a much longer period of time (weeks or months), superimposed over the twice-daily cycle of practices we continue with in our regular life when we are back in the world. Retreats accelerate progress in this way. But retreats are not a substitute for long term twice-daily practices at home. What we do every day over the long term is what will make the most difference in the end.

All of this is designed for maximum progress, making the best use of our nervous system's natural abilities for enlightenment and the time we have available to do the job.

You are in charge of your journey. These are tried and true principles of unfoldment you can use as you see fit to travel home to enlightenment.

The guru is in you.

Lesson 149 – The Eight Limbs of Yoga and Samyama – Melting the Darkness

It is time to move on to samyama, which involves moving outward with our attention in pure bliss consciousness, resulting in the cultivation of so-called yogic powers as a side effect. Before we discuss samyama, let's talk about the eight limbs of Patanjali's *Yoga Sutras*, which we have not done yet. Samyama is a combined application of the last three of these eight limbs, and ties in with the other five limbs as well, so this is a good time to cover them. All of yoga is connected, you know. It all connects through the human nervous system. In fact, all of yoga is a product of the human nervous system. Not the other way around, as we sometimes tend to think.

It took a while for people to believe that the world is round instead of flat, and that the sun is the center of the solar system instead of the earth. It took some proof. Then almost everyone believed, and the rush was on to find all the benefits in the new knowledge, the new paradigm.

Now it is time for us to come to grips with the fact that the human nervous system is the center of all spiritual experience and all divine bliss. That is your nervous system, the one you are sitting in right now. The sooner we get used to the idea that each of us is a direct gateway to the divine, the better it will be for everyone. As with the acceptance of any knowledge, it takes some proof. In this case, the proof is in you. Open a few doors here and there by doing some effective yoga practices and you will see what you are. Then the rush will be on to open it all up. A new paradigm is born!

Nothing is new, you know. Our ancient ancestors knew of these things. Much of it was written down. But communications were poor, and people lived so much in superstition. It is different now. We can find any information we want. There are so many doors of knowledge opening to everyone. The old wisdom is becoming new again. The human nervous system hasn't changed over all this time. It has been waiting patiently, like a treasure chest longing to be opened. It is time.

Patanjali's book of *Yoga Sutras* is one of the greatest scriptures of all time. Not only does it tell us what we are, but also it tells us how the doors of the nervous system can be opened. It lays out the relationships between the natural principles of opening that exist in us. This is done with the famous eight limbs of yoga.

We have been traveling through the eight limbs ever since we started the lessons of Advanced Yoga Practices. We have not gone in order, and some would call this non-conventional. We have gone in a way that is effective and makes sense, so there will be no apologies. We'll talk about that some more, but first let's review the eight limbs:

1. **Yama** – It means "restraint," and includes ahimsa (non-violence), satya (truthfulness), asteya (non-stealing), brahmacharya (preservation of sexual energy and cultivation of it) and aparigraha (non-covetousness).

2. **Niyama** – It means "observance," and includes saucha (purity and cleanliness), samtosa (contentment), tapas (heat/focus/austerity), svadhyaya (study of scriptures and self) and isvara pranidhana (surrender to the divine).

3. **Asana** – It means "posture," and includes all those asanas we have come to know and love. In the lessons, asanas are used as a preparation for pranayama and meditation. Certain asanas stimulate the rise of kundalini.

4. **Pranayama** – It means "restraint of life force/breath," and includes the pranayama methods we have discussed, plus some we are yet to discuss. Pranayama cultivates the soil of the nervous system, preparing it for deep meditation and divine experience. Particular kinds of pranayama raise kundalini.

5. **Pratyahara** – It means "introversion of senses." In the lessons, pratyahara is both effect and cause, occurring as kundalini rises and ecstatic experiences draw our attention naturally inward. Then, through pratyahara, we come to know our sensory experience as a continuum spanning the full range of manifestation from the first inner vibrations of pure bliss consciousness (*OM*) all the way out into the physical world.

6. **Dharana** – It means "concentration or focus of attention," and is the first step in taking the mind inward through meditation. In the lessons, we don't hold the attention on anything for long. We just bring attention easily to an object (the mantra), and then let it go how it will. This brings attention almost immediately beyond the beginning perception of the object, which is what we want. The mind will take us inward if we give it the opportunity.

7. **Dhyana** – It means "meditation," and is the flow of attention inward. It can also be described as the expansion of attention beyond any object. In the lessons, the mantra is used as the vehicle for this. We come easily to the mantra, and then the mantra changes and disappears. Our attention expands, arriving in its natural unattached state – stillness.

8. **Samadhi** – It means "absorption/transcendence," and it is what we experience in daily meditation. It expands over time, eventually becoming our natural state of being in daily activity. It is pure bliss consciousness, the inner silent witness. Samadhi in its various stages of unfoldment is the experience of our immortal universal Self. That is what we are.

You may have noticed that after yama and niyama, which were presented pretty much with the classical definitions (except for brahmacharya), all the rest of the limbs were given a twist according to the way these lessons have been presenting the knowledge of advanced yoga practices. This is a normal thing. In fact, every yoga teaching has its own way of presenting the eight limbs of yoga.

The eight limbs of yoga are so logical and easy to understand that virtually every teacher of yoga claims to be teaching them, which is true to one degree or another, because the eight limbs cover everything one can do in yoga. In this sense, they represent a complete road map, a blueprint and spiritual checklist of the various ways to open the human nervous system to divine experience.

Taken together as an overall system, the eight limbs have been referred to as "ashtanga yoga" and "raja (royal) yoga." But what is in a name? The Advanced Yoga Practices lessons are the eight limbs too. So is any approach to human spiritual transformation, in part or whole, including what we find in all the world's mainstream religions. If it has to do with human spiritual transformation, it is going to be found somewhere in the eight limbs. That is the beauty of the eight limbs. When you look at any spiritual teaching or religious tradition using the eight limbs as a measuring rod, you will see right away what is there, and what is not. The more enlightened traditions will have more of the limbs covered, and the less enlightened ones will have fewer limbs covered.

Traditionally, the eight limbs have been taken in sequence. The rationale has been that people have to learn to behave themselves and prepare through strict codes of conduct and self-discipline before they can begin doing more direct spiritual practices. Once they know how to behave rightly, they can begin with the body (asanas), and, later, work their way in through the breath (pranayama), and, finally, be ready for concentration (dharana), meditation (dhyana) and pure bliss consciousness (samadhi). With a traditional approach like this it can be a long road to hoe, especially if a guru (in the flesh) holds his disciples to the highest standards of performance each step along the way. Even Patanjali had this sequence of practice in mind when he wrote the *Yoga Sutras*.

That part of it (going through the eight limbs in sequence over a long period of time) doesn't work very well. This has become widely recognized in the yoga community, and Patanjali must have known it too. Maybe in his time it wasn't so easy to be jump-starting people with advanced yoga practices like deep meditation and spinal breathing the way we can do it today.

Over the years, different teachers have jumped directly into the eight limbs in different places. Some start with asanas and others with pranayama. Some focus first on devotion and then jump to meditation, or something else. Some jump straight into meditation, and then work their way back through the limbs. As you know, these lessons are of the latter approach. We start with deep meditation, and then head into pranayama, physical techniques and so on, keeping a good awareness of the role of bhakti/desire all the way through.

One thing everyone who does yoga for any length of time has found is that the limbs of yoga are connected, meaning, if we start in one limb, the others will be affected. As we purify and open, we will eventually be drawn into all of the limbs. It is common for new meditators to become voracious spiritual readers (svadhyaya), lean toward a purer diet (saucha), and feel more sensitive about the wellbeing of others (ahimsa). In fact the best way to achieve progress in yama and niyama is by going straight to samadhi with deep meditation. Then harmonious behavior comes naturally from inside, rather than having to be enforced from outside. These things are indicators of the connectedness of yoga. It occurs on all levels of practice. Sometimes it is called "Grace," because spiritual blessings seem to come out of nowhere. In truth, such blessing are being telegraphed through us via spiritual conductivity rising in our nervous system from something we did somewhere on the eight-limbed tree of yoga. Even the sincere thought, "Is there something more than this?" is a powerful yoga practice, and it is found in the niyama limb – it is surrender, bhakti. As you know from the lessons, this conductivity in the nervous system becomes "ecstatic" when kundalini begins to move. When that happens we are really getting connected through the limbs of yoga – here, there and everywhere.

If we engage in effective practices in a coordinated way in multiple limbs from early on, then our nervous system will be purifying and opening most rapidly. This is an important principle that is utilized in the core strategy of these lessons – using an integrated system of practices, having the option of working through as many limbs as possible.

Samyama is a jumping off point from the eight limbs. It is something different from any one limb that can be used to purify and open the nervous system. In Patanjali's *Yoga Sutras* it gets a whole chapter called, "Supernormal Powers."

Samyama is defined as the combination of the last three limbs of yoga used with an object. So, using focused attention (dharana), meditation (dhyana) and deep inner silence (samadhi) with an object, or objects, in a particular way we are able to develop supernormal powers, also called siddhis. Patanjali tells us that samyama is a more intimate practice and that it leads to "the light of knowledge." He also tells us to avoid getting distracted by the experiences that come up when doing samyama. We have been dealing with this in the lessons already. We see lights or have some ecstatic experiences, and we have to remind ourselves to easily go back to the practice we are doing. This is because experiences do not advance our spiritual progress. Only practices do. The same goes for siddhis when they manifest themselves. As was mentioned way back in lesson #76, we do samyama to expand pure bliss consciousness and ecstasy in the nervous system, and beyond.

If we come to samyama expecting to get some powers for our personal use, we will not get much. This is the beauty of samyama. Morally, it is a self-regulating practice. It depends on the presence of inner silence. No inner silence, no pure bliss consciousness – no samyama. It is not possible to do this practice without at least some inner silence in the nervous system. If we have some samadhi, then automatically we will also have some yama and niyama. The more samadhi we have, the more the yama and niyama, and also the more success there will be in samyama. If there is a lot of samadhi (first stage of enlightenment), there will be a lot of yama and niyama, and a lot of progress in samyama. The limbs of yoga are always hanging together like that.

Samyama is working on the deepest level of consciousness within us, and coaxing it into full manifestation by giving it a series of channels to move through in our nervous system. With samyama we are moving inner silence. We are moving the immovable, moving the rock of pure consciousness. Actually, we are expanding the rock. We are expanding it out through our nervous system. With most practices we are working from the outside inward. With samyama, we are going the other way. We are working from the inside outward. With most practices we begin with our limited ego-self and go in. With samyama, we begin with our universal divine-Self and come out. That is the difference between samyama and the other practices.

As consciousness moves outward with samyama, we experience more opening, and all of our practices move to a higher level. This is the advantage of integration of practices. Everything we do in yoga helps everything else we are doing in yoga. In this way yoga practices become like a spiral of ecstatic bliss going higher and higher.

So, as we continue to do the practices we have learned so far, we will also have the option to add samyama practice, which is opening our nervous system in yet another way. The prerequisites for doing samyama are not so many. It is a mental procedure, so there are no physical prerequisites. Unless, of course, you start flying willy-nilly through the air, and then the appropriate physical precautions should be taken.

Anyone who is meditating for a few months and is experiencing some inner silence can do samyama, with effects in proportion to the amount of inner silence established in the nervous system. Samyama expands and stabilizes our inner silence, so it is an excellent complement to meditation. In the next lesson, we will cover the particulars of samyama practice.

With the eight limbs of yoga, and samyama, we will be melting the darkness everywhere. Let's do it.

The guru is in you.

Lesson 150 – Samyama Practice

Meditation is the process of bringing the attention inward to stillness, inner silence, pure bliss consciousness, the witness state, samadhi. All of these describe aspects of the same thing. We have a particular meditation procedure that we do for set amount of time twice-daily. It works like clockwork and, over time, as we meditate each day and then go out and be active, our nervous system becomes naturally accustomed to sustaining and radiating inner silence. Our daily life then becomes calmer from the inside. We are less overwhelmed by external events. This is the rise of the first stage of enlightenment, which is inner silence present in our life twenty-four hours a day, seven days a week (24/7).

Once we have some inner silence, even just a little, we have the opportunity to begin to operate from that level of infinite potential in us. All that exists is manifested from that, and we, being that, are capable of manifesting from that infinite reservoir of life within us. So, with our toe in the infinite, we can begin to move from there for the benefit our transformation to enlightenment. It is simple to do.

You will recall that in meditation we use the thought of a sound, the mantra, to systematically allow the mind to go to stillness. It is in letting go of any meaning, language or intellectual content, and just easily picking up the thought of the sound of the mantra, that are able to dive deep into pure bliss consciousness. The nervous system also goes to silence with the mind, and our metabolism slows way down.

With samyama, we begin to go the other way. After our meditation time is up, we rest for a minute or two and we transition into samyama. We begin with an easy state of not thinking, just resting in our silence. If thoughts are coming, we just let them go without entertaining them. In samyama practice we do not entertain the mantra either. We start by not favoring anything but being easy in our silence, however much silence we have from our just completed meditation session, and naturally present in us from our months or years of daily meditation. This is the starting point for samyama – silence.

The only prerequisite for doing samyama practice is having some inner silence. For most people this is after a few months of daily deep meditation, as covered in the early lessons.

Now we are ready to begin samyama practice. Here is how we do it.

With samyama, we are initiating meaning in silence. We do it in a simple, easy, systematic way. First we create an impulse of meaning in silence, and then we let it go in silence.

Let's begin with "Love." It is a good place to start with samyama. In samyama it is suggested you use your most intimate language, the language that goes deepest in your heart, whatever it may be.

In your easy silence, pick up, just once, the fuzziest feeling of the word "Love" in your own language. Don't deliberately make a clear pronunciation, or mental images of this or that scene or situation that represent Love to you. Just have a faint remembrance of Love, and then let go into your silence, the easy silence you are in as you pick up the faint meaning of Love. Don't contemplate Love or analyze it during samyama. Don't think about it at all. Just come to it once in a faint, subtle way, and then let go into silence. It is a subtle feeling of Love we are coming to, nothing more, and letting it go. Like that.

Having thought "Love" once, be in silence for about fifteen seconds. If any thoughts come, let them go easily. Don't look at the clock. With a little practice your inner clock will tell you with good enough accuracy when fifteen seconds is up. Just be easy in silence for about a quarter of a minute. Then pick up the faint, fuzzy meaning of "Love" again, and let it go again into your silence for about fifteen seconds again.

That is two repetitions of samyama – twice picking up Love at its subtlest level of thought, and twice letting it go into inner silence.

What is the effect of this? What will happen?

To the extent we are picking up meaning on the border of inner silence (the subtlest level of thought), and then letting go easily into our silence, the effect will be very powerful. Inner silence is a huge amplifier of subtle thought. Inner silence is the only amplifier of thought. It is the source of thought. Usually our thoughts come out of silence stimulated by all that is lodged in our subconscious mind. So many habitual patterns are lodged in our obstructed subconscious mind, and these are what distort and weaken the flow of divine energy coming out from inner silence into our everyday life. With meditation we are clearing out the obstructions in the subconscious mind and developing a clear awareness of our inner silence. With samyama we are acting directly within our inner silence to produce an outflow of positive effects that purify our nervous system and surroundings in powerful ways.

During samyama maybe we will feel some energy moving out from our silence. It can be experienced as physical, mental or emotional. Or maybe we won't feel much until later in activity, and then we are more loving and compassionate for no obvious external reason. We are changing from the inside. This is what samyama is – moving intentions from the divine level of silence in us out into external manifestation.

Samyama is what prayer is when it is taken to its deepest level of communion with the divine inside us – taken within divine inner silence. Effective prayer is based on the principles of samyama we are discussing here.

Each thought/meaning we use in samyama is called a "sutra." In Sanskrit, sutra means, "to tie together, or to stitch." The English medical word, "suture" comes from sutra. In samyama, sutras are bits of meaning we give to unbounded pure bliss consciousness to amplify out into everyday life, to "tie together" our inner and outer life. So, sutras are bits of yoga we can consciously cultivate in ourselves through samyama practice.

In the third chapter, or book, of Patanjali's *Yoga Sutras* on supernormal powers, many sutras are given for many different things. All this information is not for obtaining instant results or powers. If it were, it would not be doing anyone a favor in terms of gaining enlightenment. All those powers would be a great distraction to yoga if they were so easily obtained. Fortunately, as mentioned in the last lesson, samyama is morally a self-regulating practice, which means inner silence (samadhi) is the prerequisite for success in samyama. If there is inner silence, there will also be moral responsibility and conduct (yama and niyama), due to the connectedness of all the limbs of yoga.

Samyama is having inner silence (samadhi), and the ability to pick up a thought (focus/dharana) and let it go inward (meditation/dhyana). Then the results of samyama come out from inner silence automatically. If we have the last three limbs of yoga, we will also have the other limbs, so powers from samyama will be divine in purpose. Even so, we should be clear about experiences versus practices, as always, and be mindful not to get caught up in experiences that come up. When experiences come up, we easily come back to the practice we are doing.

As with all advanced yoga practices, the real benefits from samyama are to be found in long term daily practice of a particular routine of sutras. If we keep changing sutras around every day or week, and are irregular in our practice, the results will not accumulate. If we want to strike water, we will do best to keep digging in the same place. In Advanced Yoga Practices we can do samyama after every meditation session before we go into yoni mudra kumbhaka (if doing that then) and our ending rest period. Samyama is a continuation of our meditation practice. First we are going in with meditation, and then we are coming out with samyama.

For this purpose, a balanced series of nine sutras are given here. The suggestion is for each to be done for two cycles of samyama, two times with about fifteen seconds in silence for each sutra, and going straight through the list in order like that. In a few days they will be memorized and easy to navigate through using the method of samyama, going gradually deeper in practice with each session. The sutras are:

- Love

- Radiance

- Unity

- Health

- Strength

- Abundance

- Wisdom

- Inner Sensuality

- Akasha – Lightness of Air

Each sutra is to be taken in its entirety, with the fifteen seconds in silence afterwards. For example, "Inner Sensuality" is a single sutra followed by fifteen seconds of silence. It is for pratyahara, introversion of senses. "Akasha – Lightness of Air" is also a single sutra, followed by fifteen seconds in silence.

The meanings for the sutras can be translated to your deepest or first language, as discussed above. All except "Akasha," which is a Sanskrit word meaning, "subtlest ether, inner space." We know from physics that we are ether, empty space inside, nothing really solid in here at all. Our body is that, and when we do samyama on "Akasha – Lightness of Air," we begin to feel very light.

If you do each of these nine sutras twice in your samyama session, it will take about five minutes. If there is a particular one you feel the need to do more of, then add that on to the end and do samyama with it for another five minutes. The cycles remain at fifteen seconds, and we just keep going with that for five minutes, by the clock for that last five minutes. If there is no preference, then you can do the lightness sutra for five minutes at the end. It is very powerful. It is a mental kundalini technique that brings much energy up through the nervous system. It is not uncommon to experience physical symptoms such as panting (automatic bastrika pranayama) and "hopping" during samyama with the lightness sutra. If this happens, make sure you are sitting on a soft surface like a mattress. There can be various symptoms manifested with the other sutras as well. We are moving the infinite inner silence within us, so the manifestations coming out can be very real and noticeable. Patanjali calls these manifestations "supernormal powers," or "siddhis."

For those who are full with bhakti for enlightenment and have time, samyama repetitions can be increased to four for each sutra, and then ten minutes with a preferred sutra at the end (default is the lightness sutra). This is about twenty minutes of samyama practice. Make sure to take plenty of rest when coming out of your routine of practices, especially when doing samyama. Lying down for five or ten minutes at the end is good. As always, use self-pacing in your practices. Mental techniques such as meditation and samyama are very powerful, so to overdo them is to court uncomfortable energy flows. We each will find our comfortable limit through prudent self-pacing.

Samyama greatly strengthens our presence in the silence of pure bliss consciousness. It promotes the integration of the inner and outer aspects of our nervous system. Samyama stimulates the nervous system to purify and open to the second and third stages of enlightenment, as well as enhancing our inner silence (first stage) in everyday life. Samyama makes the overall power of our desires much stronger. When we want to accomplish something that is in tune with the divine flow, resistance will be much less and obstacles will seem to melt away.

For those who live in the silence of pure bliss consciousness and develop the habit of functioning naturally from that infinite level of life, a constant stream of "small miracles" becomes commonplace.

Do samyama practice after your meditation for a few months and see for yourself. Samyama is more than a sitting practice. It is a way of thinking and doing that rises in our everyday life as we travel on the road to enlightenment.

The guru is in you.

Lesson 151 – Samyama – Settling in with Your Sutras

Q1: I am a little bit confused over how we are supposed to relate to the sutras. "Radiance" and "Unity" are for me very vague and ambivalent – for me they are pretty much context words where as "Love" is self-explanatory. Why do we choose the particular sutras? Take "Strength" – somebody would argue that "agility" can be more useful. What about pratyahara and akasha? If you've never experienced those things then they are as meaningless as mantras. Where does the eventual effect then come from? Can you add personal sutras or is this hazardous? Some people may, for example, desire more humility in themselves. I hope this will help you with filling the gaps of my understanding. Thanks for all the time you put into this group – it's a real gold mine!

A1: At first I thought to give specific definitions for each sutra, but decided not to, as each person will find their own "ecology" with meanings within their own language and culture, just as you are finding yours now. It is as it should be. Some settling in time is normal.

Someone else wrote saying they don't know what Love is, and liked all the rest. So, everyone will be different. The individual meanings are not as crucial as the overall practice, for everyone will eventually come into their own right meanings. Samyama will stimulate the rise of inner silence using the full range of sutras, which, taken all together, purify and open the entire nervous system.

As for changing sutras, it is up to you. If "humility" is not contained in "Love" for you, then add it. If "Radiance" is not clear, use "Divine Radiance" or "Outflowing Light." If "Unity" is unclear, use "Oneness." Or, maybe those clarifications will give you comfort in using the originals.

Akasha is best understood as living inner space – alive emptiness. Almost pure bliss consciousness itself. Our body is that – energy in vast empty space. There is nothing much here. Only the appearance of something. Akasha means that. Then, in the sutra "Akasha – Lightness of Air" we let it go into silence, and everything moves in us to manifest lightness. Whoosh! Don't worry too much about meanings. The necessary knowledge is inside. It doesn't take much to set the right direction.

Pratyahara is not offered as a sutra – "Inner Sensuality" is, which will enliven the senses inward. There is a lesson (#121) on pratyahara which should make the meaning of this clear. It is also discussed in the lesson before last on the eight limbs of yoga.

Picking sutras is not exact science. Commit to a good list for yourself and go with it. You can't wander too far off track if you stay with the basic range of meanings. There are plenty more in Patanjali's *Yoga Sutras*, many far more abstract than the ones given here. The idea is to cover the whole of body/mind/heart, stimulating inner silence out through it. This will purify and open the important channels (nadis) in the nervous system. Once you settle in with samyama, it is suggested you not change sutras around often. We want to go deep, and that will be difficult if we keep moving the location of our digging. For the same reason we stay stable with our mantra, except for occasional enhancements when we are ready to "shift gears" to broaden our presence in pure bliss consciousness.

As your habit of samyama develops through daily practice, you will gradually find all of your thinking and feeling during daily activity naturally originating deeper inside. This is the ultimate benefit of doing samyama practice. It cultivates the habit of living and expressing from the level of divine silence in us. Then we find increasing success and happiness in everything we do. It is a habit of thinking and doing we are cultivating. So, while the choice of each sutra is important, it is the overall effect of the full range of sutras in our everyday life we are really after.

Q2: Thank you very much for your reply. It clarified things. I just wonder, some people say that akasha has the meaning of spirit. It's the fifth tattva in the European esoteric tradition, equivalent with the fifth element spirit – ruler of the other elements. I'm not familiar with the Indian words, but it is interesting anyway.

A2: Akasha is the last stepping off point before unmanifest pure bliss consciousness, the infinite silence within us which is the essence of all that is. In all traditions there is a necessity to assign mythological deities, rulers, authority figures, to the various levels of functioning in nature. It has to do with the natural human need for an ishta (chosen ideal), which stimulates bhakti and spiritual growth. This is how bhakti works, and it is very important that we have it in some form. However, we don't want to get all wrapped up in flights of bhakti during the practice of samyama. We just easily pick up the sutra very faintly and let it go into silence. It is important not to favor flights of contemplation with the mind or rituals of worship during samyama. We can do that later. Samyama, like deep meditation, is a specific practice that we favor during the time we are doing it.

The body as "akasha" (living empty space) is the first step of the two-part lightness sutra. The second part, "lightness of air," moves inner silence, and our akasha-body with it. But it can only happen if we let the sutra go into silence. So it is with all divine manifestation, which includes everything in the cosmos. Everything we see and know emanates from vibrations flowing out from pure bliss consciousness.

John 1.1: "In the beginning was the Word, and the Word was with God, and the Word was God ... All things were made by the Word..."

The basic principles of samyama are behind all temporal manifestation.

For the sake of our enlightenment, we can enter into this divine creative process within ourselves.

The guru is in you.

Lesson 152 – Thinking about Meanings versus Doing Samyama Practice

Q: Now I'm a little confused, I thought we were to just think the word and then let it go. This recent response sounds like we should meditate or think about it. Another question – I am getting these bursts of feelings/energy within my body throughout the day. They can be localized and I seem to have some control over them. I am assuming they are kundalini. My question is this – are they just a pleasant aftermath or is something being released?

A: Yes, you are right. Just pick up the sutra as a faint idea and let it go. Then 15 seconds of silence. The discussions on meaning have nothing to do with performance of the samyama practice itself. Some people are going through some clarification, settling in with meanings, finding their own ecology. We have many languages in the group, so you can imagine what everyone is going through. As everyone settles in, the meanings go to subconscious. That is not part of the practice of samyama. It is just like, "What is akasha? ... Okay, that is what it is." Then just forget it and do samyama on the words, the sutra. The meaning is in there. We don't ponder it during samyama. We just pick up the sutra faintly, and the let go.

The pleasurable "bursts" are very good. Inner silence is moving in you from your samyama. It can be experienced in many ways. The next lesson (on becoming "super-normal") has more detail on that. Many are having similar experiences. There is no need to "control" experiences. They are natural. Let them happen, within reason. They are the release of obstructions and the emergence of divine energy. They will stabilize to steadiness over time – more natural silent bliss and ecstatic radiance in life. Samyama is doing yoga from the inside out, added to our practices that go from the outside in.

The early results many are having with samyama are very impressive. Bravo!

The guru is in you.

Lesson 153 – Yoga Sutra Translations, and on becoming "Super-Normal"

Q: Thank you again for your lessons! Two questions if I may. Could you possibly recommend a good translation of Pantajali's *Yoga Sutras*? Lastly, in working with the sutras I found my chest feel as if it was expanding, as well as my head. It was quite extraordinary. Is this normal? You spoke of the different ways of the energy manifesting and I was just wondering if this too is one of those manifestations? With love and unity.

A: There are many online translations of the *Yoga Sutras*, including in numerous languages, in addition to the dozens of English versions. Many of them have commentaries, which may or may not be consistent with the approach in these lessons. For that reason, I recommend you start with one that does not have a commentary. It is easy to find. Look under "Yoga Sutras" and "Yoga Texts" in the AYP links section on the web site.

The *Yoga Sutras* consist of four "books." The whole scripture is less than 20 pages – very concise. If you are wondering where the eight limbs are described, it starts in Book 2-29. Book 3 is on samyama and super-normal powers. By the way, the idea of becoming "super-normal" is pretty appealing, isn't it? As in very, very normal. Normal for human beings is enlightened. So why not become super-normal?

Yes, your expansion is (super) normal, a beautiful indication of your silence moving out from inside. This is samyama in action. Many different things can happen. There can be more expansion, inner sensory experiences, strong emotions, laughing, crying, physical vibrations and new kinds of breathing. It is all about obstacles being dissolved as inner silence moves out through the nervous system as a result of our practices, now with samyama added. The nervous system knows what to do as pure bliss consciousness moves through it. If symptoms become excessive, just use self-pacing in your practices. If necessary, that can mean paring back on the number of repetitions in samyama for a while. Always take plenty of rest coming out of meditation and samyama. That is important to facilitate stable energy flows in daily activity.

All of these symptoms are normal releases and are signs of the emergence of inner divinity. It is okay to let them happen. If your body wants to move or shake, let it, but not to a hazardous extreme. If breathing changes, let it, but not to a hazardous extreme. If emotions come, let them, but not to a hazardous extreme. If sexual arousal comes (and it can) let it, but not to a hazardous extreme. It is all normal as divine energy bubbles out through the nervous system from the inside.

I am reminded of a passage in Swami Muktananda's book, *Play of Consciousness*, where he described a certain stage in his journey when he'd go out of his house and roar like a wild animal. Needless to say, the neighbors were a bit concerned. There's no need to carry it that far.

At times along the path it might seem that there is not much happening with our inner energy. Maybe things are being loosened underneath without many symptoms, and later we will notice something. Or maybe we are waiting for inner silence to come up with more weeks and months of meditation. Or maybe we are not letting go with the subtle feeling of the sutra in samyama. Sometimes doing nothing is a bit tricky – just not favoring anything that comes up in the mind during that fifteen seconds in silence.

Successful yoga is not about experiences; it is about following the procedures of our practices. We are changed by practices, not by experiences. Experiences are the by-product of our practices and the resulting spiritual transformation that is going on.

Also remember that immediate responses coming up from sutras should also be let go during samyama. It is the ultimate karma yoga – divine doing while letting go of the fruit of the doing. It is built into the technique of samyama – doing and letting go of doing. So samyama is also cultivation of the outflowing of divine love which expects nothing in return. If we do our samyama that way, in time we will become radiating beacons of divine light floating in the air.

Then who will be able to deny what we human beings are? Who will not want to become super-normal?

The guru is in you.

Lesson 154 – Samyama – "Let Go and Let God"

Q: I don't think I knew what life was about until I came to this group. Your lessons on samyama have blown me away. I am filling up with light and joy every time I do the sutras, and overflowing with it. I finally know what the words mean: "Let go and let God." Namaste!

A: Yes, let go and let God is what samyama is about. We just give a subtle angle with a sutra and let go, and our inner silence does the rest. With a range of sutras, we can expand with our inner silence in every direction.

In easy deep meditation we follow the ancient maxim: "Be still, and know I am God."

Then we do samyama, letting go into our divine stillness, and it becomes clear how we are capable of expressing radiant harmony in this world.

The guru is in you.

Lesson 155 – Samyama – Lightness, Lurching and Levitation?

Q: I'm doing the sutras about a week and having good feelings since the beginning. Tonight during the lightness one I got a rise of energy that also felt good making me feel very light inside. Then I started to shake and lurch. My arms were going up and down and I was shaking and I thought I was going to yell, but I didn't. I don't know where it all came from. The next thing I knew I was near the foot of the bed and I don't know how I got there from the head of the bed where I was sitting with crossed legs. I went back to the head of the bed and started again and it happened again. This time I peeked when the lurching started after the sutra and saw my body hop from one end of the bed to the other. I did it a few more times and then lay down feeling like every nerve in my body had an enema.

Is this levitation, or is it just physical? Whatever it is it feels good during and after, so it must be an ok practice. I want to keep it up. Do you agree? But I'm afraid about going off the end of the bed. Should I move to the floor for this?

A: It came from your inner silence, and it is a wonderful start with the lightness sutra. If you feel good afterwards, then keep it up. Make sure you take plenty of rest when coming out of practices.

If you are more comfortable doing the lightness sutra on pillows or a mattress on the floor, then do that. You can continue to do the rest of your practices on the bed if you want, and then move to the floor at the end for the lightness sutra. However, you will find that there is not much risk of falling off the bed, as you will be intuitively aware of your location during the practice. It's more likely that the bed will get damaged more than you will during the dynamic beginnings, so that is a good reason to get on the floor also. Make sure you have good thick padding under you.

Is it levitation? Well, it is trying to be, isn't it? At this stage there is a lot of purification going on in the nervous system and the body is responding to the energy surging through by lurching and hopping. In time it will settle down and be much smoother, and the movements will become very subtle. There will be more energy moving inside and less external indication of it.

Movement and dramatic sensations inside (including ecstasy) are caused by friction in the nervous system as the energy moves through, blowing out the obstructions in large quantities. Karmic debris is getting cleaned out in a wholesale fashion. Hence that feeling of having the nerves purged. That's the great power of samyama. It enables us to systematically purge the nervous system from the inside with relatively little discomfort. Getting purged by using samyama is usually very pleasurable. This is because, when samyama becomes functional in our nervous system, we already have sufficient inner silence available to enable it. So it is pure bliss consciousness that is surging out through our nervous system in response to the sutras, and that's why it feels so good. It is silent bliss moving out through us in large quantities. It benefits all of our other practices, and everyone who is within miles of us as well.

With the lightness sutra, as the obstructions become less over time there is less friction and the movements refine. The same happens with the experiences with the rest of the sutras. It all becomes very smooth, pleasurable and light.

Whatever experiences come as samyama practice advances over time will be a by-product of the purification in our nervous system. By the time we are having more advanced experiences (siddhis), they will not be nearly as pleasurable or attractive as the divine love and joy we will be naturally radiating in every direction in every moment.

The guru is in you.

Lesson 156 – Muladhara/Root and Integration of Practices

Q: I am very interested in stimulating the muladhara (root chakra) physically. It is a main focus in my yoga. Can you tell me how the practices will do that?

A: Stimulating the muladhara/root at the perineum is important, but not to the exclusion of everything else. The objective is to activate the root while tying it in with the spiritual awakening of the entire nervous system.

In the lessons we use two primary physical methods for physical stimulation of the root – mulabandha/asvini (compression of the anal sphincter) and siddhasana (sitting on the heel). But there is much more to stimulating the root than physical action.

A very important method is the one that ties the muladhara up into the entire nervous system energetically – spinal breathing, which involves breath with attention cycling between the third eye and root. Deep meditation also does this integration of everything "globally" in the nervous system by bringing the mind and body to divine stillness.

With samyama, there can be some bouncing also while using the "lightness" technique. It comes from inside, a mental technique only, and the root gets bumped during spontaneous hopping. But focus on muladhara is the last thing in mind while this is happening, because the whole body is filling with light and wanting to lift up.

It can be a distraction putting too much attention on the muladhara. It is part of a much greater whole, and we should not become too fixated on it. I suggest you let the muladhara fit in naturally as part of the whole of practices. Allow yourself to go beyond muladhara, higher, through the methods of body, mind and breath. Some letting go in the lower center(s) will not hurt. Then you will be free to do more work higher up in the body. For example, have you tried the "chin pump?" It is a physical method that is very profound, and is covered here in the lessons. It is done high in the body, and ties the muladhara/root in with the illumination of the heart, throat, and head.

Let me add that it is possible to address just about everything physically necessary in the muladhara by sitting in siddhasana during practices while the attention goes to all the other methods higher up. In this sense, using siddhasana to stimulate muladhara is a "no-brainer." Once siddhasana is mastered, then everything (spinal breathing, meditation, mulabandha, sambhavi, kechari, nauli, chin pump, kumbhaka, samyama, etc.) can be done without attention being distracted. "Mastered" means able to stay in siddhasana with constant stimulation with attention not stuck on muladhara, and free to do all the other practices. It is not difficult to develop the habit, because siddhasana requires no effort to stay in once established. That is the best situation – stimulation at the muladhara with attention completely free to do all the other practices that open the entire nervous system.

Muladhara is the essential beginning of kundalini awakening, but it is not the end. Just as the basement is the essential beginning of a tall building, but the best views are definitely higher up. It is common sense, yes?

It is in the integration of a range of practices covering the whole nervous system where huge power is found in yoga. Patanjali's eight limbs of yoga support this view. Any one or two practices done to the exclusion of the others is not the most effective yoga. I suggest you avoid the trap of being stuck on one or two aspects of your nervous system. It takes integrated practices to coax the nervous system to purify and open fully. If this were not so, we would be seeing many more enlightened people in the world today. It is time for a change to more integrated systems of practice, which means balanced consideration of our nervous system and the methods for stimulating it to purify and open.

The guru is in you.

Lesson 157 – What is Inner Silence?

Q: Inner silence has been mentioned many times in these lessons, and the words seem simple, but I'd like to clarify what we're talking about. I believe it was Krishnamurti who talked about jumping into the space between mental words. Is that what inner silence means in the context of these lessons – space with no auditory content that I can extend for a while before the mind manages to start burbling again?

I have also noticed that I frequently start to have vivid mental images during samyama practice. No auditory to disrupt the silence, but clear, dream-quality images. I suspect it means that I'm falling asleep during sadhana, but therein lies another question. Is meditation and samyama performed teetering on the edge between deep relaxation and sleep? Or has mind turned off from the path of sleep and headed in a different direction?

A: Inner silence is at the heart of yoga. Without it, there can be no yoga. In the second lesson we discussed how yoga is the joining of the subject (observer) and the object (observed). The object is not so hard to find. It is everything we perceive in our heart and mind, and out through our senses. The object is everywhere. And so too is the subject. But the subject is not always so obvious. The subject is the inner silence we have been talking about here so often.

What is inner silence? It has many names in the traditions: sat-chit-ananda, the Self, the witness, unconditioned awareness, the void, emptiness, Father God, Shiva, samadhi, Tao and so on ... In the lessons we often call it pure bliss consciousness. So many names for what amounts to nothingness. But the nothingness is alive. It is aware. It is everywhere. And it is somehow blissful within itself. It is the "I" in you and me that remains constant. It is the universal "I" that expresses as all that we see, yet remains mostly hidden within, except to those who have cultivated Self-awareness through yoga. Success in that cultivation brings a state of freedom from the ups and downs of this world, even as we continue to be involved in our everyday activities.

Yoga is about revealing our "I," experiencing it in its native unconditioned state. Yoga is for answering the question "Who am I?" and consciously becoming it. Our nervous system has the ability to give us that experience, and more. This is why the human nervous system is called the "temple of God."

With direct experience through practices we can go from the philosophy/theory of inner silence to the reality of it. The leap from theory to reality is found in the ways that our nervous system manifests different forms of awareness. The nervous system operates in modes that we can identify as different states of consciousness. There are three states of consciousness we all know well:

1. Waking state – what we experience in our daily activity.

2. Dreaming state – what we sometimes experience in sleep.

3. Deep dreamless sleep state – what we don't experience much, but we were somewhere.

Inner silence is a state distinctly different from these three. We know it in our deep meditation as blissful awareness without any objects. Or it can be mixed with objects too, like thoughts, feelings, or whatever. But in its pristine state, it is without objects. So in yoga it gets it own number as a unique state of consciousness:

4. Inner silence – it is all those descriptive words and definitions mentioned already. In yoga it is sometimes called simply "Turiya," which means "the fourth state" in Sanskrit.

The difference between inner silence and the other three states of consciousness is that inner silence is unchanging and can be cultivated in the nervous system as an unending presence superimposed under, in, and through the other three states of consciousness. Those who have meditated for some time find this to be the case. It starts as some inner peace and an awareness of a silent quality coexisting with and within the objects of our perception. This happens with external observations through the senses, and with our thoughts and feelings too. We see them as the objects that they are, occurring external to our unconditioned inner silent awareness. With daily yoga practices, inner silence grows and becomes the movie screen upon which all our experiences are projected. We become the movie screen – the infinite movie screen of life.

Is inner silence is "the space between mental words" (thoughts)? Yes, it is. It is the gap we sometimes experience as we pass from one thought to another, and from one state of consciousness to another. When the music stops for an instant, we are left with inner silence, our Self. For the yogi and yogini, inner silence is also experienced behind and within the thoughts, and within all of life. So, when we let go into inner silence during samyama, there may be no mental activity, or there may be some. If we are letting go, our attention will be in inner silence, assuming we have cultivated some in deep meditation beforehand. Samyama and enlightenment (first stage and beyond) depend on innate inner silence that will be there whether the mind is "burbling" or not. It also comes up in dreaming state and deep sleep – that's 24/7 inner silence (means 24 hours per day, 7 days per week). Once we have that rising, we are becoming ready for serious yoga, union of the subject and the object, and that is the union of the divine poles within us leading to the unity condition where all is experienced as a divine flow of the One.

So, the reason why be begin with meditation in these lessons is to cultivate inner silence first, the prerequisite for all the rest that happens in yoga. Once we have that coming up, it is possible to open many doors. When Shiva (inner silence) is there, then arousing and fostering ecstatic union with kundalini/Shakti becomes possible, and then it is a joyous experience rather than a traumatic one. It is the natural next step. So after meditation is established, that is what we do here in the lessons – awaken kundalini and get down to the business of joining the subject and the object. That's yoga.

As for falling asleep in samyama, meditation, etc., from the above you can see it is not quite the same as crossing from one state (inner silence) to another state (like sleep). It is not either/or in practices. We can be in both at the same time, which is often the case during meditation especially. That is why we count time we are "lost" in thoughts or no thoughts in meditation as practice time. The purification in the nervous system is going on in these conditions. If we drift off in samyama, we just easily pick up with the sutras where we left off. In that case, we have gone from the sutra off into some blend of inner silence and the subtle flavor of the sutra. When we realize that has happened, we just easily continue from where we left off. The time for getting through samyama can be stretched out a bit if we lose track like that. If something like sleep keeps overcoming us in a particular samyama session, we can just call it done and lie down and rest. This is good samyama also. It can happen if a lot of obstructions are being released. Inner silence is being cultivated throughout the whole procedure, so, again, it is not one state of consciousness or the other. It is rising inner silence with whatever else is going on.

Keep in mind that all of this we are talking about is not on the level of the curious mind, the intellect. Only the theory has to do with intellect. The practices are not for promoting theory. Daily advanced yoga practices are for purifying and opening our nervous system in ways that are neurological and biological – a dramatic expansion of the functioning of our nervous system. The experiences of ecstatic bliss that come up are very real – ultimately as real as the most intimate lovemaking we can imagine, and it is all going on inside. So, cultivating inner silence has far-reaching implications in our lives.

The guru is in you.

Lesson 158 – Too Relaxed in Meditation?

Q: Thanks for your lessons, I am enjoying them very much. I am getting ready to use the yoni mudra in my practice next but had a question. During the meditation I almost always fall asleep while in siddhasana. Sometimes I even have to remind myself during pranayama to breathe because I start to go out then. Lots of head nodding at first, then I wake up slouched over (even drooling a few times). I try to sit away from the wall because I would nod off and thump my head sometimes. I don't feel tired when I practice or during the day. I usually wake up around the 20 minute mark. Is there something I am missing? I enjoy the way things are going but just wanted to see if you had any advice on this.

A: It is good practice you describe. It won't be manifesting like that forever. It is a special form of sleep associated with deep inner silence and purification during meditation. Once your nervous system has released those deep-rooted obstructions in there, you will experience much more clarity during practices. Your clarity in activity is evidence that good things are happening. It is a great way to get rid of lifetimes of accumulated karma. While you are "sleeping," the infinite is unfolding inside you.

I wish you all success as you continue.

The guru is in you.

Lesson 159 – Too Many Thoughts in Meditation?

Q: I thank you very much for a great service you are doing. It is good work and please keep it up. I have one question. When I do meditation, my mind drifts and it goes on thinking about different activities that I did recently and which I might be doing in the future. Because of this, instead of 20 minutes, I do meditation more time, sometimes up to 40 minutes. When I do meditation more time like this I get headache and get angry at people even on slight problems. Because of this I couldn't do higher meditation. Can you please help me to do regular meditation? How can I focus what I am doing? Also, how can I get rid of the headache?

A: Thank you for writing and sharing. Thoughts are a normal part of meditation. They come as obstructions are being released in the nervous system. If you meditate much longer than 20 minutes, you will be releasing too much in one session, and that is the cause of the irritability and headaches. So, go back to 20 minutes and follow the procedure for easily coming back to the mantra whenever you realize you are off it. Once you begin meditation, if you have nothing but thoughts for the whole time, that is okay. It is what needs to happen right then as your nervous system is purifying deep inside. It will not always be like that. Experiences change over time. Right now, your experience is thoughts – which is release of lots of deep obstructions. Good things are happening, but a bit too much with such long meditations.

If you are doing meditation according to the lessons, then I suggest you review all the lessons and Q&As on the procedure of meditation. Thoughts are a normal part of the process. It may seem very mundane sometimes in meditation. I can assure you that you are deep in meditation. If you were not, you would not have irritability and headaches from overdoing it.

Also, make sure you take adequate rest time when coming out of meditation, as instructed in the lessons. This will facilitate smoothness in activity.

Follow the easy procedure and you will be fine. If you have further difficulties, let me know.

The guru is in you.

Lesson 160 – Extreme Sensitivity to Meditation – What To Do?

Q: After 5-7 minutes of meditation, colors like orange, yellow, green and dark blue in the form of bright light appear before my eyes. This stays about for a minute or two and my head starts to ache and I can't meditate any longer. I come out of my meditation and I sleep, as my head is very heavy. At night when I sleep after meditation I am getting very violent dreams like a woman getting raped, and such destructive activities. The feeling is so real that it is scary. This kind of thing has never happened to me. The day I don't meditate I do not get these dreams. I very much want to keep my meditation going but these experiences are becoming a hindrance. Would appreciate your advice.

A: Thank you for writing and sharing. You are one of the few people who is very sensitive to meditation, with a lot of obstructions coming out very fast with just a little practice.

The thing to do is find the right balance of practice for yourself that will allow the obstructions to be dissolved during meditation rather than continuing after. It will take trying some different things to find the balance. If you are determined, you will be able to work it out. Here are a few suggestions. Feel free to experiment until you find a stable routine.

First, try and meditate for 10 minutes only in the morning before breakfast for a few days. Lie down for 5-10 minutes afterward, or longer if you feel uneasy. Taking adequate time to "come out" after meditation is very important, especially if there is a lot of release going on during meditation. See if you can get a comfortable routine going with just 10 minutes of meditation plus rest in the morning. If you can, then try adding a second 10 minute session in the early evening, before dinner, not near bedtime.

If strong sensations or headache come in meditation stop the mantra and just sit and let the attention be easily with the sensation. It is obstructions dissolving, and easy attention on it without mantra will help it dissolve. If it is too much, as you described before, then lay down and continue to be easy with the attention letting it be drawn to the sensation. Don't force the attention at all. Just be easy with it. Try not to get up until the sensation subsides. Then you will know the dissolving process has completed. Don't meditate beyond your allotted time – that includes time spent in thoughts, on sensations, etc. Everything that happens in the allotted time (10 minutes in this case) is considered part of meditation.

Make sure you have good activity during the day and during the evening after meditation. This is important to stabilize the purification happening in the nervous system during meditation. Being with people, family activities, walking, doing creative work or service – wherever your heart takes you.

Don't meditate right before bed. Always meditate before activity.

If you get it to 10 minutes twice a day with good stability and are feeling okay in activity during the day and evening (and in sleep too), then try for 15 minutes twice a day. If that is good after a few weeks or months, try for 20 minutes. If you are feeling discomfort and feel you are meditating too long, then back off to the last comfortable level you found and stay there for a while.

Self-pacing matched to your experience is what you should do. This is the key to long term success in all practices – finding stable daily practice over many months and years.

Another thing you can try is some light spinal breathing before meditation (5 minutes or so), as given in the lessons. This can help smooth out meditation. Spinal breathing is very good for balancing unruly energies in the nervous system, which includes mind and emotions. Finally, you can also try some light asanas, bending and stretching, (5-10 minutes) before spinal breathing and meditation. Maybe only spinal breathing will help at this stage. Maybe only asanas. Maybe both. Maybe neither. You will only know by trying.

Maybe you will find that only asanas once or twice a day with or without spinal breathing, and no meditation, are what you need to do for a while until the obstructions get cleared out of your nervous system a bit. Then you can try and add meditation later. Where there is a will, there is a way.

Those are some options to consider for finding a stable routine. I wish you all success.

The guru is in you.

Note: This dialog is continued in lesson #200, covering the results of the steps taken in self-pacing, and a new challenge.

Lesson 161 – Dark Nights and the Rise of Inner Silence

Q1: I'm still "on the wagon" and I guess I won't stop meditating regularly twice a day in this lifetime.

Nevertheless I have cut back my practice to "meditation only." I had progressed to meditation plus pranayama plus mulabandha plus sambhavi and things went really fine. I even made good progress in crossed leg sitting, something I found very difficult and distracting from meditation in the beginning. When things went fine the last time I was on holiday, first in the Austrian Mountains, then on a tiny island in the German Northern Sea. It was a beautiful time and I was looking happily forward to returning back home, eager to start handling my life with more fun and on a higher energy level than ever before.

Then, when I arrived back home (two weeks ago) everything seemed to crash within the first 36 hours ... I felt really, really bad and this lasted for several days (it´s not completely over right now, but better). At that time I even stopped my practice completely for 1.5 days. Nothing dramatic had happened on the outside – it was just that I tried to resume my life where I had left it before I left for holiday and that didn't work any longer.

I'm completely sure now that this crash hasn't been caused by yoga; it must have been the positive development that had taken place while I was "off duty." Maybe I've simply outgrown my former way of living.

Somewhere in the lessons you mention the advantages of a busy life for the integration of the purification and expansion achieved during practices. I can relate very well to that. Nevertheless, I'm much more a "be-er" than a "do-er." My life is certainly out of balance on the side of too much withdrawal from worldly affairs. All my lifetime it hasn't been too difficult for me to "reach high" and have sometimes quite intense spiritual experiences. But concerning "outside" day to day life I very often felt extremely overwhelmed, feeling that the world was way too rough and rude for me. A well developed sense of vulnerability...

This is why the concept of yoga you outline in the first few lessons seems to be so very attractive for me. The promise to reconcile the outer world with the inner ... I'm really longing for that.

There is so much old pain coming up while I'm typing this – it seems to be something like the ruin of my lifetime (and the basic anatomy of the separation almost every human being experiences while being incarnated). This is painful.

So I'm working my way back up in practices. I really do believe you when you say this is a reliable way out – I felt so much of it already.

Probably experiencing the "dark night of the soul."

A1: It is inevitable that highs lead to lows. It is in inner silence that we find the truth about it all. That is what meditation is for, gradually bringing up that silent bliss that is inherent in us within all the functioning of our body, mind, emotions, and the world. Then we see everything is going up and down while we, as silent pure bliss consciousness, stay put.

As for activity, yes it is good to stabilize our silence gained in meditation in daily activity. But who is to decide what that activity will be for you? Not me. It is for you to follow your heart and do the things that bring you joy. Some of us are naturally more introverted. Then "activity" may be something not constantly involved with people. Others need to be in the middle of the crush of human endeavor. Only you can know what is your right activity.

Sometimes it is facing our fears and doing things that we shy away from. Then we feel growth in having faced our fears. But neither should we drown ourselves (and our spiritual practices) in overindulgence in what is not natural to us. The important thing is that we find a way to serve life by creating something, or by helping others directly. It can be in business, charity, or doing art in a secluded studio somewhere. Whatever satisfies the inherent need we all have to flow out into the world with our hearts. You are wise to keep meditating. It will gradually bring you the inner steadiness to make the best choices for yourself. Don't rush. Just be purposeful about your life, and always try and honor the deepest longings in your heart.

As your practices advance, and with prudent self-pacing, you will find those old inner obstructions gradually dissolving. Give it time. It is the way in to permanent ecstatic bliss, and out of misery.

Q2: Thank you for your response, all your responses and your wonderful lessons ... All so very uplifting and enlivening.

I'm slowly moving out of the shit – I know I'll have to rearrange my general set-up in life and I'll do so. I'm starting to look at this rearrangement as a creative process, something I'm actively involved in, maybe even something infused with pleasure and joy ... quite a new perspective for me ... maybe I'm moving out of my default mode of feeling more or less overwhelmed most of the time without even knowing so.

Yesterday I had a very surprising experience while listening to one of my favorite CDs. I've always been touched deeply by beautiful music. But now with more and more silence accumulating in my mind something has changed. I had always wondered why I was unable to reproduce tunes I loved so very much by singing them myself. I always could feel the music inside but when I tried to sing it only something more or less similar to the original came out, if the tune was complicated, something less similar.

Yesterday I suddenly realized that I had always been trying to sing my emotions stirred up by the music which of course where not the tune itself. With a mind which is a little bit more silent now, I still can perceive all the emotions the artist expresses in the music as well as my reactions. But besides all that I can listen on a more "analytical level." I'm hearing single notes instead of big clusters of emotional reactions, I also experienced an internal "visualization" of the parallel tunes – and, most surprising, I discovered another tune in the tracks I had listened to so often before. The silence between the notes emerged like a very important new instrument I didn't perceive at all before.

All those pieces had become more "airy", somehow "thinner" with lots of empty silent spaces in them ... very surprising and very interesting.

Mmmh ... I wonder what the world will look like if this musical experience kind of generalizes, more detachment more huge empty silent spaces everywhere around and maybe more creative joy in a universe which is much easier to move around and handle?

Expecting change (and saying thank you for your continuous support).

A2: A very nice observation of silence coming up in your experience of music. Yes, all of life will become more and more like that. It will become normal and not noticed as a contrast, because you will forget how dark it was. Then there will be continuing contrasts going forward from the silence, to more silence, and then ecstasy coming up mixed with silence. On it goes like a spiral.

It comes from practices. Keep that in mind. We all tend to get a little infatuated at times with our experiences. As I have said in the lessons, progress comes from practices, not experiences, which is not to say we can't revel a bit in the fruit of our yoga.

Change is in the air, for all of us. Here come dee-light. Enjoy!

The guru is in you.

Lesson 163 – Sublime Clarity

Q: Having read the question of the person who started to listen to the music in a different way, with more clarity, more depth, somehow I could relate to it. Today is my 10th day of meditation and in the evening as I was taking my walk I felt a different emotion. It wasn't joy or ecstasy or an impulse of pleasure. It was something deeper ... sublime ... deep ... like the memories of our childhood. Then for some time there was a lingering pain which gradually went away. Then the mind started to flow again with tremendous clarity and sharpness. I never had an experience like this and was extremely excited, and wanted to share this with someone. Are such reactions normal, should these be expected?

A: Thank you for writing and sharing. It is a clear experience of pure bliss consciousness you describe in the early days of your meditation. Very beautiful. It can happen to anyone at any time along the path. It is normal. Then there can be obstructions moving out and it is not so clear, and that is normal too. That is how it goes. The light is still in there. Meditation brings us to stillness and there we can have such experiences in practices or afterward. When they do happen, it stands as evidence that there is something wonderful inside we can unfold through our daily spiritual practices.

Maybe we have clarity at the start, and then the clouds move through on their way out. Or maybe we are cloudy from the start and then the light shines through later, all at once sometimes, or bit by bit a little more each month. It can happen so many ways according to how obstructions are lodged in our nervous system and released. One thing is for sure, it will happen if we keep up our practices. In time the inner reality becomes clear and blissful like that all the time, and we accept it as normal life.

Then when people ask us how we feel about all the darkness in the world, we can only say, "Darkness? What darkness? I don't see any darkness. Only the divine light everywhere, with a passing shadow here and there."

Then we are filled with huge compassion for everyone and do all we can to help the light shine through and dissolve the lingering darkness. That is how this new age is unfolding. Everyone is helping everyone else. No one meditates only for themselves. All meditation is for everyone's enlightenment.

Of course it is very exciting when we have such a glimpse right at the beginning like you describe. Use it for motivation to stay regular in your practices. If you have some expectations in practices (normal at this stage), just continue to easily favor the mantra in meditation, your spinal breathing in pranayama and so on. If we stick with the straightforward procedures of practice we will continue to move ahead into more and more sublime feelings and clarity in our daily life.

We all have this destiny built into our nervous system. No one is an exception. It is just a matter of doing the house cleaning for as long as it takes to reveal the divine light of God always shining from inside. Our essential nature is pure bliss consciousness, beyond description. You have shown us today that it is true.

The guru is in you.

Lesson 164 – Human Power

Q: I am a new member of this group. I am a person always having faith in human power. I noted that yoga is the base for all techniques such as hypnotism, mesmerism, telepathy, etc, but I don't know the exact differences between these things. May I have an opportunity to know the answer?

A: The greatest of all human power is the divine within. Yoga is for joining (union) with and becoming that. The first priority in yoga is union with God within us.

Jesus said, "Seek first the kingdom of God, and all things will be added to you."

The powers you mention are of the subconscious mind, not very significant in relation to the pure bliss consciousness of our divinity, which lies beyond the subconscious mind and is its source. If you are interested in powers as approached in the lessons, look up "samyama" in the topic index. It is an integrated approach to powers, aimed first at expanding our deepest inner pure bliss consciousness, and then all the rest comes up as a by-product of that expansion to enlightenment. This is the correct approach to human power – seeking the kingdom of God first, and then all else is added...

Once you have checked out samyama, start at the beginning of the lessons to begin to unfold your full divine power with deep meditation, spinal breathing, and many other means, assembled into daily practice in building block fashion.

I wish you all success on your chosen path.

The guru is in you.

Lesson 165 – Desire and Change

Q: I have experienced desire very intensely to achieve my life's plan. What happens when the foundation of your past beliefs is shattered by new discoveries (yoga, meditation, reincarnation) and your desire and motivation for most things disappears?

A: Our desire will carry us through to our destination. Sometimes our desire to achieve a particular thing can lead us to surprising revelations about what is true, and we find that we are compelled to change our orientation. Change can be confusing, but isn't discovery of the truth a good thing? It is a birth. And, as in all birth, it is change of the status quo. Yet, the world need not be turned upside down. It is a fulfillment we are witnessing today, not a destruction.

There are many ways to go about handling it – as many ways as there are people, it seems, for we all react differently to our changing understandings and circumstances.

In the lessons, a gradual approach is recommended. It is actually quite fast in terms of how quickly one can take on powerful spiritual practices. But at the same time, everyday life goes on, and the lessons don't recommend throwing away our family, career, culture, or religious background. The truth is oozing out everywhere in life. We just have not been so aware of it until now. The light is coming up everywhere. If we are going to become enlightened (and we all will), then it can and will happen right where we are in our current life, family, activities, etc. Why not?

The idea used to be that we have to run off to an ashram somewhere, "drop out" of society, and give up our worldly ambitions. Paradoxically, that is an old-way strategy based on external appearances. We don't have to go anywhere. Neither do we have to give up our worldly goals, for these are spun from God also. If we look deep into ourselves, we will find that our core beliefs have room for the light of truth in them, and so does the rest of our life, just as it is today. As a matter of fact, everyday life needs what yoga brings, and there is not nearly the incompatibility it might seem. Just go into your silence in deep meditation and see for yourself.

Some would dissolve all the world's traditions to make way for the new. I am not for that. All the world's traditions will flower with the same great truth of God that spawned them in the first place. It is human desire and spiritual enterprise (daily practices) that are going to illuminate the old values, beliefs and traditions from the inside.

So don't throw away your foundation beliefs. Let them bathe in the living light that flows from within as you move into your own experiment in human spiritual transformation with meditation, spinal breathing and the rest of the advanced yoga practices. You will find that most of your foundation beliefs are good, only needing a natural tune up from within. What is not real will fade away, and the truth will shine forth from you ever brighter.

Call it a revival of who you are – a homecoming.

It is not a black or white world. Truth and untruth are mixed together in everything. Better to shine a bright light through it all with spiritual practices before deciding to make radical changes or throw anything away. After some time in daily spiritual practices, you will know what to do. There is nothing to fear...

The guru is in you.

Lesson 166 – Pay It Forward

Q: I am reading through your messages on your group and finding them very clear, informative and balanced. This is a very valuable inspiration for people taking up and maintaining their meditation practice. So thank you for the hard work you have put into this resource. I have forwarded the URL (Internet address) on your group to over 1,800 people on my distribution list and I'm sure many of them will gain help from it.

A: Thank you very much for passing the group link on to so many others. Posting the truest and most effective knowledge of practices in the lessons is the most important thing in my life at this stage. Next most important is spreading word of the existence of the lessons to as many as possible. It is at the point now where I want to encourage others to do the same as you have done.

A few years ago a movie came out in America called *Pay It Forward*. It is a story about a young boy who had a school assignment to come up with a way to change the world in a good way. His idea was to help three people in serious need, with the only condition being that if they felt helped they should do the same for three other people needing help, passing on the condition of helping three more people in serious need, and so on. He called it, *Pay It Forward*. He presented his project in class, showing the math on how many thousands, and eventually millions, would be helped by this system. Everyone, including his teacher, said, "Wow," and that was the end of it.

But that wasn't the end of it. You see, this young boy actually went out and helped three people, each who had a serious problem, and gave them the condition of doing the same for three other people. It wasn't easy, and there were a lot of difficulties, but he did it. Later on, after he did the initial helping, everything seemed to be going wrong, and he got discouraged because nothing good seemed to be coming from the effort. But it was. Unknown to him, the web of help was spreading out fast, and by the end of the story ... well, I won't tell you. Go see the movie. It is very inspiring.

Advanced Yoga Practices is a *pay it forward* project. It is my way of saying thank you to all the great ones who have gone before. It is because of them that we have yoga practices today, enabling us to purify and open our nervous system to the divine within us. Yoga works, especially if it is allowed the flexibility to be integrated and optimized to suit the needs of every individual. The guru is ever within us all.

Many have written with their thanks for the lessons. I am very happy that the lessons have been helpful to others. The helpfulness to others is my reward. Nothing else is needed, except one thing.

If these lessons have been helpful to you in some way, if you think you have received some value, then please *pay it forward* in your own way.

Maybe you have a wide network you can access, like the kind person above who sent the group link to 1,800 people. Or maybe you have just three friends you know who could benefit from the information here. Tell them about it. And tell them, if they feel helped, would they please *pay it forward* too. Like that.

Paying it forward is the only request here. It is the only prasad (divine offering). If you give that, you will receive blessings a thousand-fold in return from the rising light of the many you have helped with their yoga practices.

If you don't think this is a good idea, that is okay. It is only an idea. All are always welcome to the lessons, regardless of opinions.

Do your daily yoga practices and enjoy the results. If you got help here, even if you don't wish to pass the word about the lessons, go out and help three people in need ... help three people with a serious problem, share your good will. And then, if they feel obliged, tell them to go help three others. *Pay it forward* works with or without these lessons in the loop.

It's a good idea for everyone. It is a natural behavior that comes from daily yoga practices, the rise of ecstatic bliss, and the endless outflow of divine love. *Pay it forward* is a yoga practice that promotes unity, the highest stage of enlightenment.

So try it. Share your light in a substantial way. See how good it feels.

The guru is in you.

Note: The movie, *Pay It Forward*, is based on the book of the same name by Catherine Ryan Hyde.

Lesson 167 – Living on Air and Sunlight Alone?

Q: Have you heard of this practice or practice it yourself or know anyone who does this practice that one sustains one's body only on the essence from space or sunlight? I read many biographies of past MahaSiddhas, almost all of them have undergone austerity (fasting) and developed the ability of sustaining the physical body not on food. By the way, I am doing the sun-gazing practice rediscovered by HRM (Hira Ratan Manek) and he says he now only lives on sunlight and water.

A: I have no contact with those who exist on prana in the air or sunlight alone, and it is not an ability I am focused on developing at this time. However, the principle should be fairly clear from our yoga practices and experiences.

As we advance in yoga our nervous system purifies and opens to our inner pranic energies, fed by the kundalini/sexual energy rising from the pelvic region. As this process matures we are nourished by the active life force (prana) much more from within. So much so that breath can suspend spontaneously for long periods during pranayama and meditation, and eventually outside practices too. Even beginning meditators experience this automatic slow down and stoppage of breath. The same applies to food intake. If we are nourished from within, then we are less dependent on constant food intake also and can fast easily without discomfort, though this is a more delayed process than the immediate response of the breath.

It stands to reason that inner prana must be replenished from somewhere, normally by both air and food, and that may be where the methods of the "breatharians" and "sun-gazers" come in. Based on what was just said about inner nourishment, it would seem that these practices are not for direct nourishment, but for replenishing and storing prana in the body (probably in the lower centers) for inner sustenance. It seems to me that all this would be best served by first engaging in yoga practices to bring about the purification and opening of the nervous system that is prerequisite to such refined inner nourishment. Then it can be sustained, if desired, by harvesting prana from the air and/or the sunlight. So these practices would seem to be later stage things in the overall process of enlightenment.

The first question in the lessons is always, what does this contribute to the process of human spiritual transformation today? Is it leading to more purification and opening in the nervous system, or is it getting the cart in front of the horse? We'd all love to live as the siddha-saints do, but have we first done all the yoga they did to get to the stage we would like to emulate? Is developing the ability to live on air and sunlight so important? Or is it just a by-product ability (a siddhi) of something much more important – our enlightenment, which is the cultivation and joining of inner silence and the ecstatic energies within us. How we replenish our prana is a fairly mundane subject compared to the divine union going on inside.

No doubt higher abilities will come when required by the opening of our nervous system, and the natural rise of ecstatic bliss and divine love. This is the best, and least distracting, attitude to have about the development of any kind of siddhis. Just some food for thought (pun!).

I wish you all success on your chosen path to enlightenment.

The guru is in you.

Lesson 168 – Is Pain a Prerequisite for Inner Peace?

Q: I have been practising meditation for nearly a month now. It gives me tremendous energy and peace. However a friend of mine, a person who has a fair amount of yogic knowledge and a person whom I respect a lot, told me that if I pursue this course, I should be willing to experience pain, especially since my past is extremely painful. As a matter of fact I had started meditation to heal myself of this pain and face life, move on, live life with peace, harmony and respect for my fellow human beings. Is pain, a prerequisite for finding peace?

A: Thank you for writing and sharing. No, pain is not a prerequisite for finding peace. This does not mean we will not have any pain, or that we should assume the journey is not worth making if we encounter some along the way as our nervous system purifies and opens.

It all depends on the obstructions lodged in our nervous system, and how we manage our practices to release them. Peace and bliss are inherent inside us. There are many ways we can uncover our native state. Some are more radical (and uncomfortable) than others.

In the lessons, everything is designed for simplicity and maximum power, with minimum discomfort. In fact, Advanced Yoga Practices are designed to be a path of enjoyment from start to finish. There is no requirement that anyone overdo with any practice. In fact, it is strongly discouraged. If we enjoy the results of our daily practices, we will continue. If they are a painful drudgery, then who will want to do yoga? Only masochists. So everything is geared to balancing practices to maintain a positive experience of ongoing purification and growth. It can be done.

Advanced yoga practices are like a fine tuned automobile. You can push on the gas pedal and go as fast as you want. You can arrive at your destination smoothly and safely, or you can wrap yourself around a tree. It is all in the driving, you know. You are the driver with these practices. This is why we talk so much about "self-pacing" in the lessons. It is very important. It is the new approach in these modern times. Each person can drive themselves home to enlightenment at their own speed. Many are ready for this.

Even a good driver will hit a few bumps in the road from time to time. It is inevitable on any journey. It is part of life. So we compensate (slow down) when the going gets a little bumpy, and speed up again when the road smoothes out again, as it surely shall.

Do we have to go out of our way to drive through every pothole and ditch we see? No. This is why we say pain is not a prerequisite for peace.

It sounds like you are traveling smoothly so far, and it fills my heart with joy to hear of your rising energy and peace. You are a blessing to the entire world in your practices, for everyone is benefiting from your purification and opening. Continue with enthusiasm and prudent self-pacing, and you will arrive home to your divine Self straight away. Much is being accomplished with every sitting. Lifetimes of pain and suffering are painlessly melting away.

The guru is in you.

Lesson 169 – Is this Ecstatic Conductivity?

Q: I started yoni mudra kumbhaka two weeks ago and since then I have been feeling a strange new connection between my head and my perineum. I do sambhavi and I feel it down there. I put my tongue on the roof of my mouth and I feel it down there. It's pretty nice and sexual, but also pretty strange. Is this the ecstatic conductivity you often mention? It seems to be so. Why is it happening, and where is it leading? Where did the term "ecstatic conductivity" come from? I have never seen it in a yoga book.

A: What a beautiful experience. Yes, it is the beginning of ecstatic conductivity, and once it has begun, it will be with you to stay. A level of purification has been reached in your nervous system where your previously learned practices, combined with the addition of yoni mudra kumbhaka, have given rise to that telltale inner sensuality between the brain and the root. It is an awakening of your spinal nerve, which has led to conscious sensations between the upper and lower extremities of it. This is an excellent way to begin a gentle and loving kundalini awakening, with balance of ecstatic energies between head and root right from the start. It means you have good inner silence available to blend in a progressive and healthy way with the rise of ecstatic energies in your nervous system.

How you conduct your practices from now on will determine the rate at which the awakening will continue. If you were to stop practices today, it would likely stay at about the current level of connectedness, or "ecstatic conductivity." As you continue with practices, which I'm sure you will, the ecstatic conductivity will increase over time. It should be a comfortable and smooth unfoldment as you continue to be attentive to self-pacing in practices according to your experiences. We can thank the purifying and stabilizing influences of deep meditation and spinal breathing for our continuing growth and stability.

I confess that the term "ecstatic conductivity" is something I came up with many years ago to describe my own experiences with it, which were similar to the experiences you are beginning now. It is the awakening of kundalini, and we also use kundalini terminology to describe it. Every tradition has its own language for the experience. In these modern times, where we are able to understand such changes as an awakening of the latent capabilities in our nervous system, we can describe it as the rise of increased conductivity in the electrical circuits (nerves) in our body. That is what it is. And it is pleasurable, as you point out. The pleasure keeps increasing as the conductivity increases, eventually beyond all human comprehension, I might add. So it can be called "ecstatic" conductivity, which it certainly is.

Why is it happening to you now, and where is it leading? Well, it is your time, you know. You are doing powerful practices every day, and the time has come for your nervous system to open. It is like a second puberty that is happening in so many of us as we begin our journey into the internal divine lovemaking that leads to the unity enlightenment stage. When kundalini begins to awaken, the inner union, the marriage of our divine polarities, is in the offing. It could take only a few years, or many years, for the process to complete itself, depending on the remaining obstructions in our nervous system, and the degree of dedication we have in our daily practices. And where will it lead? Union is freedom in unending ecstatic bliss and divine love, of course. It is our destiny – it is the birthright of each and every one of us. We have explored this in discussions in the lessons on the milestones and stages we experience on the journey to enlightenment.

The fruition of the journey is also discussed in the tantra lessons from a slightly different perspective – the point of view of Sri Vidya and its *Sri Yantra* sacred diagram. See lesson #T25.

I wish you all success as you continue on your journey to ecstatic bliss and unending divine love.

The guru is in you.

Lesson 170 – That's Kundalini?

Q: After I meditated in yoga about 12 years I feel an energy in my chest, and I feel illuminated and in control. In the chest I think is the chakra. I also smell fine odors and hear some music. I feel energy in all my body. Very pleasurable. That's kundalini?

A: Very nice. Yes, all such experiences are symptoms of kundalini/ecstatic conductivity. Try not to become overly attached to them, and continue your practices. Practices will bring you steadily to enlightenment. The experiences are the side effects along the way, sometimes distracting due to their pleasurable aspects. Enjoy them as appropriate, but be sure and favor your practices. Experiences do not produce enlightenment. Practices do. You are doing very well. It is an honor to have you here.

The guru is in you.

Lesson 171 – Spinal Bastrika Pranayama – Pressure-Washing Your Karma

Now we will introduce a powerful new pranayama practice called "spinal bastrika." "Bastrika" means "bellows." It is rapid breathing, like a dog panting, done with the diaphragm only (abdominal breathing), preferably through the nose. If it is too difficult through the nose, it can be done through the mouth, as necessary.

Bastrika in these lessons is done tracing the spinal nerve quickly between the perineum (root) and the point between the eyebrows (third eye), just the same as during normal spinal breathing, only much faster. The spinal aspect brings greatly increased power to bastrika pranayama, and at the same time provides balance between the divine inner polarities in the body. Spinal bastrika charges the entire nervous system with huge amounts of cleansing prana in a balanced way.

This practice is excellent for clearing out stubborn karmic blockages throughout the nervous system by sending powerful pranic pulses up and down inside the spinal nerve, and surging out through every nerve in the body.

As with any practice, some prerequisites and cautions are in order, so let's consider them.

First, spinal bastrika is not a cure-all, not a very good stand-alone practice. It will only work well if sufficient prerequisite practices have been stable for some time. These include spinal breathing and deep meditation. Spinal bastrika is done in-between these two during sitting practices. Its greatest effects are found when it is used in conjunction with the core practices of spinal breathing and meditation.

Second, if you have any health condition that could be aggravated by this extended panting style of breathing, then please do refrain. If in doubt, check with your doctor first.

Third, under certain circumstances spinal bastrika can aggravate an inner blockage, and should obviously be tempered then. More often, it will release blockages without aggravation, and can be used more aggressively then. You only will find out how your nervous system responds to spinal bastrika when you try, which is why it is good to start out slow and use careful self-pacing. Keep in mind that there can be a delayed reaction with spinal bastrika – you will not feel all of the effects immediately.

Spinal bastrika is most useful if the ground has already been cleared underneath and throughout the nervous system with deep meditation and spinal breathing. Then spinal bastrika can help finish off the job of getting lingering stubborn karmic blockages out. In that sense, it is like a pressure washer brought in to break loose and flush out those tough obstructions that have already been loosened up with meditation and spinal breathing.

As mentioned, bastrika means "bellows." I call it "doggy panting," signifying a more gentle sustainable fast breathing approach than the huffing and puffing that bellows implies, though doggy panting can be made quite vigorous also. Sometimes it gets vigorous all by itself. It is a long series of shallow quick breaths, using the diaphragm only, and continued for the allotted time as attention goes with the breath up and down the spinal nerve between the root and third eye. It will take some getting used to. As with all practices, spinal bastrika will be a little "clunky" at first. You will find it takes some practice to have the attention going up and down quickly with the breath. Also, the lungs may tend to get gradually emptier or fuller during a long series of pants. This "drift" is normal, and it is okay to empty out or fill up the lungs as necessary several times during a spinal bastrika session to compensate for the drift. And if there is no drift, very good. Then just keep going with spinal bastrika for the allotted time.

It is recommended you start with two minutes of spinal bastrika right before meditation, after spinal breathing and whatever other pranayama you are doing then (yoni mudra kumbhaka or the chin pump). Continue with siddhasana, sambhavi, mulabandha, kechari, etc. Some uddiyana (slightly pulling in of the abdomen) can be done also during spinal bastrika. As you get the feel of the energy moving in spinal bastrika, your body will know instinctively what to do, and all of these maneuvers will refine by themselves. Once it settles in, spinal bastrika, with all of its related yogic components, is quite natural. It becomes a very pleasurable practice with long-lingering ecstatic results in activity, and makes a permanent contribution to enlightenment. When those karmic obstructions are gone, they are gone for good, and the light shines out brightly from inside.

With comfort established for two minutes of practice, after a week or two, spinal bastrika can be taken to three minutes, and eventually to five minutes, if desired. Spinal bastrika is very powerful in longer doses, so keep that (and the delayed effect) in mind as your experience advances.

You will find spinal bastrika to be helpful for deepening your meditation. With so much being loosened up during the several pranayamas before meditation, it makes the process of deep meditation to inner silence and global purification in the nervous system go much faster and smoother.

Spinal bastrika puts the overall purification process in a higher gear, loosening the nerves and cultivating the entire nervous system tremendously. Be sure to exercise self-pacing with spinal bastrika, and all of your practices. Always pace your practices so as not to exceed your comfortable limit of resulting purification in your nervous system. Take your time and find your balance with spinal bastrika in your routine of daily practices.

A little later in lessons we will look at some variations of spinal bastrika that can be used for more targeted karmic cleansing.

The guru is in you.

Lesson 172 – Spinal Bastrika Energy, Sleep and Time of Practice

Q: I've been practising 3-5 minutes of spinal bastrika in my sessions for the last few days. Amazing! Could not sleep last night I was so charged after the practice. I'll continue as is with the practices for a while with no further changes to see how stable I am in this routine. It also all adds up to 40-45 minutes twice a day now, so from a time perspective it is starting to get a little heavy for me at this stage.

A: Keep in mind that there can be some delayed reaction with powerful practices like spinal bastrika. It might feel great while doing it, and then a few hours or days later there can be a jam-up. So, it is wise to ramp up the time slowly to make sure the energy is flowing okay. Everyone will experience the energy a bit differently. And yes, the energy can be running around inside in a variety of forms (light, sound, physical vibration, etc.) for quite a while after practices, so doing your second routine before dinner and having a reasonably active evening is important to stabilize things before bed. If it isn't happening, then consider backing off a bit on practice time for a while until you find a good balance between practices, activity and sleep. From that stable balance you can explore steps to safely increase your speed. We want the energy awakening every nook and cranny of our nervous system for sure, and shall have it, but we want to pace things so as not to be wearing ourselves out. Rome was not built in a day, and we all need our sleep. Letting our rest go by the wayside continuously is not a sustainable path to enlightenment.

On the time of the practice routine getting a bit long, I recommend you keep it manageable in your overall day. Better to be doing a little less every day for months and years, than too much and burn out on it over the short run. This has been discussed in earlier lessons on time management (lessons #18 and #50). Of course, it is getting a little more complicated now with more practices in the mix, but the same principles apply.

Not much more time will be added to the practice routine in the lessons – a little more optional practice for targeted spinal bastrika near the end of the routine. The rest of the new practices will remain within in the current routine time (such as a second mantra enhancement). There is always flexibility to trim things to take a smaller bite out of our day. We will get into that in more detail once all of the practices have been covered. Then we will lay them all out and look at them as a whole, and do some further refining and optimizing.

There are many ways to skin the cat of enlightenment, including ways that enable us to get a lot of deep purification done in two economical sittings each day. I know this is important, having spent many years in the business world myself. In a fast-paced culture, an efficient use of yoga practice time can make all the difference. So we will deal with it. Where there is a will there is a way!

The guru is in you.

Lesson 173* – Spinal Bastrika Cycle Time

Q: Thanks for your lesson on bastrika, the fast vigorous spinal breathing pranayama. Kindly just mention what should be the ideal number of bastrika breaths per minute. Also, I am doing bastrika for about 5 minutes. Is this ok?

A: The bastrika pace is like a dog panting comfortably. No cycle time is ideal. What is comfortable for you is ideal. Sometimes it will speed up or slow down by itself. The nervous system knows what it needs. Go with it as long as it does not become uncomfortable.

Five minutes of spinal bastrika is much too long starting out. If you are new to this practice, do only two minutes until you know your experience in practice and daily activities is smooth. Then you can inch your time up, monitoring your experiences along the way. You may wish to review the lesson on spinal bastrika again.

Wishing you much success in your practices.

The guru is in you.

Addition – Here is another Q&A on some of the practical aspects of spinal bastrika practice.

Q: I have started bastrika and a few questions about it came out. I have been doing the following sequence:

1. Spinal breathing (10 minutes)
2. Chin pump kumbhaka (aim – up to 5 minutes)
3. Spinal bastrika (aim – up to 5 minutes)
4. Meditation (20 minutes)
5. Samyama (5 minutes)
6. Yoni mudra kumbhaka (aim – up to 10 minutes)

Is this right order? I know you warned me before about not overdoing pranayama. I progress carefully. Moreover, I have been doing pranayama for a couple of years already, but in more "free-diving" fashion. In many yoga books the advice is to perform bastrika before kumbhaka. What do you think?

In most sources, bastrika is 40-60 cycles per minute. Is this what I should aim for? During bastrika we use "shallow quick breaths, using the diaphragm only." What happens with the belly? Do we expand it filling with air like balloon when inhale and contract muscle on exhale (in Taoism it is called "fire breathing"), or keep the belly muscles more or less under control using the diaphragm only?

A: Yes, your routine is okay. Ramp up to your target times carefully one practice at a time, as previously discussed. You can add asanas on the front end if you wish. Don't forget rest at the end of practices, 5-10 minutes at least. Ending rest is very important to assure smoothness in activity. Rest can be done lying down, if desired.

Spinal bastrika is at one's own pace, as fast as is comfortable. The example of "dog panting" was given. Each person will find their own rhythm. It will become automatic yoga – slower sometimes, faster other times. Counting breaths is not recommended during spinal bastrika, because it can divide the attention as it oscillates quickly between brow and root. Bastrika can be done before spinal breathing or chin pump if you wish. You are right about that being more traditional. The reason we have bastrika after spinal breathing is because it will be much more refined after spinal breathing and some kumbhaka. Then there is more kumbhaka later on with yoni mudra. It is the practitioner's choice. It is not possible to make big mistakes moving pranayamas around a bit like that. Just keep the spinal breathing in front of meditation. That is important. Also, be very measured in the length of all your practices. That is important also. Otherwise, it will be easy to overdo and run into excessive energy flow problems, which we don't want. Maintaining stability through a good balance in practices is essential for steady progress.

Diaphragm breathing is the same as belly breathing. It is the diaphragm that makes the belly move in and out. So, yes, the belly can move. Other times the belly may pull in and up a bit during bastrika due to automatic yoga. The diaphragm will still be doing the breathing, but the belly may be pulling up too. This is a combination of bastrika and uddiyana/nauli. We should not aim for this in practice, but if it happens due to automatic yoga sometimes, we don't fight it. Both ways are good. With the belly moving during bastrika, the lower centers are stimulated. With the belly pulling up during bastrika, the energy is being drawn up. There will be a time for both during spinal bastrika. The nervous system knows. Without a clear inclination one way or the other, we go with the belly breathing.

Best wishes for your continuing practices!

Lesson 174 – Sex and Sambhavi

Q: As I practice yoga following your guidance, some additional questions come up regarding certain matters. I was hoping you could relate to them:

Sexual arousal during meditation – During meditation and pranayama I experience great sexual arousal. I know this is a usual symptom, but I believe I experience it in a rather extreme way; the sensations are very strong at times, and moreover – at times I even experience ejaculations during meditations (I do not notice it while it happens, only after the session is over). I don't even practice siddhasana yet – it simply happens while following the mantra. Isn't it a horrible waste of prana? Is there any recommended way to avoid it?

Crossing eyes during sambhavi – the act of directing the eyes towards the point between the eyebrows quite worries me. Obviously, this is not a natural activity for the eyes, and is (even when done gently) very straining and stressing for them, especially considering the effect of accumulating effort during long periods. Isn't it hazardous to the functioning of the eyes? Couldn't it affect one's eyesight?

A: Actually, sexual arousal is not a common symptom during meditation and spinal breathing without siddhasana. It is a sign of good things happening though, as it is an advanced experience of purification. The emissions will not last, so don't be overly concerned about them. Consider it to be a stage, like wet dreams. In this case, wet spiritual dreams as you travel through a second puberty of the spiritual variety. Genital arousal and emissions will stop as the obstructions come out and normal ecstatic functioning of your lower centers in conjunction with your higher ones evolves.

When you do get into siddhasana, it will be more of a help than an aggravation to the situation. First of all, it will gradually coax your sexual energy inward and higher, and the tendency to go down with the energy will become much less. Secondly, siddhasana can be used to block emissions. When the heel is properly and comfortably placed in the soft area behind the pubic bone, the urethra can be blocked by leaning forward slightly. Not that saving a few emissions is so crucial, but the ability is there in siddhasana and can be used for that as desired. Before you bombard me with questions on that one, please go and check out the tantra lessons, if you have not already. There you will find detailed lessons covering the management of sexual energy in relation to yoga.

Regarding sambhavi, all practices we undertake have a "clunky" stage in the beginning, and any of the practices might seem a bit unnatural starting out. As they settle in, that perception changes. As their role in purifying and stimulating the opening of higher experiences in the nervous system occurs, the idea of unnaturalness goes by the wayside. Then we know that the practices are doing exactly as they are supposed to – bringing up natural spiritual abilities contained within our nervous system. By the time it gets to that point, the practices are as natural as breathing, because we immediately experience bliss and ecstasy from their use. The cause and effect of them in our nervous system becomes an integral and automatic part of our neuro-biological functioning.

Don't force sambhavi. Be very easy about directing your eyes, favoring the sensation created by the slight furrowing of the brow at the point between the eyebrows. In time it becomes pleasurable and then easily becomes automatic. Your eyesight is not at risk. Thousands of yogis, sages and saints have been using sambhavi for thousands of years without negative effects. Just the opposite; sambhavi opens our inner sight, expanding our vision through our increasingly ecstatic nervous system to encompass the cosmos. You may want to check another lesson on doing sambhavi (#131) which gives further detail on the technique, including an exercise to aid in coordination of the eyes during spinal breathing.

Interestingly, your question on sambhavi is related to your question on sexual arousal. The reason I say this is because the rise of a direct sexual connection between the physical brain and the lower centers is how the awakening of the third eye and sushumna (spinal nerve) is experienced. Sambhavi is one of the key players in this, along with spinal breathing, mulabandha, siddhasana, kechari and kumbhaka, plus a few others. Sambhavi in one form or another is prominent in all of the spiritual traditions. When the third eye/sushumna is awakened, sambhavi becomes a primary means for promoting "ecstatic conductivity" at will in the nervous system (see recent lesson #169 on ecstatic conductivity). A simple intention with the eyes is enough to produce waves of ecstasy in the nervous system of the yogi and yogini. What a treasure sambhavi is!

When the conductivity begins to come up by all the means mentioned, the sexual implications are unmistakable. From there it evolves from sexually erotic to spiritually ecstatic. The two experiences are related, being different expressions of sexual energy evolving higher in our nervous system.

You are having some shades of this already from meditation and spinal breathing only, and no doubt your fledgling sambhavi is getting into the act too. It is a sign of good things to come. Don't worry, everything will work out fine. There is nothing to fear.

The guru is in you.

Lesson 175 – Suspending Breath and New Experiences

Q: Today while practising breath awareness during slow breathing, I started to feel the breath backwards from the nostrils – top of nose – throat – chest cavity – upper stomach. I decided to probe further and started to go further down to the navel point and below it. Suddenly I realized my breathing was almost nil! Very, very faint as though I am not breathing at all; I could feel air in the lower abdominal cavity, then I continued concentrating and to my surprise:

Though I was stunned about faint breath and not thinking about sex, the sexual organ was getting very aroused. Also during pranayama if concentration is on the forehead I can feel energy flowing from the chakra, but this time it was flowing upward from the lower abdomen (I'm not sure about the chakra's name). Strangely, only while in siddhasana I felt the intense energy, but not while lying down. The first time while practising I saw a vision of a hissing snake around a shiva lingam.

Why did the above things happen?

A: Thank you for writing and sharing. All of those experiences are signs of purification and eventual full opening of your nervous system to divine experience. It is normal for breath to reduce in meditation and spinal breathing, even just beginning. The symptoms indicate your nervous system is spiritually sensitive and that you will likely continue to respond well to daily yoga practices such as deep meditation, spinal breathing pranayama and other practices designed to stimulate the nervous system toward greater openings.

You did not mention if you are doing sitting practices from these lessons, or elsewhere. Your experiment with breathing and attention, while interesting, is not something that will promote your spiritual growth very much. If you are not doing regular daily practices, you may wish to consider going through the lessons from the beginning. Not only will you learn solid practices, but you will also see many similar experiences discussed, and how to handle them.

All experiences are signs of purification and opening, and the experiences themselves do not produce the spiritual progress. The practices do. If we find experiences coming up during practices, we just easily go back to the practice we are doing. Analyzing, trying to manage, or getting overly involved with physical sensations, visions and other inner sensory experiences during practices will be a distraction from our progress. So this is why we just favor the practice we are doing. This produces maximum results. The business of favoring practices over experiences is very important. It was first mentioned early in the lessons, and is revisited often, like now. Enjoy the scenery as it goes by, but don't take your eyes off the road so as to compromise your good driving (practices).

All you are seeing now is normal, and there is nothing to worry about. Good things are happening. Experiences come and go. Ecstatic bliss and rising enlightenment from practices come and stay, which is what we are all born to live. I wish you success on your chosen spiritual path.

The guru is in you.

Lesson 176 – Dissecting Samyama

Q: The question that arises is about the coherence and definition of samyama. Without these two, we don't have teachings, right?

I think that the *Yoga Sutras* on the eight limbs mean that dharana, dhyana and samadhi are levels that our consciousness passes through in practices. So, while practicing dharana, I am not yet in dhyana and samadhi. Once my dharana reaches dhyana, I am not in dharana or samadhi. And when my consciousness attains samadhi, I am no longer in dharana or dhyana, is that right?

How can I apply these three disciplines together? Probably only if I attain samadhi, so I can lower my consciousness to produce thoughts as objects of dharana to bathe the practice with the permanent state of being that is samadhi. Dhyana will occur as a melting of the two (dharana and samadhi). Is that right?

Bringing the focus to our samyama practice, is the inner silence after meditation on mantra a kind of samadhi? But if it is, what kind of samadhi is described in chapter 1 of Patanjali's sutras? Does this inner silence fit?

I know that this will be different in each person depending on how deep one goes in meditation, but the second question is that the levels of samadhi of chapter 1 of Patanjali's sutras are not easily identifiable.

Probably we don't need to understand this.

A: Your last statement is correct: "Probably we don't need to understand this."

When we get in the car to drive, we don't have to understand all that that is going on under the hood of the car. We just press on the gas pedal and go. Good integrated advanced yoga practices are like that. We just need to know where the easy-to-use controls are, and we use them and go. All the practices in the lessons are like that.

Keep in mind that Patanjali was trying to dissect and describe the inner workings of the human nervous system. The nervous system is there, and he (or you and I) do not define how it works. We can only try and describe it, understand its underlying principles, find the controls to open it, and use them to our advantage.

Dharana, dhyana and samadhi are words to describe aspects of the process of conscious mind that can go in two directions: Inward from attention on an object (dharana on right mantra in this case), to fading away (dhyana), to pure inner silence (samadhi). And outward from inner silence (resident samadhi – it can be any level and we don't split hairs on that), to attention/subtle feeling of an object (dharana on sutra) which is let go (dhyana) in silence. Then a flow of divine energy comes out from inner silence – samyama producing purification and siddhis.

We don't have to understand all these elements to do the simple practices of meditation and samyama. The practices themselves are enough to activate the machinery of the nervous system. The dissected elements Patanjali has identified are occurring mostly at the same time, overlapping in time. Some inner silence is there all the time once meditation has been going on for a few months. Dharana is a very little thing on a sea of silence – an instant of attention on something that is letting go immediately by the developed habit of meditation in the mind, and that letting go is dhyana. It is all a mental process involving cultivating and utilizing the natural state of stillness/inner silence in the mind. In doing that, we change everything in the body too, providing the foundation for the rise of ecstasy in our nervous system, and the joining of silence and ecstasy to produce the unity stage of enlightenment – ecstatic bliss and ever-flowing divine love. This is what we are designed to become on this earth. This is the "car" we are driving.

The practices are all we need to know. The rest is automatic. The primary purpose of intellectual understanding (the dissection of the process into named elements/limbs) is to remain confident of what we are doing so we will continue daily practices. Other than for that, we don't need to know the inner workings. It's all under the hood. Just press on the gas pedal and go. It is that simple. So simple that many have missed it for thousands of years. It is time for everyone to be informed on what we all have – this human nervous system, the gateway to the divine, easily opened if we know where the simple controls are. That is what the lessons are about. Only that – nothing else. Spiritual science is interested only in reliable results that anyone can produce using the most efficient methods. And spiritual science is always looking for even better ways to utilize natural principles in the nervous system to open to the infinite within.

The guru is in you.

Lesson 177 – Advanced Siddhasana

Q: What is happening when I put my heel under our perineum in siddhasana. Can it be harmful? It feels ok when I'm doing it but I have noticed my sex drive has declined or is maybe more controlled. Is control of sex drive a part of the spinal breathing and siddhasana? I just wanted to be sure I'm not cutting off blood circulation or doing anything harmful. I'm not complaining. I do feel great doing the spinal breathing, yoni mudra, etc... It has really helped my practice! I feel like a new person.

A: Spinal breathing, siddhasana and other practices that cultivate our life force (sexual energy) up into the nervous system do not reduce our ability for sex. Rather they expand our use of sexual energy beyond the reproductive function, up into the awakening spiritual neuro-biology throughout our body.

It is correct that this expanded role of sexual energy in our nervous system gives us more "control" over sex. Actually, it is less dependency we experience, and less obsessive need for sex. We finally have a choice, and we can relate to our sexual energy and our lover in much healthier ways, even as we are steadily rising into the ecstatic bliss of enlightenment in our daily life.

Siddhasana plays a key role in this transformation. As taught in the lessons, it is a safe and healthy practice with huge long-term benefits. I have been using it with good success every day for over twenty years.

It so happens that a new lesson on advanced siddhasana was just posted in the tantra lessons, covering enhancements that can be made to basic siddhasana by mature practitioners. It also addresses fundamental questions regarding the what and the why of siddhasana.

The lesson is #T28, "Advanced Siddhasana for Women and Men." It should cover your questions about siddhasana, and then some. It is okay to read it without going back to the beginning of the tantra lessons. But if you want to read more on tantra, it is suggested you start at the beginning of those lessons.

It looks like you are doing very well there. I wish you all success as you continue along your chosen spiritual path.

The guru is in you.

Lesson 178 – Dharma

Q: I have been an outdoor painter for many, many years. Though I have never sat to purposely meditate, I can not recall once while in the "painting process" consciously "thinking." There is the "stillness" of being in right brain mode, which I always felt was my meditation. I'm not far into the lessons, but finding them interesting and will probably try "meditation without painting."

A: Your "painting meditation" is beautiful. Everyone should be so blessed to find inner silence in the work they do. I'm sure it has brought you much peace and spiritual growth over the years. It is called our "dharma" – activity we do which supports our spiritual unfoldment.

Adding sitting yoga practices such as deep meditation and spinal breathing will broaden and stabilize your presence in silent pure bliss consciousness. One of the wonderful characteristics of yoga is its connectedness through our nervous system. By this I mean that your painting meditation will help your sitting meditation and vise versa, and so too will breathing (pranayama) methods interconnect with the other practices you are doing. All yoga practices connect through our nervous system, producing a leveraging effect, taking us ever higher.

By the same principle, one kind of practice will often lead us to additional kinds of practice. The nervous system instinctively knows what it needs once the inner doors begin to open. So, it is likely that your painting meditation has increased your receptivity to other methods of yoga.

I wish you all success on your continuing inner journey. Enjoy!

The guru is in you.

Lesson 179 – The Star Revisited

Q: I am reading the previous posts and feeling the desire to return to yoga practice and most especially meditation.

About 4 years ago I was meditating regularly at night and this is what happened: I always see a purple cloud like object that begins to pull my consciousness through the tunnel as I call it. My mantra is usually the word or image of the word God. When I go through the tunnel – I see what looks like the universe of stars – filled with little white beams that seem to be stars in the heavens. I just linger there.

But, this one time the little star or light beam began to move towards me (my pineal, as I call it – the third eye). At first I felt somewhat alarmed and then I just said, "Let only that which is of God come to me." And I continued my mantra of "God." When the light became close I realized it was a huge white sphere of beautiful and light, and attached to it and flowing out of it was a multitude of dancing ribbons. The movement was beautiful, as was the light of the sphere.

Eventually, as I observed it, the light completely merged with me – that is my pineal. For many weeks after that, I would get what I call "light flashes" in the front part of my cerebrum and I could see them as I was going about normal business.

I have always heard people who practice meditation say: "Do not focus on these events." My response to that is: It is pretty hard to not remember, feel and think about such a powerful phenomenon. It is not that I gave it power over me – it is just that I was amazed at the beauty and effect on me that the experience had!

Thank you for your thoughts.

A: Thank you for writing and sharing. That is a beautiful experience, and it is natural as the nervous system reaches an increasingly purified state.

You may want to review lesson #92, "The Star," which goes into some detail on the kind of experience you described. It can give you some additional perspective on your inner anatomy. Reported experiences of group members are discussed in many places in the lessons as they relate to practices.

Experiences are the "scenery" we notice on the way to enlightenment. We are certainly entitled to enjoy the visions that come. At the same time, it is important to recognize that experiences are a product of the purification occurring in our nervous system due to daily practices. As with any journey, we can enjoy the view along the way. But to reach our destination, obviously, we must keep on traveling. That means gently favoring the practices we are doing over experiences that may come up during our routine. After our practices, during the day, if we have visions, we can enjoy them, or favor the work we may be doing at the time. It is our choice. Inner experiences will become a regular part of our life, and we will go on to ever-higher expressions of the divine shining out through us. In time, we become pure channels of divine love in the world.

This is where humanity is heading – to more enlightenment coming up in everyone in everyday living. It is happening as more and more people engage in daily practices, and everyone doing practices is helping everyone else energetically. No one has to go anywhere for this. We are opening right here in the life we are presently living.

If you are ready to resume practices it is suggested you go through the lessons from the beginning. They give a step by step build-up of integrated practices that stimulate steady purification and opening of the nervous system. I think you will find lots of interesting information relating to your spiritual unfoldment. If you are using a system of practices from another source, then just use the lessons as "food for thought." You are in charge of your journey.

I wish you all success as you travel along your chosen spiritual path. Keep your hands on the wheel, and enjoy the ride!

The guru is in you.

Lesson 180 – Off to a Good Start in Meditation

Q: I just wanted to tell you how glad I am you started this group. I will be the first person to admit how skeptical I was of yoga. I decided to at least read and educate myself. But after my very first meditation session, I have to admit that I have never felt so relaxed. It was very strange, yet comfortable. The time flew by, my meditation lasted about 26 minutes and it seemed like 5 minutes. A few things did happen that I did not see mentioned in the lessons. I felt "tingly" and numb. I even had small visions, if you want call them that, of light "dancing" and forming into small balls of light. Anyway, I just wanted to tell you how "At Peace" I feel with myself after my first lesson. I have a very stressful life and a lot of things that need to be "flushed" out, and I will be continuing your lessons as long as it takes. I am smiling right now, something I have not done in I do not remember how long. Thank You! You have made me a believer.

A: You are off to a great start with meditation, and this is wonderful. As you get further into the lessons you will find more information that will help broaden your understanding of the process of purification and opening of your nervous system to the reality within. The inner lights and tingling you have experienced right away are symptoms of good things happening – inner openings. When experiences like this come up during meditation, and you realize you are off into them, just easily go back to the procedure of meditation, which is easily going back to the mantra. There is a lot of discussion throughout the lessons on how to handle experiences during practices. Experiences are a good sign of progress on our journey to enlightenment, but it is practices that move us forward, and this is why we favor the practice we are doing during the time of our routine. That doesn't mean we can't take a look out the window once in a while as we cruise down the road and enjoy the beautiful scenery.

While you have had an exceptionally good start in meditation, I must tell you that it will probably not always be idyllic like that. We all may not start out with such a smooth experience, and this is no reflection on the progress, peace and joy we will experience as we continue to meditate. As the nervous system is being purified during yoga practices, sometimes the experience can be very clear and blissful. Other times it can be a bit murky as obstructions are being loosened deep inside and coming out. Whatever the experience is, good progress is happening as we follow the procedure of meditation. It is important to understand the mechanics so we will be clear about the effectiveness of our practice during both the idyllic and the murky experiences. Both have their fascinations and their distractions, and both will yield more clarity in our activity in daily life as we undergo gradual purification and find more blissful silence coming up from within. The most important thing is that we continue with daily practice for as long as it takes. If we have that attitude, enlightenment will not elude us.

This is why "desire" was the first topic covered in the lessons after the brief introduction on yoga. The cultivation and direction of desire is repeatedly touched on, and then covered in its full implications as the rise of "bhakti," which means, "love of Truth, or God."

All of this is to say, once we learn to rely on our ongoing spiritual desire (bhakti) and commitment to cultivating the divine union within ourselves, then we can sustain our daily practices over the long haul, no matter what. Then our motivation is not dependent the ebbs and flows of daily experiences, even as they steadily grow to become unending (and sometimes overwhelming) ecstatic bliss over the course of our journey in yoga.

Of course, this experience of enlightenment is what we are all after. The paradox is that the best way to cultivate it is not by focusing on the experience, but on effective practices that cultivate it over the long term.

You will find many new things coming up as you move forward in yoga. One of the most interesting and useful is the natural "connectedness" of the different aspects of yoga through our nervous system. This means that while spiritual desire leads to meditation, meditation also leads to more spiritual desire, yogic breathing methods and a range of other practices. Then all of these new practices lead to other yoga connections. It is like we are living in a glass house with dirty windows. As we clean one window, we can better see all the other windows that need to be cleaned, and we can also see more cleaning tools and are drawn to use them. The yoga methods are about cleaning all the windows. The more cleaning we do, the more ways we find to do the job faster and better.

Once the nervous system starts to become purified from within, it knows what it needs to hasten the process, and all we have to do is go with it. The lessons are designed to accommodate this rising connectedness of yoga we experience. As you continue to meditate you will notice this phenomenon occurring in many areas of your life. It is like waking up to a whole new luminous world that was right here in front of us all the time. Enjoy!

The guru is in you.

Lesson 181 – Expectations and Our Time Line

Q: I have recently joined your group. In Sept 2003, the root knot of kundalini opened. I was practising kriya yoga for one year before. Since then with any spiritual gathering or intense worship my heart chakra opens and I feel the spinal flow going upwards, coming out through the top of the head, fontanel. I believe that is Satya Sai Baba, as I am his devotee. Still, full enlightenment is eluding me. Can you help?

A: Thank you for writing and sharing. Your experiences of opening are very beautiful, but probably do not represent the end of your journey to enlightenment – more like the beginning of a new and wonderful stage.

There is the idea out there that kundalini energy moving to the crown is the end of the enlightenment process. It rarely is. In fact, if it is premature, before adequate preparation is done, it can signal a long and difficult ordeal (see "crown opening" and "Gopi Krishna" in the topic index). If you are consistently using spinal breathing between third eye and root, you will likely be spared the greatest difficulties of kundalini imbalance that can happen due to premature focus on the crown (sahasrar). We will be covering more on opening the crown in future lessons.

More importantly, it is essential to be cultivating inner silence (pure bliss consciousness) through deep meditation to round out the neuro-biological transformation going on inside. If you read through all the lessons, you will see the importance of this discussed from many angles. Enlightenment is a union of divine polarities within us, and kundalini/Shakti is only one half of that equation. Inner silence/Shiva is the other half.

As for having the blessing (and shaktipat) of a great one such as Sai Baba, it certainly can't hurt. Even so, the obstructions in your nervous system will have to come out to reveal your enlightenment, and no one can hasten that process beyond the physical limits you can tolerate. In other words, for most it is a long and gradual journey of unfoldment. It can be done in a lifetime, but not likely in a few years, unless you are of avatar stature (a savior born nearly enlightened), which we would all welcome, of course.

It is more likely that you have more work left to do. The good news is that there are plenty of good integrated yoga tools available, and you have the blessing of a great one besides. It is just a matter of bringing your expectations in line with your actual time line, and proceed with gusto from there.

It is suggested you settle in for the long haul and focus on doing a routine of good integrated spiritual practices every day. Then you have the best opportunity for rapid progress. You may wish to review the lessons from the beginning and check for elements of practice you may not be using yet that can help accelerate your progress.

It is wonderful to have the blessings of saints and sages, but in the end it is we who must follow through on our spiritual transformation with the daily use of yoga practices.

I wish you all joy and success on your chosen spiritual path.

The guru is in you.

Lesson 182* – Healthy Skepticism

Q: I like your writing – both the content and the style. Your approach is sane and practical. But some aspects don't satisfy me. Isn't the "spinal breathing" a hyperventilation with attention on an imaginary spinal nervous channel? How does the mix of breathing physiology and mental phenomenon really purify the "nervous system?" Are the so-called impurities physical (physiological) or mental? You rightly point out that visions, etc. don't mean "realization." Nobody knows how the body-mind interaction works. But the yogic lifestyle of meditation, contentment, "yama-niyama," does alter one's world-view. How do you characterize "divine love?" Is it "karuna" compassion? Maybe you can shed some light on these questions.

A: Thank you for your note. It is much appreciated. Healthy skepticism is good because it reduces the tendency toward blind faith and superstition, which are not good for yoga or spiritual progress – as long as skepticism does not become extreme and kill our desire to seek the truth altogether. Then skepticism becomes a kind of superstition itself. A good intellect is one that is inquiring and balanced, and willing to accept the demonstrated truth of things, even if it means dissolving the intellect (and ego) in the process!

As you can tell, I have a scientific orientation and view yoga as both an ongoing experiment and the application of known causes and effects. For this reason you find minimal theory and philosophy in the lessons. The lessons are not to entertain the curious mind. They are to offer solid means for us to change what we are on this earth for the better, if we choose to. There is a lot we don't know. But we are here, and we can grow in our experience of life in remarkable ways if we are willing to do what is necessary to stimulate our nervous system to go in its natural evolutionary direction.

If you find the explanations of things hard to believe, that's okay. They are just explanations, just ideas. The practices are something else. If we do them in the ways suggested, changes will happen in us. No one has to take anyone else's word on that. It is a personal experience each of us can have in the privacy of our own room, and in our daily activities. The experiment of yoga is one everyone can do, and that is the first and last word on yoga for all of us. So, consider the experiment and see what you find in yourself. It can be a wonderful surprise – one so attention-grabbing that it can give us a belief in our divine possibilities. The best yogis and yoginis are both believers and skeptics. They believe there is a destination, and they will accept nothing but the most effective means for traveling there. They leave cults and dogmas behind, after they have harvested the seeds of truth from them. And they are constantly on fire to carry on the journey.

Having said all that, I'll take a shot at your questions. Keep in mind that, if you give the practices a fair try, your own experience in these things will outweigh anything that I, or anyone else says about them. You are the playing field. Everything else is just information and advice.

On spinal breathing, hyperventilation is too much oxygen in the bloodstream. That is why people who are hyperventilating are advised to breathe in a paper bag for a few minutes until they can reduce the over-oxygenation. Spinal breathing and most other forms of pranayama are the opposite. Pranayama means "restraint of life force (breath)." So with pranayama we are systematically and safely restraining oxygen consumption. Why? It stimulates the life force stored in the body (mostly in the pelvic region) to compensate, to move up into the nervous system to nourish us. It is a neuro-biological phenomenon. This produces both calming and energizing effects in the body and mind.

Can this life force substance/energy be directed with the attention? Experience indicates that it can. By directing it up and down through the spinal nerve between the point between the eyebrows and the perineum, something happens. In time, it is no longer an exercise of the imagination. An awakening occurs and it becomes a neuro-physical event. I call it the rise of "ecstatic conductivity." In any case, the spinal nerve can be induced by the attention used with breath to produce a permanent awakening that produces a wide range of neuro-biological and psychic effects. I can't tell you exactly why this is so. But I can tell you that it is so from experience. Many others can verify this, and you can find quite a few examples in the Q&As. It is also described in writings going back thousands of years. Not that we have to take anyone else's word for it. It is what it is – a path to somewhere that the human nervous system can take us.

Enterprising humanity is such that whenever there is someplace new to go, someone will go there. If the place is good, then many will go eventually. Maybe we are on the verge of many people going to this wonderful place called "enlightenment." It is only a matter of describing the place and marking the route. Many have done so. These lessons are another attempt at it, leaning toward a more open scientific approach.

The purification aspect you ask about is mysterious, I admit, yet does happen in those who do yoga practices. It happens in mind, emotions and body, and these are intertwined. We know that the human body will purify (and also heal) itself when given the opportunity. This happens during rest. It also happens whenever normal loads are taken off the body or mind. Fasting has been shown to produce purifying effects in the body. Pranayama is a kind of fasting, involving air – and is found to produce physical effects. Meditation is also a kind of fasting, involving thinking – systematically allowing the mind to become still. We don't force the mind to stillness. It just happens automatically when the right conditions are set up in the mind. Generally, purification happens in the body when we allow something to reduce or stop – food, air, thoughts, metabolism, etc. When any or all of these come to be less, or completely at rest, then purification happens.

Purification from yoga can take on many forms – ranging from seemingly random streams of thought, to unusual emotions, inner sensory events, and physical indications such as involuntary body movements, perspiration, physical sensations, etc. In rare cases, rashes, fevers, pain and other extreme physical symptoms can happen. A big part of yoga is about managing practices in such a way so as to keep the level of purification going on as stable and comfortable as possible. I get emails every day from people who are trying to balance practices with various symptoms of purification. The variety of physical, emotional and mental symptoms of purification that can come up in yoga seems endless. The neuro-biological process of purification and opening is very real, and is at the heart of the journey of yoga. That is why there is so much emphasis on self-pacing of practices in the lessons.

"Divine love" is what happens as the nervous system purifies and opens to the point where our consciousness is much less identified with the body as self. Then everyone is becoming part of our own rising sense of oneness. Divine love (unity) is born of a neuro-biological union involving deep inner silence and ecstatic energies blending in our nervous system. Then, somehow, it expands beyond our physical body and we become the other. When we become the other and the other is as dear to us as our own self, that is love, yes? Everyone feels this intuitively. Peace, wisdom, compassion, conscience, selfless service and sacrifice are natural qualities we possess within ourselves. We may be in touch with them, or not, but they are there latent inside each of us.

The ongoing human drama is about revealing the light in ourselves as we overcome the darkness. Just about every story ever told has been about that, either literally or metaphorically. Why does this theme have such a universal appeal? Is it because we know instinctively that we are the light?

As we continue with yoga, the positive qualities in us do become stronger. This implies that as we continue to clear away the inner obstructions, something "divine" shines through from inside. Is this really true? Are we inherently divine? Again, it is cause and effect. If we continue in yoga, this is what eventually comes out. It is the experience of many throughout history. It has been written down for thousands of years. It is part of the human experience that is available to anyone who is willing to undertake the means to let it blossom out.

Don't take my word for it. Do the full investigation of yoga and find out for yourself. I wish you all success in your endeavor to uncover the truth.

The guru is in you.

Addition – Here is a Q&A from another skeptic who is feeling the divine desire coming from within. We all have had this conflict at one time or other in our life.

Q: In my last email, I asked you to explain the spinal breathing, and you referred me to the lessons. I looked at the specific lessons you mentioned, but I still seem to be having trouble understanding it all.

I am extremely skeptical by nature. Yoga is often said to be an experiential method whereby belief is not necessary, but again I have trouble with this. I am sad to note that I find psychic phenomena dubious, which includes the kundalini. I'm usually told that a little skepticism is good but this doesn't seem to satisfy me.

The spinal breathing that you teach is basically kriya yoga, isn't it? Now, I wanted to know exactly how this works physically on the body. I've heard of people that have done kriya for years and nothing happened for them, despite the fact that it is called the "airplane route to God." How can this be? It is also called "scientific" which I take to mean that if I follow the instructions, I should get the results. But this simply doesn't seem to be the case.

Please, can you put my doubts to rest? I want to believe in God, I want to believe in yoga, but it just all seems too confusing.

A: I know it can be tough to "keep the faith" if the experiences are not there as much as we would like. Then it is bhakti (desire for truth) alone that keeps us in the game. Bhakti will be more than enough, if it is cultivated. Then the rest will come.

The explanations you are looking for are in the lessons, but maybe they don't jump out if the corresponding experiences aren't there to attach them to. For the same reason, the *Bible, Bhagavad Gita* and other scriptures make much more sense to those having rising inner silence than to those who don't. That's just how it is. Spiritual practice is what will make the difference, even if it is just resolving to live a purer lifestyle and do daily deep meditation.

Spinal breathing pranayama has two aspects – the restraint of breath aspect, and the movement of neural energy through the nervous system with attention aspect.

Restraint of breath is pretty easy to explain in biological terms. We gently restrain the availability of oxygen in the body, either with slow breathing and/or suspension of breath (kumbhaka), and the body compensates by drawing energy up from the sexual essences stored in the pelvic region. This corresponds to the raising of kundalini, and it is, first and foremost, a physical experience, with a full range of physical and sensory symptoms, both inside and outside. So, kundalini is a neuro-biological experience before it is a spiritual one. Actually both are occurring at the same time – neuro-biological and spiritual are two sides of the same coin. That is what we mean by spiritual transformation of the human nervous system.

The movement of neural energy up and down the spinal nerve with attention is less easy to explain, yet is experienced directly as sensory sensations inside when it is done, once there has been some inner neuro-biological awakening from pranayama practice. However, that isn't all that is necessary. Some inner silence is necessary to provide a "screen" of silent awareness upon which all of this plays, which is where meditation comes in.

Yes, spinal breathing comes from kriya yoga, and kriya yoga comes from a much older tradition involving spinal breathing. The deep meditation used in AYP does not come from a spinal breathing/kriya-style tradition. It comes from mantra yoga. AYP is an integration of these two simple, yet powerful, methodologies, and many other powerful practices. This broad integration of practices increases the effectiveness of all the practices. The whole is greater than the sum of the parts, you know. A lack of broad integration of effective methods in some systems of practice may explain a lack of results.

All that has just been mentioned is in the lessons, admittedly, spread around a bit.

Rather than reaching to believe things you are not experiencing yet, maybe the best course is to follow your own desire in these matters. Your feelings are real, and can't be denied. You are obviously experiencing something, or you would not even be asking. Go with that, your own longing (bhakti), and do what it calls you to do, adding your common sense to the process. Cultivate that longing, and use it to inspire your conduct. Then you will have the inspiration you need to move forward. It is in your hands, no one else's.

The lessons are tools for you to use, if you wish. They are there to inspire also. With so many coming to the table with their experiences, challenges and successes, there can be little doubt that there is much to be gained by undertaking the spiritual journey in some form or other. What it is for you will be unique. You are doing it right now. I encourage you to carry on with your research.

Believe in your own deepest feelings about these things. They are the truth.

Lesson 183 – Movements and Automatic Yoga

Q: I have started to do yoni mudra kumbhaka and dynamic jalandhara along with spinal breathing and meditation. During meditation I find sudden jerks in some parts of my body like my hand moves involuntarily, and most times the upper part of my body moves towards the ground. These movements are sometimes distracting. I just want to know if this is normal, or am I doing anything wrong.

A: Yes, the jerks are normal. It is energy opening inner pathways. The movements will reduce as the pathways open and offer less resistance.

Sometimes movements point to "automatic yoga" positions. For example, if you feel compelled to go down to the mat with your head and torso while sitting, this is the sushumna (spinal nerve) wanting to stretch itself for more purification (it is called "yoga mudra"). If you do some "maha mudra" and "yoga mudra" as part of your asanas before pranayama and meditation it can help pre-empt the tendency during sitting practices. These are covered in the addition to lesson #71 on asanas. If your head and torso irresistibly want to go down during sitting practices, then let them for a few minutes. Or you can let yourself go into it for as long as necessary at the end of your sitting practices. It is a natural expression of the connectedness of yoga through your nervous system.

Obviously, we don't want to interrupt our sitting practices too much with spontaneous yoga positions, but sometimes these things happen, so we let them if the urge gets to be strong enough. The best way to minimize movements in pranayama and meditation is with a good set of asanas before we start. If the hands or arms are moving during sitting practices, using the jnana hand mudra can help (review lesson #135).

If the movements become too much, we do as we always do when symptoms of purification become excessive. We use self-pacing in our practices and back off for a while until we find stability in our routine, and continue from there. When we hit a few potholes in the road, we slow down until the road smoothes out again.

The occasional jerks are common at certain stages of development, and a sign of purification going on. Milestones on the road to enlightenment!

The guru is in you.

Lesson 184 – Teleportation, Samyama and Siddhis

Q: I was wondering what information you could provide me with this – teleportation. Currently, various siddhis powers have been developing, but none of them interest me. I understand that they are just by-products of a much larger picture. However, this has been a concern of mine. I have been aspiring to see a friend of mine who I haven't seen for many lifetimes.

Recently, I've developed "the power to" (as with many things), just not a method/understanding. Each time I try, I feel strong energy sensations throughout the entire body. Is it just a phase?

Thank you in advance for any advice you can give me.

A: The strong energy you feel on the way to siddhis is the real fruit of the performance. The siddhi itself is not the fruit. The fruit is the purification in our nervous system that facilitates our enlightenment, and that is of much greater value than any power we might develop as a consequence. If you are moving the energy toward siddhi without prerequisite practices and a balanced routine, it can be uncomfortable, too much for the nervous system in its current condition. It could also create karmic aberrations in your nervous system if too much attention is going for a particular siddhi. In other words, there is a cost for developing a particular power at the expense of our overall enlightenment.

Samyama is the means for purifying the nervous system from the inside (inner silence) outward, with siddhis being a by-product. As you review the lessons on samyama here you will find powers and their relationship to yoga discussed in detail, including referrals to the *Yoga Sutras* of Patanjali (available in the AYP links section on the web site) where more information on powers can be found. In the lessons, the method is given for practicing samyama to systematically promote balanced purification and opening of the nervous system to enlightenment. Before you use the samyama technique, I suggest you review all that comes before in the lessons – deep meditation, spinal breathing pranayama, mudras, bandhas, etc. Then you will have the means for preparation, and can see samyama, siddhis and your unfoldment in their full context. You may choose to add practices from the lessons that can accelerate your progress toward enlightenment. It is up to you.

As for seeing your long absent friend, if you have this desire, it will happen in due time. Making it a primary goal of your yoga could be a distraction to your spiritual progress though, and could generate more karma (future consequences) than it would release. My suggestion is to focus on your spiritual practices, with the goal for enlightenment, and let the rest happen naturally. Then all of your actions will become an expression of the divine within, which is what you are.

Jesus said, "Seek first the kingdom of God, and all else will be added to you." I wish you all success on your chosen spiritual path.

The guru is in you.

Lesson 185 – Role of the Intellect

Q: I have been reading the lessons present in this group from about a month or so ... It's really wonderful that I see people are experimenting and experiencing the yoga practices and finding fruits for their practices. I would like to bring a topic to your concern.

In all of these yogic practice lessons that I have gone through I have found that people mention visions of light and other things connected to their visions. What I feel about their vision is that they tend to have a pre-conceived notion about having a vision of light, or what they believe to be an experience of kundalini expansion in the nervous system even before they start their yoga practice. What I would like to get clarification on is: Is the duration of just one or two years of yoga practice enough to awaken the kundalini within us? I believe that they might be correct only to an extent of 10%, though I have personally never seen their experience. I am making this statement based on the fact that for good yogic practices it is very much necessary to have a good disciplined life of non-drinking, non-smoking and diet which will keep our body, especially our nervous system, free of any addictive effects.

The point I am trying to make here is that practising yoga without any jnana (intellectual understanding) could be a futile practice (I am not saying they are not knowledgeable).

The very term yoga means union, and union cannot be achieved by mere practising of asanas (I am not being sarcastic or skeptical here). Yoga of karma only when coupled with jnana (intellect) will help us achieve the ultimate nirvana or mukti (liberation).

The reason that I am mentioning about jnana is because jnana, according to me, is the inquiry of Self, which will kill our ahankaara and other egoistic views about the world we see. It enables a good yogi or yogini to not only find the real meaning of yoga but also attain mukti from the materialistic world.

I would request you to write more lessons concerning the jnana yoga (path of the intellect) which will clear the maya (illusion) that we live in and help us see the real light of the world.

A: Thank you for writing and sharing. In the lessons we start with meditation going immediately to inner silence, and through the connectedness of yoga this enlivens the yamas and niyamas (restraints and observances), which are the behavioral elements you mention as preparation for kundalini. So we approach those conduct things by going deep right away, and the conduct changes naturally. Instructions on diet and personal habits are not required much because the nervous system goes for that automatically with inner silence coming up.

Then one is ready for stimulating kundalini soon enough. Can it be done in a few years? Probably not awakened fully without previous experience in this life or another, and many do come wired for it like that, so their early experiences are real – not pre-conceived or imagined at all. Spinal breathing and associated mudras and bandhas are good for everyone, and will lead to awakening of ecstatic energies in due course. Everyone has to work from where they are at their own pace, and the lessons are designed for that. So you find people at many levels of experience here, all opening to their inner truth. It is wonderful!

Jnana (role of the intellect) is woven all through the lessons in the form of the primary inquiry, "Who am I? Is there something more?" and the decision to engage in practices as a result. Both the inquiry (which feeds bhakti) and decision (which feeds action in practices) begin as acts of intellect. Beyond those two basic yogic functions, the intellect has a tendency to build huge castles in the air, which is not much of a help to yoga. So the focus is on fanning desire to practice, not so much analysis, except for inspiring practices. It seems simple, doesn't it? It works.

If you try daily deep meditation as given in the lessons for a few months you will see how the intellect naturally fits in with this efficient approach to yoga. We have deliberately avoided building an edifice to jnana yoga in the lessons. For most of us it can end up becoming a distraction – going outward into a maze of ideas instead of inward to the simplicity and power of pure bliss consciousness, and up into endless realms of ecstasy.

As for the many spiritual experiences, if they inspire continuing daily practices, that is good. If experiences are lacking, that can also be used to inspire continuing daily practices. Inspiring practices and the importance of pacing practices so as not to overdo purification (discomfort) are the two main reasons why experiences are discussed. Beyond that, experiences can be a distraction also, and we mention that a lot, as you have probably seen. So we enjoy experiences as passing scenery if we are having them, and then easily go back to the practice we are doing.

The bottom line in the lessons is daily practices to stimulate the nervous system to purify and open. The heart and mind are used to inspire and sustain practices, and not much else. We don't worry much about our personal habits or lifestyle. If we have the desire to meditate, yoga is already happening, no matter what we are eating or smoking! Once meditation begins, the impurities (including non-yogic behaviors) start to drop off. The practices do work, and all the goodies come along naturally, including steadily increasing intellectual understanding of the intricacies of the process. It happens by direct observation.

Our purifying and opening nervous system is a very interesting book to read. Each day brings a new page filled with sacred knowledge. We are that.

The guru is in you.

Lesson 186 – Meditation – Second Enhancement of Mantra

As we meditate over many weeks and months we are releasing lots of obstructions that have been lodged deep in our nervous system for a long time. As our subconscious mind is gradually cleared out we find an underlying inner silence becoming more apparent in our daily life. It is, in fact, our true Self emerging as we clear out the muck that has been blocking us from experiencing our own true nature. As the process of meditation and deep purification in our nervous system continues, we become spiritually empowered by our rising inner silence, and are able to accomplish much more in illuminating ourselves (and all who are around us) with ecstatic bliss and divine love naturally flowing out through us.

Meditation is the core practice to stimulate our nervous system to yield all these wonderful spiritual results. The mantra is the vehicle we use in meditation to systematically bring the mind to stillness. As we do, we unleash our innate pure bliss consciousness, which dissolves and releases the obstructions in us.

We began with the powerful universal mantra, *I AM*, which takes us deep into the silent reaches of the mind effortlessly as we practice the easy procedure of deep meditation. As we became intimately familiar and smooth with this process of using the *I AM* mantra, we introduced the first mantra enhancement. This gave us the option to broaden our presence in pure bliss consciousness during meditation. The result of using an enhanced mantra is to stabilize more inner silence throughout our daily activities.

Now we are ready to cover a second enhancement to the mantra. But before we do, please go and review the discussion included with the first mantra enhancement. It is lesson #116, "Meditation – First Enhancement of Mantra."

This will save us from having to cover again here the basic concepts involved in mantra enhancement, and the analogy of stepping up the mantra in a way similar to how we skillfully shift gears in an accelerating car.

Now, if we are ready, we have the opportunity to shift gears again with a second enhancement of the mantra. We will still have the same root syllables of *I AM*, and also the syllables that were added with the first enhancement. And something more will be added now.

The second enhancement is a further expanded mantra. It is:

… SHREE OM SHREE OM I AM I AM NAMAH …

This mantra is used with the same procedure of meditation we learned in the beginning.

Note: As has been discussed on several occasions in past lessons, the *I AM* component of the mantra can also be spelled *AYAM*, with the exact same pronunciation.

You can see that this is quite a long mantra with many more syllables than the simple *I AM* we began with. It is important to understand that this is not a beginning mantra, and that no one will be served if it is used as such. If you are a new meditator, or have been using the first mantra enhancement for only a short while, undertaking this new mantra will not be in your best interest. It could bog you down and retard your progress, just as shifting to a higher gear in a car can bog us down if done too soon.

How will we know when it is time for us to shift to a more enhanced mantra? First, we will be smooth and stable meditating using our previous mantra for at least several months, with some steady silence being experienced in both meditation and in daily activity. Second, our bhakti (spiritual desire) will be compelling us to move forward. Both smoothness in our present practice and bhakti are necessary for us to make the shift.

With our present mantra, if we are having a lot of thoughts and sensations happening in meditation without a lot of silence, this is very good also. It means we are doing a lot of purification, and many obstructions are coming out. However, this is not the time to shift gears to a more enhanced mantra. Imagine you are driving up a steep hill in your car, and your engine is doing okay in the present gear, but not having power to spare either. Would you up-shift at that time? Of course not. It is the same with meditation. If we are unloading lots of obstructions with our present mantra, then this is not the time to shift to a higher mantra (gear). We just keep on going with our present mantra, and at some point we will see some clearing in our meditation process, with more silence coming up and fewer obstructions coming out. After some time in that situation, at least a few months, then we can go for the shift if we want to. If we don't want to, that is okay too. The entire journey can be made with *I AM*, or with the first enhancement, if this is our preference.

If we have shifted to an enhanced mantra too early, we will know it soon enough. We will feel like we are slogging through mud. We will be bogging down and not having good results in daily activity. It is not the end of the world. If we find ourselves in this situation ongoing, the solution is simple. We just shift back down to our previous mantra and go with that for a few more months, or however long it takes us to reach the point when we are ready to shift up. Self-pacing, remember?

A false start with a mantra enhancement can happen, but we should avoid it if we can. The reason is it takes time for a new mantra to settle in. If we have shifted too early and are trying to settle in with the new mantra, and then decide to go back to the previous one, it will take time again to change the pattern of the mantra deep in the mind. For this reason we do not change mantras often, up or down. We want to be going deep with our mantra in one place. These enhancements are for facilitating that process. Beyond these basic shifts we do not switch our mantra around. Neither do we try and use multiple mantras, not with the approach in these lessons. We want to cultivate the ability to go deep in every sitting. To do this, we will be best served by using a single vehicle, our mantra.

So let's take our time, and do everything we can to produce good progress while maintaining stability and comfort in our routine.

Regarding this second enhancement to the mantra, no doubt there will be some questions about what the components are for. Why this particular mantra?

For starters, as has been previously discussed, the mantra is not about language or meaning. The mantra at every stage is for stable and progressive vibrational quality deep in the nervous system. The quality of vibration is for maximum purification with comfort, and this can be clearly perceived with different mantra syllables by anyone who has ecstatic conductivity coming up in their nervous system.

This is why we started with *I AM* as the beginning mantra instead of something else. *I AM* is very balanced, stable and progressive deep in the nervous system. If we had started with *OM* for deep meditation we would have had a progressive beginning mantra also, but not such a balanced and stable one deep in the nervous system. In fact, *OM* can wreak havoc deep in the nervous system if prerequisite housecleaning has not been done. *OM* is not a good beginning mantra for this reason. As with so many things in spiritual life, this is a paradox, because *OM* can be seen and heard everywhere. It is even written on the subway walls! Yet, *OM* is not a good choice for a beginning mantra for deep meditation. *OM* is not so good in a first enhancement either, where we want to expand on *I AM*, beginning to develop another dimension of inner polarity in our nervous system. We do this with *SHREE*, which is also progressive and stable, and going in the desired new direction. With that in place, we are finally ready for *OM*.

Note: *OM* is fine for traditional chanting and kirtans (devotional singing), which do not go as deep into the nervous system as we do in our sitting meditation. So don't take this lesson to mean *OM* should not be used in the traditional ways.

Some might be thinking, "What is the big deal? Is the build-up of the mantra really so delicate?"

Yes, it is. As we facilitate the process of the mind going to stillness, we are entering the silent level of greatest power inside us. Recall that this is where samyama and siddhis (powers) originate also. If we are premature in our evolving practice with an angle of vibration with the mantra, it can produce a lot of upheaval as obstructions are released either too fast, or in the wrong order. In dealing with the inner workings deep in the nervous system, there are easy ways to do house cleaning, and there are hard ways. We will always opt for the easy ways whenever we can find them. We will get into more detail on the design of the mantra in another lesson.

Now you have the second enhancement of the mantra available for use whenever you are ready. Don't rush into it prematurely. It will be here when you need it, and I know you will find great inner joy using it then.

The guru is in you.

Lesson 187 – Establishing and Maintaining Daily Practice

Q: I came upon these lessons last week and have started the mantra twice a day. However, I missed last night. I got back at it this morning. I am very undisciplined, I don't sleep well and my days get off track sometimes. Do you have any suggestions for people like myself? Thank you

A: If you keep up with daily meditation for at least a few months, that will bring more steadiness and pleasurable feelings, and better sleep. Regularity in daily practice comes from the recognition of this "cause and effect" of meditation.

In the beginning, it is a matter of forming a habit. If you view meditation to be part of your regular routine of hygiene and nourishment, then it will fit into the normal sequence of morning and evening activities, and will be sorely missed if not done. Like bathing, brushing teeth, eating, etc., meditation is something we will do automatically. If we take that attitude about it, then the habit will be established and stick. It is our all-important spiritual hygiene and nourishment.

In the beginning and in the end it is about our desire for more in life. It is a chicken and egg thing. We want to meditate to feel good, and feeling good inspires us to meditate. Once we get it rolling with meditation, and experience some rising inner silence and clarity, then we have more continuous desire for daily practice – this is "devotion." Devotion going higher is called "bhakti," which is love of Truth or God. Once we have that we are always burning inside for spiritual progress, and the best way to achieve it is by doing our daily practices.

Going into more advanced yoga practices (spinal breathing, mudras, bandhas, etc.) happens from bhakti also. Then there is more blissful inner silence and also the rise of ecstasy in the nervous system. That makes us even hotter for daily practice, and we run to our meditation seat when we get home from work. At that stage our desire for daily practices is fed by the living light in our heart and the ever-increasing joy welling up from within. Our commitment to daily practices rises along with the spirit within us.

If you form the habit of daily meditation and keep going you will catch the bug. Actually, the bug will catch you. In time you will find your ordinary wants and desires transforming naturally toward maintaining your daily practices. Once the nervous system starts opening, it knows what it wants – more opening. So our motivation naturally goes for that.

Beyond knowing the most effective methods of yoga, establishing and maintaining daily practice is the greatest priority. This is how enlightenment grows in us.

The guru is in you.

Lesson 188* – Mantra Design 101

Q: You stated, *I AM* can be pronounced as *AYAM*; this is very similar (if not the same) as the tantric beeja mantra, *AYEIM*. Are these two the same?

What is the basis for the first and second enhancement to the *I AM* mantra? I mean you have probably written this on the basis of several years of experience with these mantras, and experiential knowledge is very hard to intellectually convey in many instances. Still I would like to know how you arrived at this mantra – I have never seen this mantra or anything similar in any of the classic tantric texts on mantra shastra. How is it that the mantra is *SHREE OM SHREE OM I AM I AM NAMAH* and not something like *SHREE OM I AM I AM NAMAH*? Why are there two *SHREE's* followed by *OM*?

And why does not the *SHREE* end in M (i.e., *SHREEM*) as is usually how it is used in mantras?

A: Thank you for writing, especially on this topic. I have been looking for an inspiration to post a lesson on mantra design. We can call it "Mantra Design 101." As with many things presented in these lessons, traditional approaches are respected but not necessarily adhered to strictly if direct experience guides us to a more optimal solution in yoga.

If the pronunciation is the same as for *I AM*, then *AYAM* and *AYEIM* are the same from the point of view of mantra. There may be different meanings for the different spellings in Sanskrit, but that does not matter. It is the vibration we are using. If you do a web search on "Sanskrit ayam" and also on "Sanskrit ayeim," you will find both used in various mantras. There is also a Muslim version spelled *AYYAM*.

If *AYEIM* is pronounced *AYEEM*, then it is not the same. *AM* and *EEM* go in opposite directions in the nervous system. With some ecstatic conductivity coming up it can be easily felt by anyone. This "feeling" is the basis of design of all the mantras in the lessons. They are not based solely on scriptures. In fact, no scriptural authority is claimed. Of course, nothing is conjured up out of nowhere either. The syllables are familiar, and have appeared in venerable scriptures, though the order of use may be a bit different here.

Mantra syllables are like tuning forks in the nervous system. Each vibration resonates in a different part of our inner circuitry. This is true with or without ecstatic conductivity previously awakened. The difference is that, when the nervous system is ecstatically awakened, the effects become experiential, and can be observed in the body. The effects are experienced with the inner senses and have an ecstatic overtone. The resonating effect of a syllable deep in the silence of the mind loosens obstructions in a particular way unique to that syllable. With that experience-based feedback, and knowing the most effective and safest order of awakening the nervous system, especially the spinal nerve, the mantras can be suitably assembled. Let's get more specific.

I AM (by any spelling) resonates in the full length of the spinal nerve from the third eye to the root.

This has not been said before in the lessons. It has only been hinted at. It has not been mentioned because I don't want to encourage anyone to think the mantra in any particular location in the body. The mantra resonates naturally with the particular part of the nervous system it is attuned to. We don't have to help it by directing it here or there. In fact, we can interfere with the natural resonance by doing that. So, don't locate the mantra, okay? Just pick it up easily and effortlessly wherever it may be, as always, and let it refine. If *I AM* is coming up in the feet, or anywhere else, it will resonate from the third eye to the root. Just as a tuning fork will vibrate the corresponding string of an instrument if brought anywhere in the vicinity.

Having said that, now you can do an experiment and observe if you want. If you think the sound *"I,"* maybe you can feel the subtle neurology in the head reaching out through the center of the brow. If not, no matter. That is where it naturally vibrates. No need to help it or feel it. That is where it is. Now, if you think the sound *"AM,"* maybe you can feel it going naturally down through the center of the body. If not, well, no matter. When ecstatic conductivity comes up you will. Feeling it has no bearing on the effectiveness of the mantra. Feeling it is only a symptom of the degree of purification we have in the nervous system, and the degree of ecstatic conductivity (kundalini) we have coming up. It will come to all of us as we continue with daily practices. When we do feel the mantra ecstatically like that, and notice our attention off in thoughts about the sensation, location in the body, etc., we treat it like any other experience that comes up in meditation and easily go back to the mantra. Nothing changes in the procedure of meditation. Only the experiences change to become more ecstatic and divine, so we have to be mindful not to get preoccupied with them during meditation and our other practices.

As has been said in earlier lessons, *I AM* is a "dual pole" mantra. The resonance of it in the spinal nerve is the reason why. *"I"* is the Shiva component, and *"AM"* is the Shakti component. With this mantra we are bringing the mind to stillness in such a way so as to purify the full length of the spinal nerve. By using a mantra that resonates between the third eye and the root, we are following the safest and most balanced path of awakening, just as we do in spinal breathing pranayama. The two practices are parallel methods, both working to purify the spinal nerve on their respective levels in the nervous system. Both practices, done in sequence (spinal breathing and then meditation), awaken and stabilize our ecstatic energies and inner silence. Together, these emanate out naturally from the spinal nerve.

With the first mantra enhancement (*SHREE SHREE I AM I AM*), we are doing two new things. First, we are increasing the number of syllables of the mantra. This broadens our sweep through the subconscious, purifying a wider path through the nervous system. It also slows down our descent into pure bliss consciousness, and brings more of it out with us as we come back out. So, more syllables do more purification and stabilize more inner silence in the nervous system. Why not one *SHREE*, or three *SHREE's*? We could have built up slower, beginning with one *SHREE*, and then added another one later. That way we'd have two enhancements instead of one. I did not think it was necessary to make the steps that small. Will we go to three *SHREE's*? It is not anticipated at this time. With the second enhancement added to the two *SHREE's* it is quite a good and long mantra already. More than enough to get the job done.

The reason for *SHREE* itself is for a new direction we are taking in the purification of our nervous system, expanding our mantra beyond the familiar third eye to root spinal nerve resonance for the first time. Expanding where? To the crown. *SHREE* takes us straight up the spinal nerve to the crown. In the center of the head the spinal nerve (sushumna) has a fork. It goes in two directions from there. First is the route to the third eye at the point between the eyebrows. Second is to the crown, straight up into the middle of the corona radiata, above the pineal gland and ventricles of the brain. Right up through there. With the resonance of *SHREE* in the crown we start to purify that area in relation to the entire spinal nerve. *SHREE* is a phonetic spelling of *SRI*, so it is not the same as *SHREEM*, per your question.

That is the first enhancement of the mantra.

A note on the crown: Way back when we first started discussing kundalini, it was mentioned that going to the crown prematurely could create all kinds of problems in the nervous system – the example of Gopi Krishna's well-documented nightmare-ish journey to enlightenment was given. Opening the third eye to root spinal nerve is the safest and most enjoyable way to go about purifying and opening the nervous system, and fast too. This is recognized in some of the traditions, and not recognized so well in others. Being wise travelers, we have gone the third eye to root path, both in spinal breathing and in meditation. And for most of us it is very progressive and smooth. As we are opening the third eye to root spinal nerve, we are also affecting the crown. It is inevitable, because the two are connected in the middle of the brain. Anyone who experiences the rise of ecstatic conductivity in the third eye route will experience an ecstatic crown opening as well. The difference is that, with the third eye leading, the process will not spiral out of control into excessive kundalini symptoms, as can happen when the crown is leading. So we go along that way, opening the third eye with gusto, letting the crown follow along safely. Then, at some point, the crown is purified enough "by osmosis" from the third eye opening so we can take a more direct approach to the crown. That is why we add *SHREE's* (and also *OM's*) into our mantra, and we will be taking a more direct approach to the crown with pranayama as well a few more lessons down the road. So, you see, we are getting around to the crown in our own time and in our own way, prudently avoiding the long-term havoc that a premature crown opening can bring.

The third eye is like our window to the divine and we can accomplish a lot going in and out through there. It is controlled (ajna means "command/control"), safe, very ecstatic, and it must be opened. The crown, the sahasrar (the thousand-petaled lotus) is like our roof, and once we open it up, we are easily dissolved into the divine. There is some control in this, but no where near the control we have working through the third eye. By the time we have purified the crown, both indirectly through the third eye, and directly later on by going straight up, we are ready to surrender ourselves on the altar of our crown, and then we find ourselves gone into ecstatic bliss. When we come back, we are no longer working for ourselves. We are then working for the Self in all – we have become That. It is not an instantaneous transition. It happens over a period of years – decades even. It is human spiritual transformation. So, I wanted to make clear that we never intended to avoid the crown forever – only until the time is right. You will know when that is for you in your heart, and these practices are designed to give you some guidelines on the matter, and the tools.

The second enhancement to the mantra (*SHREE OM SHREE OM I AM I AM NAMAH*) adds more syllables for the same reason as before (a much bigger sweep through the subconscious), and introduces the powerful *OM* component. *OM* resonates naturally in the medulla oblongata, the brain stem, spreading out everywhere through the nervous system, and beyond. Please be reminded that we don't try and localize the mantra in any particular physical part of our body. The tuning fork effect will work best if we are easy with the mantra, following the procedure of meditation as originally instructed early in the lessons. The nervous system already knows how to respond to the mantra in the appropriate way. All we have to do is use the mantra correctly, and everything will be fine.

OM lives up to its reputation of being the "mother of all mantras." It is the deeply ecstatic primordial sound of what we are, manifesting from pure bliss consciousness. As explained in the lesson on the second enhancement, we have to prepare for it before using it in deep meditation. Otherwise, it can wreak havoc. Under the best of circumstances, *OM* is "devastating ecstasy" in deep meditation, especially once ecstatic conductivity is coming up. It will be too much for anyone who goes to the second enhancement prematurely, so don't rush into it. You will know when you are ready. For deciding when to "shift gears," use the guidelines given in the lesson.

OM is paired with *SHREE* for a reason, and it is second instead of first for a reason. It is paired to maintain polarity between the crown (*SHREE*) and the rest of the nervous system resonating with *OM*. This is another dimension of the Shiva-Shakti balanced relationship, in this case between the crown and the medulla oblongata. It is a more dynamic and far-reaching manifestation of the Shiva-Shakti pairing than *I AM* (which also continues). *OM* is placed after *SHREE* for more longevity in the vibration of *OM*. *SHREE OM* is coming into the body, and *OM SHREE* is leaving the body. It is a distinction with a noticeably positive difference in effect when seen through the inner senses of ecstatic conductivity.

Finally, *NAMAH* is added for its syllables and as a traditional transition in mantra repetitions. It resonates ecstatically in the heart, cultivating bhakti, and has a purifying effect throughout the nervous system.

I realize that we have all had to take our mantras on faith from others who are supposed to know, who get them from scriptures. You know, I think it is going to change as ecstatic conductivity comes up in more and more people in this rising new age. We already have some people in this group with awakened kundalini who can no doubt judge for themselves how the mantra syllables are resonating in their nervous system. In other words, if you are taking my (or anyone else's) word for it now, you won't have to in the future. All it takes is awakening ecstatic conductivity through the practices. Anyone who has will "see" the effects of the mantras inside and know for themselves. Then the proof will be found right there in the pudding, and you won't have to take anyone else's word for it anymore.

Well, that is quite a lot of information. I sincerely hope that it does not distract anyone from the simple procedure of favoring the mantra and letting it happen naturally in meditation. None of what has been written here is necessary to do correct meditation, and it could indeed be distracting. So file all this under "food for bhakti" and continue to enjoy your journey homeward to enlightenment using the easy practice of deep meditation.

The guru is in you.

Addition – A third enhancement to the mantra is offered in this lesson addition. It should not be undertaken until the second enhancement of the mantra has been fully digested, and meditation is smooth. The enhancement is simple enough, adding two more syllables in the form of another *NAMAH*. So the third enhancement of the mantra is:

… SHREE OM SHREE OM I AM I AM NAMAH NAMAH …

This broadens the footprint of the mantra in our awareness one more step, making a wider cleansing stroke through the mind and nervous system as we use the mantra to facilitate the mind's natural march toward stillness. With this mantra, once we have arrived in stillness, we will find more inner silence staying with us as we go out into our daily activities. That is the purpose of meditation – to infuse our nervous system and all of our activities with the quality of inner silence, which is pure bliss consciousness. Then we come to know who we are in relation to all that is going on in the realm of time and space. We are That…

Lesson 189 – Where is the Third Eye?

Q1: You said the third eye was between the eye brows but many say it is the pineal gland area and some say the third eye is actually the medulla. Could you clarify?

A1: It is all of those, and more. The third eye is the spinal nerve (sushumna) going from the medulla oblongata through the general areas of the pineal and pituitary glands, and out the front at the center of the brow. It is more of a functioning zone in and around the spinal nerve than a specific organ. It could even be considered to extend down the spinal nerve below the medulla, because inner seeing is there also, but that is stretching it. Traditionally it is looking outward, as an eye would be, so that is why the external point between the eyebrows gets labeled as the third eye most often. The ecstatic relationship between the pineal gland, pituitary gland, and brow is probably the most common esoteric labeling. The medulla often gets labeled as part (or all) of the third eye too. It is pretty fuzzy yoga because labeling physical counterparts for the spiritual neuro-biology is not precise. There's nothing fuzzy about the experience of the ecstatically awakened third eye though. When it happens there is no doubt about what it is, or where it is inside. It is just a little difficult to describe it in physical terms.

The awakening of the third eye is an awakening of the entire spinal nerve all the way down to the root. As mentioned in the previous lesson on mantra design, the awakening third eye also is awakening the crown. So, awakening the third eye is ecstatically awakening the entire nervous system. That is why the Sanskrit word for the third eye, "ajna," means "command" or "control."

Q2: So are you saying it is just as correct to put your attention on the medulla where you say attention in-between eyes?

A2: No, the eyes go to the point between the eyebrows (gently favored), with a slight furrow of the brow in the middle. This is a physical positioning of the eyes to create a particular stimulating effect in the brain, which reaches instantly down the spinal nerve all the way to the root. At the same time, our attention goes with our practice, up and down the sushumna with spinal breathing. See lesson #131 – "Coordinating Sambhavi and Spinal Breathing" for a detailed discussion on this separation of the physical eyes from attention.

There are no instructions anywhere in the lessons to fix the focus of our attention in the medulla oblongata. The medulla is a "pass though" during spinal breathing, and is also stimulated by the resonating effect of the mantra in deep meditation, without deliberately focusing the mantra there. Mudras, bandhas and kumbhaka stimulate the medulla in a big way too. So the medulla is constantly being stimulated, but not by a sustained focus of attention on it in practices. The medulla is part of the greater whole of the awakening nervous system, and that is why it is addressed the way it is in practices.

We have been discussing the several ways how the third eye has been labeled in relation to the physical body. No particular techniques are intended in the labeling. The lessons themselves are very specific on techniques. Pardon me for any confusion on that point.

The guru is in you.

Lesson 190 – Sambhavi During Meditation?

Q: I know you do not instruct developing sambhavi during meditation. I have got it pretty well developed in spinal breathing, and now it is happening in meditation without any effort. Is this okay?

A: Yes, this is how it should happen. Meditation is a much more delicate process than spinal breathing, so we use our spinal breathing sessions to do our development work with mudras and bandhas. We make a habit of sambhavi during spinal breathing, so we don't even have to think about it. With the habit in place, as soon as we sit and close our eyes, they go toward the point between the eyebrows. Then we begin our spinal breathing with attention going up and down in the spinal nerve and the eyes automatically continue to favor that direction toward our slightly furrowed brow. When ecstatic conductivity comes up, then we have great pleasure coursing through the whole nervous system as a direct result of sambhavi, and it becomes a habit of ecstasy we do very naturally.

In meditation, the process of favoring the mantra is easy but delicate, and so we are stingy with our attention, not volunteering it for developing or doing other practices while we are meditating. While we are meditating, we just meditate. Even so, if we have developed good yoga habits during spinal breathing, things will occur during meditation without our attention being used to sustain them, and we can let them be there.

Siddhasana is a good example of this. Once we have the habit of siddhasana, it takes no attention or effort to sit in it, even as it is naturally energizing whatever practice we may be doing while we are sitting in it, including meditation.

Sambhavi becomes like that too. In fact, once sambhavi becomes a habit, tied in with the pleasure of ecstatic conductivity between the third eye and the root, then it becomes a natural part of all our practices, including meditation. Let's not fool ourselves on this though. If we find ourselves favoring the development of the "sambhavi habit" with our attention during meditation, then we should easily come back to the mantra. That is always the procedure. When we notice our attention has gone off to anything else during meditation, then we easily come back to the mantra. This does not preclude automatic habits developed in our spinal breathing sessions from naturally arising in meditation. In this way, over time, we find non-distracting habits of siddhasana, mulabandha, sambhavi, kechari and other mudras and bandhas occurring naturally during meditation. This is how it happens. Always follow the procedure of meditation, easily favoring the mantra over whatever else that draws the attention, and the rest will happen naturally.

This is how our inner silence and rising ecstatic energies come to blend in the dance of divine lovemaking. The persistent nudging of our nervous system in these ways through yoga leads to a transformation of our experience of life to unending ecstatic bliss.

Enjoy!

The guru is in you.

Lesson 191 – How to Cultivate Ecstatic Conductivity

Q: What must I do to experience ecstatic conductivity?

A: The experience of ecstatic conductivity can begin with any practice, depending on the amount and location of obstructions lodged deep in our nervous system. The more practices we have worked up to in a stable daily routine, the more is ecstatic conductivity being cultivated.

Whenever we do practices, the awakening is always happening by degrees. When we sit to meditate the very first time, feeling some peace and bliss, this is a step toward ecstatic conductivity. When we take up spinal breathing, and feel some pleasant tingling all over, this is movement toward ecstatic conductivity. It is the gentle stimulation of kundalini in our pelvic region that happens with all practices, beginning with the global techniques of meditation and spinal breathing. If our nervous system is already "wired" for ecstatic conductivity due to yoga in our recent or distant past, then the energy will begin to move noticeably right away. If it does not seem to be moving much as we meditate and do spinal breathing, never fear. It still is moving quietly underneath. The ground is being prepared as obstructions are being dissolved within.

As the ground is being prepared with meditation and spinal breathing, more targeted practices are added along the way. With each new practice the pressure for awakening ecstatic conductivity (kundalini) is increasing. It can move through us at any time as waves of pleasure, and be felt as a connectedness between our head and our root. Siddhasana and the mudras and bandhas in combination are for promoting this. So is the powerful practice of samyama.

There is one practice that stands out in its power for stimulating the awakening of ecstatic conductivity. This is kumbhaka (breath retention), which we use with our practice of yoni mudra. It is also used with dynamic jalandhara (chin pump). Finally, though it is not called kumbhaka there, the restraint of breath that occurs in spinal bastrika produces a persistent kumbhaka-like effect, combined with the rapid pulses of pressure up and down the spinal nerve. Even the most stubborn obstructions can be loosened and dissolved with the aid of spinal bastrika, and luminous ecstatic energies come flooding up to fill our liberated nerves.

Once we have developed a stable twice-daily routine involving all of these practices, if we have not noticed the rise of ecstatic conductivity, then it will only be a matter of time. With a routine of such powerful advanced yoga practices, the obstructions are dissolving by the truckload and must yield to the inner light.

Continue with daily practices. Ecstatic conductivity will grow steadily in the nervous system to accommodate the infinite divine love surging up from within.

Every flower bud is destined open and bloom gloriously.

The guru is in you.

Lesson 192 – Tips on Kechari

Q: Can you please clarify the following regarding kechari: When I try kechari I keep my mouth closed and try to suck my tongue in with the base of the tongue touching the roof of the mouth. Is this the right way of doing it? If so I am unable to follow your instruction of pushing the tongue to one side to enter the nasal passage because as soon as I open my mouth to put a finger, suction is lost and the tongue doesn't go as far as it did while sucking.

A: No, using suction to get to stage 2 is not part of kechari. It is done with the tongue muscles – helped with the finger in the beginning stages.

Opening the mouth helps with entry up into the nasal pharynx. Later on, opening the mouth and finger help are not needed to go up.

Try an experiment. Put the tip of your tongue back on the roof of your mouth (stage 1) with your mouth closed. Then open your mouth. The tongue goes a little further back with the mouth open, right? So, open mouth, finger help, and going to the left or right side of the soft palate is the way up into the nasal pharynx. The frenum under the tongue is the only limiting factor then.

There are two approaches for dealing with the frenum – tiny snipping and/or milking (stretching) of the tongue. Of the two methods, tiny snipping is the quickest and least uncomfortable, but more controversial. Both methods can be used over a period of time.

Please review the detailed lesson on kechari (#108) just to be clear on everything.

Getting into stage 2 kechari and stabilizing in it will be a big boost to your practices and experiences. The connection of the tongue with the sensitive and spiritually erogenous edge of the nasal septum is a huge leap forward in yoga. It is an important contributor to the ongoing cultivation of ecstatic conductivity in the nervous system.

I wish you all success.

The guru is in you.

Lesson 193 – Extending Practice Time Safely

Q: Last Sunday, I had much spare time. During meditation, I doubled the duration. At last, I could feel and hear the heart beat in my head. Should I always meditate longer than 20 minutes for better result?

A: Thank you for writing and sharing. Your spiritual enthusiasm (bhakti) is wonderful, and you can use it to enhance your practices for sure. However, it can be hazardous to suddenly lengthen your meditations greatly beyond the 20 minute guideline. Any change should be done very gradually, only five minutes at a time, with each step stabilized and sustained as part of your regular routine over weeks and months. It is not good to jump the meditation time around every day and week. If you overdo in that way, you could have too many obstructions coming out and run into discomfort, irritability in daily activity, etc. See lesson #159 for an example of this kind of difficulty in meditation time management.

There is a way to systematically increase meditation and all practices if you have no responsibilities on a weekend, holiday, or are retired. This is to repeat your entire routine a second time in the morning – adding one routine of practice for one or two days on a weekend or holiday, or possibly doing this ongoing if retired or on extended retreat. This adds huge purification and deeper momentum in spiritual progress. Being free of responsibilities is very important to do this, or it can also lead to discomfort and unpleasant experiences because so much is being released from inside. If you do three routines in a day (two in morning, one in early evening) it is important to have some light activity, like easy walking and gentle (social) satsang during the afternoon and evening. This light activity helps balance the process of release of obstructions from the nervous system.

For two morning routines, the sequence of practices is asanas, pranayama (all doing to date), meditation, samyama (if doing), yoni mudra, rest (at least 10 minutes lying down) ... and then start over.

In the evening only one routine should be done, so it is three full routines of practice in a day.

So, if you are ambitious, you can try that. Don't be surprised if a lot is coming loose inside. Advanced yoga practices are deceptively simple and very powerful – especially deep meditation. If releases are ever too much, then back off practices to a more stable routine immediately.

Always keep self-pacing in mind, especially when you are undertaking new practices or stepping up to longer times of practice.

I wish you all success on your chosen spiritual path.

The guru is in you.

Lesson 194 – More Flashing Lights

Q: OK ... I've been doing the advanced yoga practices from the beginning. Tonight I just read lesson #179, "The Star Revisited."

In this Q&A, the writer said they see flashes of white light during their day. I was wondering if this is in fact related to doing the advanced yoga practices. I started noticing the flashes about five weeks ago. I didn't think too much of it and thought maybe it was the beginning of some eye problem. I had lasic surgery about two years ago. I kinda just ignored it and decided if it got worse I'd go see the doctor.

Well it pretty much has stopped and then tonight when I read this Q&A, I read that person had the same experience. So now it's got me wondering if maybe it is related to the advanced yoga practices. Is it some flushing out of blockages that just happens to occur during the regular day? My natural instinct was to not worry about it. Just curious now, I guess. It's the human in me...

A: Yes, those kinds of symptoms of purification in (inner) vision can come with yoga practices. On the other hand, if something like that becomes a chronic difficulty for you, then it is good to get it checked out medically, especially if you have some history there.

Keep in mind that your view of the world will naturally change over time to become more luminous, and there will be these sort of energy jerks of purification going on from time to time along the way. In the end, the flashing lights will give way to steady vision, and a luminous world will then seem to be perfectly normal.

It sounds like you are moving right along with your practices. Bravo!

The guru is in you.

Lesson 195 – Mantra, Thoughts and Attention

Q1: For 13 years, I have done japa of a few mantras several hundred thousand times. One such specific mantra is "Om Namo Naaraayanaaya" – you may know this as the mantra directed toward Lord Vishnu. Due to the constant practise of mantra chanting, I find a particular problem in the *I AM* meditation: The moment I start *I AM*, my mind which is used to chanting something always, picks up the *I AM* and continues with it. However my mind also wanders into other thoughts, even without giving up the *I AM*. Now, should I consider that my mind is with *I AM* because it is chanting it, or should I consider that my mind if off *I AM* since it is into other thoughts? If I consider that my mind is off *I AM* and therefore I should bring it back, what should my mind think of? You have said that I should not think on the meaning of *I AM*. What else is there to think on, since my mind is already chanting *I AM*? What do you mean exactly when you say, "Meditate on the sound *I AM*."

A1: The mantra and thoughts can be in the mind together. The mantra can be going on even while we are thinking about something else. If we have the mantra going on in the background while we are sorting out our grocery list, is this meditation? Not if we are consciously favoring the groceries over the mantra. Having the mantra going like a motor in the mind without favoring it with our attention is not deep meditation. Meditation is about favoring the mantra with our attention, not about having the mantra going on automatically while we are focusing on other things. What we want to make automatic is bringing the attention easily back to the mantra when we realize attention is off the mantra. So, if we have thoughts and mantra going on at the same time, meditation is determined not by the presence of the mantra, but by our favoring it with attention. Other thoughts may still be there as we favor the mantra. It doesn't matter. It is attention that determines the process. It we have the habit of favoring the mantra with our attention when we realize we have not been, that is right meditation.

This should answer your question about what to be thinking about while "chanting" the mantra inside. It does not matter how many times we repeat the mantra inside. Deep meditation is not mental chanting. It is a process of using attention and the mantra together to create a condition in the mind that enables it to go to stillness. Just habitually chanting the mantra in the background inside while going about all sorts of other mental business with the attention is not deep meditation. In deep meditation, the attention is for favoring the mantra. By doing this as a procedure for our allotted time of meditation, the mantra will fade and become very refined over and over again. At whatever level we find ourselves in the mind we come back with attention and favor the mantra in that fuzzy refining journey. Before we know it, our attention is without objects, not even the mantra. It is a pleasurable feeling. This is samadhi, the eighth limb of yoga. As this happens the breath refines, the metabolism slows down, and obstructions throughout our nervous system are dissolved from the inside. It is inner silence (pure bliss consciousness) we are going to in deep meditation. All the good results come from that, and it comes through a process of managing our attention easily and rightly in meditation.

Q2: I have a doubt: You have mentioned in your lessons that the mere sound *I AM* removes the obstructions in the nervous system. In later lessons, you have also elaborated that the sound *I*

AM starts from the third eye and goes all the way down to the perineum through the spine. Such being the case, as long as the sound *I AM* is there in the mind, the cleansing should take place with or without the attention, isn't it? Over and above the cleansing done by the sound itself, is there additional cleansing done by the "attention" part?

A2: Consider the mantra to be a tool. If we have a hammer and keep it with us at all times, will it build a house for us? Of course not. Something more is needed. We need to apply the hammer with some skill. A mantra is nothing if not applied with some skill.

I know that may go against the background of many, where mantras are said to have magical powers and all that. Well, different sounds do resonate differently in the nervous system and that is why different mantras have different effects. But they are still just tools, and won't do much unless applied with some skill. The mantra is a tool that can be used to bring the mind and body to stillness. That requires a method of using attention in a particular way with the mantra. If we do, then attention will repeatedly be left standing alone without any objects, including no mantra. That is as still as it gets, and then the inner obstructions dissolve in that state of deep silence in the nervous system. Once the obstructions are going, then the inner silence is with us more and more in daily activity.

That is why we meditate using a particular procedure. The mantra alone without correct application of attention is like a hammer with no carpenter around. You are the carpenter!

The guru is in you.

Lesson 196 – Refining a Sound in the Mind

Q: What will be the effect of meditating on objects (such as an image of *OM*) and also ideas and meanings (such as that of God) when compared to meditation on sound (such as *I AM*)? It looks like my mind clings to an image sooner than to sound. Which do you advise for faster purification of the nervous system?

A: We should use only one object for deep meditation – our mantra. And we do not cling to it. We only favor it, and we allow it to change and refine as we go inward. Sound is particularly effective because it refines easily in the mind to finer and finer vibrations, and can be picked up easily and gently with the attention very deep inside. Meditating on physical objects, symbols, pictures, or meanings of things is not as effective as sound for going deep. This is not to say it can't be done with these other objects. It is only that we should choose one way and use that with effectiveness. The sound of the mantra is very easy to refine to penetrate our depths of inner silence, using the procedure described early in the lessons. Then we are quickly cultivating inner silence in our nervous system, which is the cornerstone of all enlightenment.

The guru is in you.

Lesson 197 – Kechari Sensations

Q: Thanks again for your lessons. A point of interest is that several times I have been on the verge of asking a question only to be answered by one of your Q&As before I had a chance to ask the question.

I have a question about kechari mudra. Whenever I have tried it in the past, after a little while I get such a burning sensation in my tongue and palate. Like I have stuck my tongue in a power point (electric socket). After this happens I have to stop the mudra; it's just too much.

Any thoughts?

A: It is interesting how answers come to us when we are ready for them. They can come from these lessons, or from anywhere else. It is our desire that attracts spiritual knowledge. Our spiritual desire is enhanced by yoga practices, so there is an incentive to keep going higher in practices.

A burning sensation like that in kechari is transitional purification of the nerves and biochemistry involved, and it will not last. I assume you are speaking of stage 1 kechari, which is the tongue lifted and pulled back comfortably on the roof of the mouth.

In stage 2 kechari, with the tongue behind and above the soft palate, there can also be stinging or burning sensations in the early stages. Even much later on it can sting a bit sometimes. This is a cyclical thing having to do with the ongoing process of purification. Most of the time the nasal pharynx is conducive for stage 2 kechari. Sometimes it is not. So we go with what is working at the time. That goes for stage 1 or stage 2 kechari, and any other yoga practice for that matter. We don't force things.

So, as you pull away from the intensity of the experience you are doing the right thing. You will be invited back soon enough.

All these symptoms and perturbations pass as the course of purification in the nervous system advances. We keep applying that gentle persuasion in our yoga practices, moving forward when we can, and holding back when there is some limiting symptom occurring. Like that, we keep pressing forward comfortably on the road to ecstatic bliss and enlightenment.

Going into kechari is an important part of the evolution in this process. It is a move toward whole body ecstatic conductivity, and happens automatically when the nervous system is ready. Our bhakti takes us up.

The guru is in you.

Lesson 198 – Targeted Bastrika – A Laser for Karmic Cleansing

Back in lesson #171, we introduced the powerful practice of spinal bastrika. Before proceeding with the current lesson, it is suggested you review that lesson.

Now we are going to consider additional applications of bastrika as a discretionary targeted tool. Why?

Sometimes we may run into a really stubborn obstruction somewhere in the body, and with focused bastrika we can put a lot of pressure in a localized area and literally burn the karma away. It is like using laser surgery in a small area of the body. This is in great contrast to the "global" methods of meditation and spinal breathing we use as our core practices.

It is important that we have met the yoga practice and health-related prerequisites for spinal bastrika before we add targeted bastrika. This cannot be over-emphasized. Targeted bastrika is not a shortcut to enlightenment. In fact, it could land us in substantial discomfort if applied prematurely. If we are new to yoga, and try targeted bastrika without the prerequisite global cleansing provided by meditation and spinal breathing, we could create an unpleasant energy imbalance in our nervous system.

So, keep in mind that targeted bastrika is for cleaning out stubborn residual karmas. It is not for going into an area for the first time, thinking it is all we need for a good cleaning out. It doesn't work like that.

Targeted bastrika is a close relative of spinal bastrika. We are still working in the spinal nerve with targeted bastrika. The difference is we are tightening the range of attention moving up and down in the spinal nerve with our rapid bastrika panting.

For example, let's say we have been doing meditation, spinal breathing, associated mudras and bandhas, and spinal bastrika for quite a few months. All is going fairly smoothly. We are experiencing some ecstatic conductivity, which is detected by a pleasurable reaction coming up from the root when we do sambhavi. Still, we still feel some resistance in the area of our third eye between the center of our head and the point between the eyebrows. This is possibly a good candidate for some targeted bastrika. I say "possibly" because we will only know when we try. If we do try, and find too much obstruction there to remove comfortably with targeted bastrika, we will have to back off and rely on the less intensely targeted means for some more time, i.e., meditation, spinal breathing, sambhavi, yoni mudra kumbhaka, etc.

When we use targeted bastrika we do it at the end of our sitting practices, after meditation, samyama and yoni mudra, but before rest. We set up just the same as for spinal bastrika (including associated mudras and bandhas), but we limit the cycling of attention during rapid breathing to the area we are targeting. So, if we are targeting the area between the center of the head and the point between the eyebrows, then we let our attention cycle quickly there during bastrika. Attention goes in the same direction as in spinal breathing and spinal bastrika – up with in-breath and down with out-breath.

When first learning targeted bastrika, we only go for two minutes, and then do our normal rest period at the end of our sitting practices routine – preferably lying down for at least 5-10 minutes. Then we monitor how we feel during our daily activities. If there is no undue roughness, then we know the targeted bastrika is probably okay. But we won't know for sure for a few more sessions, so be cautious about ramping up targeted bastrika to more time until you know you are stable with it. Once we know we are stable, and still wish to focus on a particular area, then we can creep the time up to three minutes, and then five minutes, monitoring for stability in daily activity each step along the way.

As with spinal bastrika, targeted bastrika can be very pleasurable, and we should be careful not to overdo if we get into a reverie with it. It can happen. When it does happen we may find ourselves in the position of having ecstatic sitting practice and crabby daily activity – that is not what we want happening over the long term, because it is in not sustainable. Better we should have enjoyable sitting practice and enjoyable daily activity. That is the balance we are looking for. Our friends and loved ones will appreciate it too.

Targeted bastrika is the most discretionary of all the practices we have covered so far. It is for those who are well established in their daily practice routine, and who have a clear recognition of their inner silence and ecstatic conductivity in relation to localized obstructions in the nervous system. Some ability for "inner seeing" should be developed before using targeted bastrika. Without some inner sensory ability, using targeted bastrika is like using laser surgery without the magnifying glass that is necessary to see to aim it accurately. Then who knows what will be burned up with the laser beam? Inner seeing comes with ecstatic conductivity. Then we will know where the obstructions are and can target them accurately with attention in the spinal nerve oscillating in combination with the power of bastrika. Even then it could be too much upheaval, and often those with inner seeing have to back off too. It is not a perfect world inside, not until we have gotten all the obstructions loosened and out. That is what all of these advanced yoga practices are for, working on many levels in our nervous system.

What are some of the areas where targeted bastrika can be used?

We mentioned the third eye area (ajna). This is a very important one because the purification of the entire nervous system ultimately depends on the region of the third eye becoming fully functional as the "command and control center" of our rising enlightenment.

Other areas where targeted bastrika can be used, according to our inner seeing, include the throat, the heart, the abdomen and the pelvic region. In advanced yoga practices involving pranayama, we are always best off to be in the spinal nerve. So we will be working in the spinal nerve on whatever level in the body we may find the need for targeted purification. The spinal nerve is the foundation for all spiritual purification and opening of the nervous system. As long as we are working in the spinal nerve, we will be in cooperation with the natural process of evolution going on within us, and this is how we keep our journey of spiritual transformation both progressive and smooth.

Another area where targeted bastrika can be used in a discretionary manner is the crown – the sahasrar. This is a completely different situation from any other part of our spiritual neuro-anatomy, and will be covered in the next lesson. There are huge repercussions to doing any practice at the crown, so please don't start doing targeted bastrika at the crown until you review the next lesson and understand the delicate dynamics that are involved there.

Always err on the side of caution when considering the use of targeted bastrika anywhere in the body, and always use it in the spinal nerve. It is a powerful practice that will be effective only when the necessary prerequisites have been met. Once the right conditions are in place, targeted bastrika can be used with good effectiveness, and it will greatly enhance our steadily rising experience of ecstatic bliss.

The guru is in you.

Lesson 199 – Managing the Opening of the Crown

Once we are underway in yoga it is not difficult to open the crown. The trick is to open it in such a way so as facilitate a smooth and progressive journey on the path of yoga. If we are premature in opening the crown, before there is adequate purification in the nervous system, we can be in for a lot of difficulty with kundalini excesses, as everything inside us strains to catch up with the huge pull of energy going up through the crown. So, it is very important to understand something about the dynamics of the crown in relation to the purification going on in the rest of our body, and to engage in practices in such a way so as to purify the entire nervous system while opening the crown at the same time. This is not as difficult to do as it sounds, once a good integration of practices is being used. In fact, if you are using advanced yoga practices as laid out in the lessons, you have been doing it for some time already. This is the best way to open the crown – indirectly, without focusing on it until much later in the game.

The crown is also known as the "sahasrar" – the thousand-petaled lotus located on top of the head. Physically, it corresponds to the corona radiata, a mass of nerves located near the top of the head above the two main ventricles of the brain. When inactive, the energy rests there in a "skullcap" shape, not noticeable to us. When it is aroused by the attention, the skullcap turns up to form a cup, or flower shape, the thousand-petaled lotus. When it is up like that it is said to be awakened, or opened. We can't miss it then, because when the crown is in full swing it draws us up inside like a spiritual vacuum cleaner. This drawing up can be felt deep within our loins. Kundalini can't resist the temptation of an opened crown and lurches up toward it. The problem is that, if our nervous system between the root and the crown is not purified enough, kundalini energy will begin tearing through everything to get to the crown. This is what produces so-called excessive kundalini symptoms, which can include a counterpart of emotional difficulty as well.

A number of traditions encourage going to the crown with practices early on the journey of yoga. A few even go there first. The results are predictable – people with kundalini problems, and there have been quite a few folks that have come to these lessons looking for relief. Others experience what is called a "spontaneous awakening" of kundalini. While I cannot prove it, it is my opinion that spontaneous awakenings are also the product of yoga practices that have gone to the crown prematurely, but in a past life rather than in this life. Such people are born in this life "wired" for a spontaneous awaking due to those long forgotten practices and imbalances stored deep in the nervous system. Premature awakening of the crown is the number one cause of excessive kundalini symptoms. It may be the only cause.

Fortunately, good practices for awakening the crown in tandem with purifying the rest of the nervous system also aid in smoothing energy imbalances that are a hangover from the past. So there is good news here for all of us – we who are stable with our energy who want to finish the journey, and we who have fallen off the wagon with kundalini difficulties and want to recover the situation and move on to finish the journey also.

Let's talk about the dynamics of the crown in relation to the rest of the nervous system. In the recent lesson on mantra design, it was mentioned that the sushumna has a fork in it in the middle of the head. One fork goes forward to the point between the eyebrows, and the other one goes up into the center of the crown. In spinal breathing we take the front fork with our attention and traverse the spinal nerve repeatedly with our breath, going between the root and the point between the eyebrows. In doing so, we are cultivating and purifying the spinal nerve along that route. The result is a radiation of purifying life force (prana) going out in all directions in the nervous system from the spinal nerve.

This radiation of energy from the spinal nerve also goes up the other fork to the crown. We don't even think about it. We don't put attention on the crown. Nevertheless, spinal breathing between the brow and the root purifies the crown in this way, just as it purifies all the rest of the nervous system.

A similar effect happens with deep meditation. With the *I AM* mantra the crown is naturally permeated with inner silence and is gradually purified along with the rest of the nervous system. With the mantra enhancements we gradually expand the mantra in ways that serve several functions. One of those functions is to bring more purifying influence to the crown without focusing attention directly on the crown. It is done through the resonance of the mantra vibration deep inside us. Samyama amplifies the influence of inner silence in the nervous system by moving silent awareness out from the inside in various directions through the nervous system, and the crown receives its fair share of this moving siddhi silence.

Over time, we add many other practices to stimulate the purification of the spinal nerve – mudras, bandhas, siddhasana, yoni mudra, kechari, chin pump, spinal bastrika and so on. All of these practices are opening the crown by indirect influences. By awakening the spinal nerve between the third eye and the root, we are automatically awakening the crown.

A milestone on our journey is the awakening of ecstatic conductivity. This is a gentle, gradual, and ecstatic awakening of kundalini. It is easily recognized by the direct connection that arises between sambhavi and the pleasurable sensations stimulated at the root. From there, ecstatic conductivity proceeds gradually with our continuing daily practices. Once ecstatic conductivity is occurring, we are in the position to clearly observe for ourselves what the connection is between the gradually awakening crown and the rest of our nervous system. If we put our attention up into the rising flower cup on top of our head, we will feel it pulling us ecstatically upward inside, from the root all the way up. Don't make an extended practice of this, because even with ecstatic conductivity awakened it is possible to overdo and experience excessive energy flows and an emotional letdown afterward. In other words, ecstatic conductivity is not a license to go straight to the crown. But we can experiment a little now and then and get the feel of what is stable and what is not. Usually any slight excess at the crown experienced in this way will only last a few hours, or a day, before the energy balances again.

We can touch the crown with attention for short periods in this way when ecstatic conductivity is awakened, because we have also awakened the third eye. Having the sushumna awakened between the third eye and root gives us a stability we did not have before, and a natural inner energy balance that can be stimulated at any time simply by letting go into the conductivity occurring between the third eye and the root. This is the power of a third eye awakening. There is little that can destabilize it once ecstatic conductivity comes up in the third eye to root spinal nerve. That is why the third eye (ajna) means "command." With ecstatic conductivity rising in the sushumna between the third eye and root, we are in command of the kundalini process, and having a very good ecstatic time with it too.

As mentioned, this does not mean we can go all out in the crown. Even a small mess we make at the crown will not be fun, so why do it?

Some have asked, "Why can't I just shift my spinal breathing from the third eye to root to the crown to root?" Two reasons: First it curtails the continuing activation of the third eye to root awakening. Second, it shifts the emphasis of attention to the crown, which will increase instability in the energy flows. So don't shift your spinal breathing to the crown. It will not be stable, even for advanced yogis and yoginis. Just keep going with third eye to root spinal breathing, deep meditation and all the rest that has been given, and all the openings will continue to progress rapidly and smoothly, including at the crown.

With occasional "testing" with awareness placed at the crown from time to time along the way, eventually those tests will become more stable. Putting occasional brief awareness at the crown will not be the cause of this stability. It will only test to see how far the crown has come in tandem with purification in the rest of the nervous system. Any stability that comes will be from our integrated advanced yoga practices. Once some stability does come, we will be able to put our attention at the crown for a few minutes without falling into energy difficulties, or an emotional letdown afterward. Then, and only then, we can have the safe option to let our attention rest at the crown for a while at the end of practices, before our rest period. We can be reclined or lying down if we want, and using sambhavi as we let our attention enter the gorgeous raised crown flower with the shaft of the radiant sushumna coming up through the center. Sambhavi adds a layer of both ecstatic bliss and stability, because it activates the third eye at the same time while the crown is being stimulated with attention. Maybe we see the crown as a flower. Maybe a cup. Maybe red. Maybe silver or white. Maybe violet. It comes in many colors. Some may see it as a cobra with a great flared hood going up. However we see it, it is how we feel it drawing us up that will be the in-common experience. As the crown opening and nearly purified nervous system mature, we are drawn up without the chaos and mayhem that is so common in premature awakenings. We are drawn up into pure ecstatic bliss. Then we can surrender...

We may be gone and not know where we were. Or we may have some celestial visions. When we do come back, we are somehow new, illuminated, radiating like never before. That is the beginning of the experience in the awakened crown.

Once we become stable in our visits to the crown, then we can take a more active role there. Still, we keep all of our advanced yoga practices the same. But we can add something. It was mentioned in the last lesson on targeted bastrika. Once our nervous system has been purified enough to carry the flow of energy stimulated by an open and active crown, then we can do additional targeted work there. One of the most efficient ways to do this is by using targeted bastrika between the crown and the root. We can do it with the crown raised and open, or closed. The former is more intense. We can use sambhavi and other mudras and bandhas while we do targeted bastrika between the crown and root. One thing we do not do, and that is do it without having met all the prerequisites of targeted bastrika, and also the testing and gradual development of crown awareness described above. If we are premature with anything involving attention at the crown, we will know it within a few hours. This applies especially to targeted bastrika, which is all-out stimulation of the crown. So, when targeted bastrika at the crown is undertaken it should be very sparing at first – not more than a minute at a time in the beginning. If the result is stable and good in activity, then it can be stepped up a minute at a time. This practice is done at the same time that any targeted bastrika is done – at the end of sitting practices, before rest. The effect of this practice is to bring the environment of the crown into our daily life. What is that like? "Heaven on earth" is a phrase that comes to mind.

So carry on with practices, and be mindful not to get too far ahead of yourself with anything. If you do, you will know soon enough because it will be uncomfortable. Then the thing to do is back off immediately to a stable platform of practice. Sometimes we can go forward faster by going backwards a bit.

It is good to be stubborn about keeping up our routine of twice-daily practices. It is not so good to be stubborn about overdoing practices. That applies especially for anything we do at the crown.

Keep moving forward at a smooth pace, and you will arrive in time at your destination – endless ecstatic bliss and outpouring divine love!

The guru is in you.

Lesson 200* – Follow-up on a Sensitive Meditator

Note: This is a follow-up on the same person who was having difficulty in lesson #160, "Extreme Sensitivity to Meditation – What To Do?" This series is a good example of prudent self-pacing in meditation, and then moving on to spinal breathing to stabilize some kundalini symptoms. This interaction is with the husband of the practitioner, who is assisting her.

Q1: My wife had taken up meditation but seemed very sensitive, so she does only deep meditation for about 15 minutes twice a day. The dreams and all she used to have after meditation are now gone. A few days back she started to get small peanut size rashes on her stomach, upper arms, back and chest. They are red, don't pain or itch, and go away after few days. Also, since the day before the rashes started she gets very sexually excited during meditation.

She has been doing only *I AM* meditation for the last 1.5 months and I suggested to do spinal breathing also. I am not sure if the rashes are some blockages coming out. We will be taking medical advice too. But I thought I should ask you just in case you can throw some light if they are in any way related to cleansing process.

A1: I'm glad your wife's scary dreams have subsided. That would indicate some purification was happening, and some balance has been reached in the process. Good job on self-pacing!

More purification is probably what is happening now with the rashes – which can happen in the early stages of kundalini awakening. It is amazing she is having all this with only 15 minutes of meditation. She must be a yogini from way back, and now is sorting out some old imbalances deep in her nervous system. These can be latent inside from extreme yoga done in the distant past. If the rash subsides in a few days or a week or so, then you can conclude it is yoga related. Seeking medical attention would be prudent if the rash becomes serious. If medication is given it can complicate the process of yoga, so make sure it is necessary.

On the sexual symptoms, this can happen as part of purification and awakening of the nervous system also. It too will find balance. Rarely will such episodes of extreme arousal during practices last a long time. On the other hand, sexual energy has an important role in the process of human spiritual transformation, so there will always be something going on with sexuality moving upward from the root in the nervous system once ecstatic conductivity (kundalini) is permanently awakened. If you and your wife have not, it might be good to review the tantra lessons, so sexuality and sexual relations can be viewed in yogic context.

Spinal breathing offers the possibility of balancing all of these things more quickly and progressively. Kundalini symptoms (probably what these things are) usually are caused by Shakti energy coming up into the nervous system without enough counter-balancing by Shiva energy coming down. Spinal breathing can correct this, and then progress can go very fast with much less chance of uncomfortable kundalini symptoms. Maybe try 5 minutes of spinal breathing before meditation and see how it goes for a few days. If it doesn't help, or if it aggravates the symptoms, then back off. If it helps, then give it a few weeks of stable practice and then consider going to 10 minutes of spinal breathing.

Rashes can be related to pitta (inner fire) imbalance that is aggravated by kundalini awakening. It can also be experienced as excessive heat or acidic sensations in the digestion or anywhere in the body. Ayurveda (the Indian system of medicine) can help with this. A "pitta pacifying diet" with a pitta pacifying routine is one of the first things to look at. If you search the web for that, you will find much information. You can also find information in the AYP links section on the web site under "Ayurveda."

Beyond diet and routine, an Ayurvedic physician can advise on additional remedies. Anyway, the chances are good that your wife's symptoms will pass naturally as her energies come into balance and move ahead with the process of yoga. Even then it is good to be mindful of bodily constitution and not be aggravating it with inappropriate foods or routine. Maybe hold off on the spicy foods for a while...

With prudent application of practices and good self-pacing, I'm sure that smoothness and steady blissful progress can be achieved. Good things are happening.

Q2: My wife has started spinal breathing and the rashes started to subside from day one. Now they have almost faded away. It's amazing how the practices work. Thanks for all your advice.

One more amazing thing was that my wife's sight has improved from using lenses of 2.75 to 2.5 since she has started meditation. She had to change her lenses. I can't stop from thinking that this incident and her practices are related. Does meditation help in correcting physical problems apart from cleansing the nervous system? Curious to know!

A2: That's great news on your wife's spinal breathing and disappearing rash. It is a wonderful practice with many long-term benefits, and one of the most effective internal energy balancers there is. It is the perfect companion for deep meditation. And these two practices together make an excellent foundation for enhancing yoga practices further to transport us quickly and comfortably along the road to enlightenment.

It is not common for yoga practices to suddenly reverse external physical dislocations, such as correcting eyesight. For that reason yoga is not presented as an instant cure-all for everything that can be ailing us. We do yoga for enlightenment, and perfect physical health is not always a prerequisite for that, though overall health will certainly tend to improve as the nervous system becomes purified. There is no question that sudden cures do happen sometimes. Is it the yoga? It could be if the ailment is tied to obstructions being dissolved deep in the nervous system where yoga is working.

Whether or not we are being physically cured, we can be sure we are being spiritually cured through yoga, and that cultivates in us a deep sense of wellbeing that is independent of the condition of the body. Inner harmony always becomes outer harmony, but not always in the way we might expect. Over time, we develop an inner perspective on things that enables us to cope with whatever may be going on in the body or around us, often with laughter. That's liberation.

The guru is in you.

Addition – And a few months later, this follow-up occurred regarding the same practitioner:

Q3: This is regarding my wife's meditation experience recently. She had started the first enhancement of mantra a week ago. A few days back she felt a burning sensation over her navel region but it wasn't very significant. But yesterday during her meditation the burning sensation was very strong and the region over her navel became very hot. Also, her fingertips became numb as if losing any sensation. Is this some kind of blockage and does she need to do something about it? Please advise.

A3: It's good to hear from you. It is much like when your wife first started. More energy is moving with the mantra enhancement, so her sensitivity is showing up again. The thing to do is back off a bit on meditation time (keeping the new mantra) for a week or two until things settle in, and then creep up again according to comfort. Based on her previous experience, it is a good bet that she will be able to acclimate to the increased energy flow okay. If it does not work out after a few weeks of adjusting, then maybe it is premature for the mantra enhancement and she should go back to the first mantra, and try the enhancement again 6-12 months later. Switching the mantra back is not the first choice though. It takes the mind significant time to adjust to a change in mantra, so we don't want to be jumping back and forth between mantras unless it is absolutely necessary. Like the well analogy says: "If you want to find water, better to keep digging in one place."

Q4: Thanks for your advice. I asked my wife to do as advised by you, i.e., to reduce the time of deep meditation. Now she is doing deep meditation for 10 minutes and the burning sensation and numbness of fingers is gone. Thanks once again for your advice. Looking at all these experiences and your guidance I now understand why the yogic scriptures talk about a need of a guru.

As for me. I am doing the enhanced mantra and recently am having jitters in my body during meditation. I do 10 minutes of spinal breathing, dynamic jalandhara (chin pump), 20 minutes of deep meditation, and sambhavi. The jitters happen at least once or twice during meditation and it feels as if some strong wave has passed through my body from head to toe. I have been doing the enhanced mantra for the last three months and the jitters have increased over the last week. Please advise me.

A4: I'm glad to hear your wife has stabilized the situation. She can consider creeping her practice time back up in a week or two, if she wants.

In your case, if odd experiences come up now and then, that is normal purification and opening. Don't mind them too much. On the other hand, if an experience keeps building over weeks and months, like your jitters, it could be a sign of inner energy movements exceeding your nervous system's capacity to adapt to them. In that case the same advice given for your wife applies to you too. If energy is building up, becoming more uncomfortable, and you don't see it cycling back down, then it is time to slow down a bit. You know the procedure.

Often times a rising instability is related to the last practice or additional time of practice added, and that would be the first one to pare back a bit. If it isn't that, then the thing to do is go back and trim other pieces until a stable platform of practice is found. Once things are stable for a while, then creeping back up can be considered again.

For all the reasons we have observed, self-pacing is a very important practice in its own right.

Yes, it is tricky stuff, but it can be managed with the right knowledge in hand. I hope it can be systematized in writing to the point where anyone can do this with much less outside help. Much more self-sufficiency in yoga – that is the goal of the lessons.

Q5: Thanks for the advice. Instead of reducing the meditation time I increased the spinal breathing time to 15 minutes. The jitters did not happen. I will continue with the practise and see if it works.

A5: Good job. By using spinal breathing to stabilize the energy imbalance (it's very good for that), you not only solved the imbalance, but you are adding to forward progress. Just keep an eye on your experiences, and make adjustments as necessary.

Lesson 201 – The Drama of a Premature Crown Opening

Q: You most probably don't need confirmation on the information that you're sharing but I thought I'd let you know my personal experience as a confirmation anyway.

I'd had a slight fascination with this "New Age" stuff since an early age but didn't delve into it much until a life crisis in the early 1990's. For health reasons I decided to meditate to reduce my stress and unintentionally ended up in a small meditation group that went into Tarot readings, personal growth and "chakras" which I had never heard of before.

My first contact and first meditation with this neighbourhood group totally scared the heck out of me – coloured hues on the walls, coloured lights, bouncing balls of light off the ceiling, seeing auras, clairaudience, special messages for me, etc. Looking back now it was all positive – pink love beams, religious figures, loving all encompassing compassion. But I didn't know at that time. I couldn't help but follow it through, mainly out of fear and trying to get it all to stop. Luckily (destiny?) I had intelligent and wise people to help me along. When the student is ready the teacher "does" appear. I jumped ahead so fast – psychometry, channeling, lucid dreaming, astral travel, guides, angels, God, all paths, all religions/beliefs, clairaudience, clairvoyant, darkness and hauntings, past lives, etc. It happened only once for each experience and I was told repeatedly I didn't need to learn it in this lifetime, I had already achieved it before. This was just a "remembrance" for me to experience in my life where I was now.

Following common teachings at the time in the Western world of "Spirituality," I constantly meditated on the chakras, raising the energy and my vibrational levels from the root to the crown chakra. This was all I knew. I didn't know of kundalini and Eastern methods.

My growth and experiences were so rapid that it caused some problems, because I soon advanced past whoever was teaching me, and sadly sometimes there was jealousy and disbelief, causing me to leave and most of the time feeling isolated and alone – unaccepted. I reached levels within a couple of months that they had taken years to achieve and they just couldn't accept that it was so "easy" for me. It was a very hard time for me and also very confusing as I needed support to help me through what I didn't understand. I didn't ask for what was happening to me; I felt unfairly judged at times, and also adrift and lost with what was happening.

Then the spontaneous awaking of kundalini happened about 1995-6, which threw me into further turmoil. Then I looked at Eastern teachings and understood more about the chakras. Unfortunately, meditating so many years on raising the energy to the crown and not the third eye is what caused my problems.

Without being egotistical – and I'm sure you're one of the few people who can understand this – I obviously have been born close to this stage specifically in this lifetime because of what I've achieved in lifetimes before. This has been made clear to me for many years now; its just hard to find someone who can accept this and not look at me weirdly or believe I have a extreme narcissistic personality. You really are a breath of fresh air for me.

As I mentioned in my previous email I've finally found some relief in focusing on breathing up and down the spine from the root to the third eye. It's difficult to "re-train" the energy this way but it is happening.

I don't go anywhere near the crown chakra but can feel certain areas of it tingling or pressures there sometimes. I'm also uncomfortable about getting my hair cut and feel like a ponytail affect at the back, which I don't physically have. I just let it all go without worrying too much about it. If anything, I'm more worried about being too active with it and spend a lot of time just balancing and calming down the energy within.

I'll also admit after having such strong energy and emotional reactions for so many years that I've developed a fear of even looking anywhere near the crown. I hope this isn't detrimental in any way to the natural flow of awakening. The last couple of weeks has had a lot of activation in the heart chakra. I don't know why. I've read somewhere that the heart is one of the last to open because it can be very emotional and physically draining. Do you know of this?

A lot of my breathing has been happening at the throat and nose which I believe is balancing, as I usually breath in and out through the mouth, something I did from the beginning as this is what I was told to do for chakra work. I allow it all to happen naturally now, with some direction mentally. I have found the nose and back of tongue energy directing itself now. It's all a new experiment for me.

I also understand why many of the yoga/kundalini teachings where kept secret from the general population. Unless there is an experienced teacher on hand to help, many problems do arise. The Western world looks upon yoga and the chakras as a form of exercise or general meditation without realizing the power and potential it has to impact the human energy field so much.

Thank you so much again for all that you're doing and the help you have given me.

A: Thank you for your generous sharing. All confirmations (and disagreements) are welcome. Your experiences fit right in with what we are talking about in the lessons, especially now that we are discussing the crown. Let me add a few more perspectives on it, which will tie in with the wise adjustments you are currently making in your daily practice.

Premature opening of the crown creates so much release throughout the nervous system that we can easily get caught up in the drama of it, and you are doing a great job of looking beyond the fray. All the visions and feelings that come up are difficult to resist. The same thing goes for any siddhis (powers) we might experience. With the nervous system still needing a lot of purification, much of what we experience is colored by the "smoke" of innumerable karmas being burned up, often in a random fashion. So the experiences can be a mixture of the real with the unreal. It is no wonder that a severe premature crown opening can lead one to a psychiatric ward, or worse.

Here is the kicker. Visions and revelations, while often part of the journey, are not primary indicators of progress toward enlightenment. In fact, enlightenment can occur with very few, if any, visions at all. To the extent we have visions and revelations, we can be distracted from the practices that assure our continued steady and stable progress. We have talked about distracting visions a lot in the lessons, but so far not much from the perspective of the extremes of a full blown premature crown opening. It is not an easy thing, because it can become a world unto itself – the ultimate distraction.

None of this is to say that visions or revelations are bad. Indeed, we should enjoy the scenery as we travel along the road to enlightenment. But if the scenery becomes the path, with our sense of self wrapped up in it, then we will be heading off course. With extreme premature crown awakenings the risk of this is greater than average. Extreme awakenings are sometimes ecstatic, often hellish, and always seductive. Right practices can gradually put an end to the flights of fancy we might be drawn into, and bring us into the peace and joy of the divine reality within us. Then we will see our visions from a different perspective. They might even go away – replaced by an abiding sense of peace and happiness that does not constantly fling us from pillar to post.

So what is happening with a premature crown opening? Are we getting anywhere? Are we getting enlightened? Well, yes and no. Yes, obstructions are being released willy-nilly. And no, the chaos of it and our identification with the chaos can create karma also – a weird kind of karma that can lead us into a cycle of premature spontaneous crown openings, life after life. If we continue working at the crown in this situation, we perpetuate the whole thing, and spiritual progress can be elusive, even as our visions continue. It is only by our conscious intervention in the form of stabilizing practices that we can get off this wheel.

There are only two sure signs of rising enlightenment. In fact, there is really only one sure sign, because the second one does not go very far without the first. The first, and most important sign of rising enlightenment, is the emergence of inner silence – an unshakable blissful inner awareness – eternal peace taking up residence in our nervous system. The second sign is the rise of ecstatic conductivity in the nervous system. Not necessarily ecstatic visions or revelations. Just simple neuro-biological ecstatic pleasure coursing up through our body. Together, inner silence and ecstatic conductivity in the nervous system make up the foundation of enlightenment. As they merge into one we see the journey coming to its fruition in endless ecstatic bliss and an outpouring of divine love. It is very simple, really. If we view our progress through these two parameters, which are readily cultivated with specific yoga practices, and easily observable, then we will be on the right track. At the same time, we will be quelling the storms of any premature crown awaking we might have gotten ourselves into in the recent or distant past.

The great nineteenth century kriya yogi, Lahiri Mahasaya, said that enlightenment is "the merging of emptiness with euphoria." This is the merging of inner silence with ecstatic conductivity. That's it. It is very simple. Nothing else is necessary. So, if we are inundated with visions and revelations, we will be wise to easily go back to our practices, the ones that cultivate these two modes of functioning in our nervous system that lead to our liberation.

In the lessons we concentrate on cultivating the two components of enlightenment with a variety of practices. The two main practices are deep meditation (for inner silence) and spinal breathing (for balanced ecstatic conductivity). Many other practices are added to build on the ongoing progress cultivated by the two core practices. Taken all together, it is an integrated system of practices.

At the heart of smooth and progressive purification and opening of the nervous system is the spinal nerve (sushumna) between the third eye (ajna) and the root (muladhara). With all practices naturally working on purifying and opening the third eye to root spinal nerve, we are able to avoid the drama of a premature crown opening, even as we are nudging the crown open indirectly all the while. Then, in time, we can go to the crown directly. When that time arrives, further crown opening does not lead to chaos. It does not lead to a lot of visions or revelations either. Why not? Because there is much less karmic smoke floating around in our purified nervous system. The visions we do have are not extreme, not overwhelming, yet profound, and not needing to be mentioned. In short, a crown opening when the time is right creates no upheaval at all – only a channel of ecstatic bliss and divine love flowing into the world.

This condition of a mature opened crown and nervous system is its own source, and its own justification. And it too is a very simple thing.

So, that is a round-about way of saying, yes, I think you are doing the right thing taking up spinal breathing. Besides being a world-class stabilizer of wayward kundalini energies, it is a core practice for cultivating ecstatic conductivity in the third eye to root spinal nerve. Awakening the third eye (ajna) like that is the way forward. I encourage you to take up deep meditation also. Pranayama, with all of its benefits, does not cultivate the deepest level of inner silence in the nervous system. For this, the mind must be systematically brought to stillness every day – that is deep meditation.

As for breathing through the mouth or nose, using the nose is generally better if it is not a strain, because important aspects of our spiritual neurology are located in the nasal passages and sinuses. Nasal breathing during spinal breathing stimulates these, as do other "targeted" practices we cover in the lessons, i.e., sambhavi, yoni mudra kumbhaka, kechari and the bastrika pranayamas.

Once you have developed some comfort and stability in third eye to root oriented practices, I think your fear of the crown will subside. It will just be a place you can touch occasionally to see what is happening there. It will not be "practice" at the crown until there is stability in whatever you do there, as discussed two lessons ago. And there is no need to rush it, because the crown is being opened safely every time we meditate, do spinal breathing and the rest of our integrated advanced yoga practices.

Yes, I have heard also that "the heart is last to open." But I think it is more involved than that. In the lessons, we begin with the heart because desire is the engine that drives all yoga. Desire that is intensified and directed toward spiritual unfoldment is bhakti, and this is all heart work. Practices feed back into the heart, increasing bhakti every step along the way. So the heart is opening all the time, along with the rest of the nervous system. Then ecstatic conductivity begins to rise and we are melting in love inside in the face of so much ecstasy and rising inner sensuality – more heart opening. Finally, when Shiva (silence) and Shakti (ecstasy) are merging and we finally go directly to the crown, then it all pours down and the heart goes all the way into overflowing pure divine love. Maybe that last step is what is meant by "the heart is last to open." But the truth is, yoga begins with the heart, the heart is opening every step of the way, and it ends with the heart, as we finally become an expression of divine love on earth. And all of these steps of the heart will not be traumatic, as long as we do the yoga practices that cultivate smooth purification and opening of the nervous system. This is what the heart calls us to, and this is what opens the heart.

If there is discomfort in the heart (non-medical), it is a symptom of energy imbalance and we should look to our practices and good self-pacing to resolve it. This is a path of joy, not one of discomfort and fear. So we always are using practices in a way that cultivates smooth progress and pleasurable experiences. That way we are always motivated to continue, and our arrival at our destination is certain.

Keeping yogic teachings secret may have been appropriate in the past, but I don't think it is appropriate now. There are so many people running around these days with intense desire for God and practices, spontaneous spiritual experiences, etc. Burgeoning worldwide spiritual need does not favor such important knowledge being locked up (in fragments, I might add) in a few overly protective esoteric traditions. We are in the midst of a massive shift in world consciousness. Now is the time for everyone to have access to the complete means for safely and effectively purifying and opening their nervous system. That is what these lessons are about.

I wish you all success as you continue along your chosen spiritual path. It's good to have you here, and I hope the lessons will be a continuing help to you.

The guru is in you.

Lesson 202 – Free-Form versus Structured Practices

Q: I love reading your lessons. I have not caught up and read them all, but I print them and will get to them.

Most of the practices you have written about seem to happen to me spontaneously over time during my meditations. I do not consciously do any of them. I have this energy that comes upon me almost as soon as I sit down on my mediation cushion. I simply surrender to it and let it have its way with me. I have learned to simply surrender with trust and gratitude.

Four years ago at a ten-day vipassana silent meditation retreat, I experienced a profound kundalini opening. I have been meditating every day since, usually for one hour. I have done this usually only once a day.

I had to learn to deal with this new energy that was out of control and totally in charge of my physical body at first, creating various problems for me. I had to learn to ground myself, protect myself and learn to function in a new way. There have been many profound experiences during this ongoing process. I have learned to simply trust that I am being purified.

I have incorporated several techniques in my daily practice. I use incense, because I like it, and I often listen to Sanskrit chants while I meditate, but I really feel more like I get meditated. I sometimes repeat chants in my head; I have found the full *SHREE OM I AM* works better for me then simply *I AM*. But I often just disappear into nothingness.

My question has to do with my practice. It seems to work for me. Sometimes in reading your lessons, I recognize the techniques you talk about as having happened to me at some time during my meditations. Since what I am doing is working, I wonder if it benefits me to change to a more conscious doing of the various techniques?

I often feel like I am simply the witness to what is happening in my body. I simply surrender, and observe. I become the witness, I do not judge, I simply let go. Sometimes I have a profound emptiness, at other times there are many thoughts, colors, lights, visions, etc. I feel like the energy has been moving through my body, healing me, clearing away blocks. There has been much physical movement at times and at times it has been painful, but I just let it happen. I often experience various yoga postures or mudras spontaneously. There have been times when I would simply cry for the full hour, not even sure of why I was crying. The energy would simply get to a part of my body and I would be crying. It always feels like a tremendous release, and I feel wonderful thereafter. I feel like I am becoming Lighter and Lighter. I am very sensitive to energy, and quite empathic. I keep learning how to deal with those issues. It has been, and continues to be a journey.

Any comments or suggestions? I find your lessons to be very helpful.

A: Thank you for your kind note. It is much appreciated. Your experiences sound very progressive and smooth (wonderful!), so who am I to suggest alterations? It sounds like you are having fun on your journey, and that is how it should be.

On the other hand, meditation and most other practices produce the most efficient results if the technique in use is favored for an allotted time. "Efficient" means maximum forward progress with the least discomfort. It takes some doing, and I'm not sure how it can be done without measuring practices in some way.

A structured program of practice might seem restrictive if you are in a long time habit of using a free-form approach. Still, structure has its advantages. It keeps us on course, especially when there are influences that can distract us. It keeps us from fooling ourselves into believing we are doing practices at times when we may only be coasting. Structure is also useful when we are using an integration of powerful advanced practices that move a lot of ecstatic energy through our nervous system. It is easy to overdo when there is so much ecstasy being generated, and then we need a way to measure our practice for optimum application and comfort. Using the clock for each practice becomes important then. There are plenty of examples in the lessons on the importance of self-pacing. Self-pacing is an essential part of most people's practice here. This is a very fast path – as fast as the practitioner wants to go. Without prudent self-pacing, we'd have folks burning out left and right. Even with self-pacing it gets a little hairy sometimes.

So it is a question of how fast you want to go, while keeping safe (and sane) at the same time.

Maybe a compromise would work for you. Certain practices you could do by the clock, and then another part of your routine could remain free form. A steady dose of spinal breathing could be especially helpful to you if you are experiencing delicate emotions at times, which can indicate an inner energy imbalance.

It is a matter of traveling as quickly and smoothly as we choose. It is up to you.

The guru is in you.

Lesson 203 – Reflections on Some Dramatic Experiences

Q: I am going to an ashram in India for almost a month. My guru will be there, the one who I truly resonate with.

I want to talk to you about some things that have been going on. I am grateful to have someone who will respond with something other than a hearty laugh at my "goings on." (My guru always just smiles or laughs.) He told me less than a year ago that I was resisting. I do not wish to resist Truth. Why live in ignorance? But still, I must have some resistance.

I have had all sorts of crazy things happening. I'm the one who'd written you a while back about always having the kundalini – even as a little child – seeing the lights, feeling the buzz, hearing the hums, etc. But what's going on now is even more. I need to tell this to someone who does not know me, not to anyone around me. A lot of it is stuff I've already experienced, but some of it is new. I'll list it:

Seeing flashes of light of all colors now and then – especially around animals and people and some trees.

Feeling energy coursing through my body – highly erotic, but not sexual (not exactly...)

Stiffness and pain around the bottom, back of skull and into the back of the neck and jaw. Lots of popping going on along the spine there – especially during the spinal breathing you gave me (which I incorporated into my yoga pranayamas).

My right hand has been doing a lot of sporadic shaking and if I get any extra energy surges, I start squeezing it and then releasing it by flexing it backwards quickly – as if the energy were just pouring out of it. A lot of vibrating in the hands and feet.

A general feeling of excitement.

Sobs come when I think on my guru's compassion. People keep telling me what you have told me, that the guru is within ... that brings me to the next thing … I hear my gurus in my head. Yes, I know it sounds crazy, but they tell me the answers when I need them. I could actually go to them with all of this – but I want external validation.

If I need an answer, I open up *Beyond Words*, and it speaks of exactly what I need to hear – in the precise words.

My guru's picture seems to move and the expressions actually change while I am looking at it, communicating with him.

I can tell what people are feeling – and seem to know before them why they are feeling this way.

If someone asks me a question on spirituality, I can move aside and someone else seems to answer through me.

At certain times, it's like I'm detached, like a balloon, floating in the air, watching myself down below. During these times, if I look at the ground, it seems so far down there ...but there is a general unconcern during these times about most things.

Things are seeming to manifest – without any stated intention on my part. I only have to sort of unconsciously think it, and it happens.

I am meeting people on "the path" a lot now.

I am still having fits where I shake – especially if I go inside to certain places where I feel a lot of intensity.

I started having those things again where energy explodes through my system (that I've had my whole life off and on) where it shoots out everywhere, but my solar plexus is disturbed and I feel like I have to swallow a lot, and I also feel like I need to use the bathroom, and often have to find a restroom very soon afterwards. I am then tired and have a hard time communicating anything – sort of in a daze.

When I'm talking to people that I feel free with (at my church or in my yoga group), I've found that my body starts doing things to express its bliss. It will start waving its arms in the air in a dance, or doing tree posture, or outright dancing!

When I meditated with a man from our church – doing a tantric meditation – I started a lot of the shaking – energy going up the spine and out the top or around the mouth or third eye.

If I ever just lie there, still, my awareness of the energy increases heavily. During meditation, I feel surges coming, Grace from above, descending down, down, down, through me. (Thank you God and guru!)

Third eye is doing a lot of whirring about.

Often, lately, in the car, I will begin feeling my guru(s), or having a conversation with them, and this inwardly exciting thing starts happening, and I feel I have to scream! So I scream a scream that is penetrating and shrill and sort of blissful. My right hand starts doing its thing and/or my spine starts lurching about – but I'm perfectly OK and still in control of the car.

At times, I will move my hand in a certain fashion, or flip my hair, and I feel as if I am my guru. Yes, strange, I know. Is this something to do with merging? It's literally as if I can't tell the difference between him and me for that short instance. It's nothing I'm thinking about, really; it's more like for a flash, I feel no difference between us.

I'm feeling like I need to meditate with others a lot lately.

During my meditations, I used to be able to go into them without even remembering anything. Now, though, I have jerks in my body often. I have had two dreams/visions, where I am not at all afraid of death. One, while standing on a plastic tarp in the middle of the ocean as large waves rolled around. The other, a man was burying my orange dress. The dress stood for spirituality and seemed to be synonymous with my skin. I did not feel anything as I watched him covering it with dirt. I am willing to drop every concept I have had of "spirituality" and begin anew.

I seem to have picked up a hoard of spirit guides or teachers on the astral plane. I don't even know how I am aware of this.

I have recently spoken with an "Indigo." I could feel him very strongly over the phone, although I've never met him. Beautiful.

I'm picking up vibes of lower entities, and also seeing one in my classroom door. He lurks about there often as a dark silhouette Indigo opening my cabinet door, etc. to get my (and my students') attention.

Longing is intense. I feel this "place" which I've known before, but cannot seem to find and hold. It visits like a flash and then is gone. My guru told me, "You have not done this before."

Anyway, I'll be seeing my guru coming up, but I am unsure if I should tell him about these things and talk with him about them. I don't know what will happen next. Never do. I don't care. I am here for it to happen. If it is unnecessary emotion and commotion which helps nothing other than convincing me, then I want to fast forward to the part where I no longer need these things to be convinced.

As Llewellyn Vaughan-Lee says of the two year old girl's prayer, "God, I know." and God said, "Yes, and I know."

My guru knows. But I could use some sort of explanation, still. Do you have one for me? Or is it all part of the mystery and will be spoiled by another telling me? Or will I not understand anyway?

Should I be doing meditations? I've met a new man who I want to do meditations with. He goes to my church. Also, should I do Reiki swap outs? Or is this not good for me at this time?

I was speaking with someone who I know has been working on himself for a long time. He is one of the very few I confide in, and actually I'd not told anyone this outright, but I was telling him that I could communicate with my teachers in my head and that one of them comforts me and another is more of a motivator, but that the essential core of them felt the same. (It gets confusing. Are they me?) And he said he does not have this. I doubted for a second my experience when he said it because of him and you – always telling me the guru is within. I don't know who I am anymore – I seem to be expanding into something else. Maybe my guru and others are within as aspects of my inner guru...

Maybe it's the pranayamas, meditation, and asanas that are speeding things up. I still don't feel as if I've reached where I once "was."

Despite all of this, my life is pretty balanced/ordinary. I'm still teaching and planning to make more trips to India. I'm testing the waters on this trip. If it feels right, I'll come back for a while, and then move to India for two years (as my guru has suggested.) On the other hand, I'm having to do extra alternate nostril breathing for inner balance. The family still doesn't like my yogic stuff, but my church and yogic family does. I still have some time for my dog and 3 cats.

I also make time to read your Advanced Yoga Practices often. Still not anywhere near finished with them...

Sorry such a long letter! I had a lot going on and I needed to release it! We are all so blessed to have someone to respond to us and give us the attention you have given us.

A: It's good to hear from you again. Much of what you are experiencing falls under the category of purification in the nervous system. As such, it is a mixture of truth and the karmic "exhaust" of obstructions being dissolved and burned up. That is perhaps why your guru is not responding on the details. It is impossible to do so and make sense of everything that is happening. Nor will it matter for the karmic combustion parts of it. And what is true will stand on its own. Truth is what is left when all the rest has been burned off. There are a few points I'd like to mention.

To the extent you are doing practices, you are hastening the process. That is good, but excessive practices can lead to excessive symptoms, and then prudent "self-pacing" should be applied. There is no point to be doing practices to the extent where life becomes chaos and one cannot function. I know that is not where you are, but if you press too hard with extra practices, and all the other things you are considering, it could become like that. So, a little moderation and measurement of daily practices would not hurt. We want to go fast, but not so fast that we shake to pieces or burn up.

Keep in mind that the most balancing practice you have from the lessons is spinal breathing. Too much or too little of it can leave you either short on balancing or short on progress. Doing the same amount of spinal breathing at each twice-daily sitting is important, whether it be 5, 10, 15 or more minutes, depending on your comfort level. The same goes for meditation. The rest of the practices in the lessons wrap around those two. If you are "doubling up" on practices in each sitting, like doing two or more kinds of meditation, or multiple pranayamas beyond what is recommended in a single approach, or adding additional group practices on a regular basis, all that will contribute to the potential for excessive releases. So it is best to stick with a steady routine of complementary practices, paced for maximum progress with good comfort. I mention all that just as food for thought. You seem to be doing okay, though you are pushing the envelope a bit there. No doubt the envelope will get pushed even more in India, though you will be under good supervision there, right?

The two most important experiences you mentioned from my perspective are the witnessing, which is the rise of inner silence, and the erotic/ecstatic sensations moving up through your body. These two are at the heart of the enlightenment process, its foundation actually, and are what advanced yoga practices cultivate. To be honest, all the rest is just a passing show, and ought not be given more than casual notice, and definitely not favored over practices. A recent Q&A covering this in detail is called, "The drama of a premature crown opening." With limited inner silence/witnessing, one can be prone to identify too much with experiences. Enlightenment is not about experiences. A few lessons earlier is one called "Managing the opening of the crown." You might find these two discussions pertinent to your situation. Not that all of it applies to you, but you will see some of the same elements, benefits, and risks you have had or are facing now.

On seeing the guru(s) inside, that is along the lines of what is described in lesson #57, "The Guru is in Me?" The guru begins in us as desire, goes out to link with outer knowledge and/or physical guru, and then goes back inside and is seen there. So seeing your guru(s) inside is a natural part of the bhakti process. Eventually, he/they will dissolve into your rising enlightenment and it will be your own Self that is radiating out. All of this is part of the process of purification also, so your guru may not focus on it because the details of karmic release are unfathomable. It is all going on in you, leading inevitably to your enlightenment. That is the most important thing.

It sounds like you are doing very well. Just favor stability in your routine of practices, and try to avoid jumping whole-hog into new ones until you develop an understanding of how they will complement your overall practice. Otherwise you could be "doubling up" on things and overdoing. It takes a certain amount of ordinary everyday activity to stabilize the energies we stimulate in practices, so sometimes less practice and more activity can bring more progress. You have all this in your busy routine already, of course. These are just reminders.

Have a wonderful time in India! I'd love to hear from you when you get back.

The guru is in you.

Lesson 204* – Summary of Principles, Abilities and Practices

We have covered a large amount of information so far, and now we have come to the point where all of the main advanced yoga practices have been shared. Does this mean there is nothing else to add in the way of practices? I don't think we could ever get to that stage, because yoga is a vast subject with innumerable details that we could discuss indefinitely. There are many supporting and incidental practices we can get into. Maybe we will as the discussion continues. But the primary ones have been covered already here in the main lessons and in the tantra lessons. Using the advanced yoga practices given so far, so much purification and opening deep in the nervous system can be achieved that everything else that is necessary for enlightenment will come automatically through the connectedness of yoga.

That is the goal in these lessons – to provide the essential means to stimulate the nervous system to purify and open itself, which it is very inclined to do when given the opportunity. Once the ball gets rolling, many aspects of our natural inclination toward human spiritual transformation will kick in. The goal here is to assist you in becoming self-sufficient in yoga like that.

Way back in the beginning of the lessons, we talked about natural abilities contained within all of us that only need some stimulation to move us toward conscious inner openings to the infinite. These abilities are rooted in several fundamental principles that are inherent in our nervous system. We are all designed and built to experience unending divine ecstatic bliss!

In this lesson we will review the fundamental principles, the natural abilities that stem from them, and the practices that have been given that stimulate these natural abilities. The essence of yoga science is discovering and applying the simplest and most powerful means for leveraging the natural abilities we have to hasten our spiritual transformation. That is what these lessons have been aiming to do.

The fundamental principles of human spiritual transformation are simple enough, and we have touched on them often in the lessons, discussing them from many different angles. There are five of them:

Fundamental Principles

- Attraction – To Truth and/or God, expressed as desire – It is Love.

- Purification and opening – A process every human nervous system is naturally inclined to go through.

- Inner silence – Pure bliss consciousness, our native state that shines though our nervous system as purification and opening occur.

- Ecstasy – Experienced when our nervous system is stimulated by the awakening our inner life force.

- Union – our transformation to a permanent state of compassionate unity, the fruition of the merging of our inner silence and ecstasy – It is Love.

These fundamental principles of enlightenment begin with love and end with love. It is love that leads us through human spiritual transformation involving the purification and opening of our nervous system, which reveals the principles of inner silence and ecstatic conductivity in us, and their merging. To accomplish this, love employs the methods of yoga, which take advantage of natural abilities we all have that are associated with the five fundamental principles. Let's list those abilities now:

Natural Abilities

1. The ability that desire, consistently applied toward an objective, has to move our inner and outer expressions of energy (life force) in ways that fundamentally change our experience of life.

2. The ability our mind has to move naturally toward stillness. This is awareness without any objects – also called inner silence, or pure bliss consciousness.

3. The ability of the mind to effortlessly refine the thought of a sound, naturally bringing the mind to stillness over and over again. Certain sounds resonate with certain aspects of our nervous system. These sounds can be used selectively to stimulate the nervous system toward an orderly transformation.

4. The mind-body connection that enables naturally cultivated stillness of mind to induce stillness of our body, metabolism, and breath. This is the connectedness of yoga, experienced in many ways through our opening nervous system.

5. The ability of our nervous system to naturally sustain the quality of stillness, our silent blissful inner consciousness, even when it is not being cultivated. This is called a state of "silent witnessing," among other things.

6. The ability of restraint and regulation of breath to influence the flow of life force in the nervous system, producing a sensation of relaxation and, ultimately, feelings of ecstasy in the body.

7. The ability of inner silence and the flow of life force in the body to remove obstructions lodged deep in our nervous system, purifying and opening our awareness gradually to an expanding experience of inner peace, creative energy, happiness and love.

8. The ability of restraint and regulation of breath to "awaken" the vast storehouse of life force located in our pelvic region – sexual energy that is drawn upward in our nervous system to compensate for a reduced intake of oxygen when the breath is gently restrained.

9. The ability of attention to influence the flow of the life force in the body, especially when combined with restraint and regulation of breath.

10. The ability of certain nerves and nerve plexuses to be stimulated physically to enhance and direct the flow of life force in the body.

11. The ability of the neuro-biology in the center and front of the head (the third eye) to connect with and direct (control) the neuro-biology near the base of the spine and the vast storehouse of life force (sexual energy) in that region.

12. The ability of the nerve in the center of the spine to conduct the life force and ecstatic energy between the pelvic region and the third eye. This is called the spinal nerve.

13. The ability of the spinal nerve to radiate life force and ecstatic energy throughout the entire body, enlivening every aspect of the higher neuro-biology within us in a smooth and orderly way. This is the rise of permanent ecstatic conductivity.

14. The ability of the nervous system to amplify the power of a thought when the thought is initiated deep in inner silence, yielding great purifying effects in the body and surrounding environment.

15. The ability of inner silence and ecstatic energy to merge and be sustained as one self-conscious presence in our nervous system. This is experienced as ecstatic bliss. This we come to know as the expression of our Self.

16. The ability of ecstatic bliss to flow out from us to our surroundings as divine love. Then we find our Self in the form of all we encounter. This is the natural flowering of divine love in service to all beings.

All of these abilities exist in us, and only need some nudging to begin to manifest changes in how our nervous system is functioning. With the full range of advanced yoga practices, we can do a lot of nudging, stimulating every natural ability we have that can move us along the path of human spiritual transformation.

Everyone reacts a little differently to the processes of stimulation through yoga practices, due to the differences we each have in the structure of inner obstructions that are to be steadily and safely dissolved. We all can make the journey of transformation through yoga. It is only a matter of managing the conduct of our practices. This we call, "self-pacing."

We have built up an integrated system of practices that stimulate the activation of the abilities listed above, bringing to our conscious experience the fulfillment of the five fundamental principles.

Let's now list the practices for review.

Practices

1. Cultivation of desire for practices – bhakti (love of Truth and/or God in the heart). Bhakti/desire is the engine that drives all yoga practices. We accomplish it by favoring a chosen high ideal (ishta) with all of our desires and emotions, whether they are positive or

negative. In this way, a huge momentum driving us toward enlightenment is created within us and around us. Then everything we need to progress on our journey is drawn to us magnetically, including the willpower to engage in daily advanced yoga practices for as long as it takes to complete our journey.

2. Deep meditation with the mantra *I AM* (plus several mantra enhancements along the way). Meditation involves easily favoring the mantra to bring the mind (and body) to stillness over and over again twice-daily, stimulating deep purification in our nervous system, and yielding permanent inner blissful silence.

3. Spinal breathing pranayama – the primary practice for awakening and balancing the life force in the spinal nerve between the third eye and root. The life force is also called kundalini.

4. Enhancements to spinal breathing using throat opening on inhalation, restricted epiglottis (ujjayi) during exhalation, and tracing ascending cool currents and descending warm currents in the spinal nerve during inhalation and exhalation. These enhancements increase stimulation of the life force in the spinal nerve.

5. Mulabandha/asvini – manipulations using the anal sphincter muscle to awaken the life force (kundalini) at the root.

6. Sambhavi – a means for producing direct physical stimulation of the neurological mechanisms of the third eye in the head, involving raising and centering of the eyes toward the point between the eyebrows, and slightly furrowing the brow. Controlled and stable stimulation of kundalini at the root and throughout the nervous system is achieved in this way.

7. Asanas (postures) – systematic bending and stretching of the body that is a natural complement to spinal breathing pranayama and deep meditation. Asanas help cultivate and purify the nervous system.

8. Siddhasana – a powerful way of sitting during practices for awakening kundalini at the root. The heel is placed firmly at the perineum, and constant stimulation of sexual energy is achieved. Over time, the entire nervous system is illuminated by this procedure, performed effortlessly during all sitting advanced yoga practices.

9. Yoni mudra kumbhaka – a practice that helps open the third eye with air pressure in the nasal passages and sinuses, and awakens the life force/kundalini in the entire nervous system through kumbhaka (breath retention) and associated mudras and bandhas.

10. Tantric sexual relations (the holdback method) – similar to the dynamics of siddhasana and used during sexual relations with or without a partner. Tantric sex is a powerful way to enliven and distribute the life force (kundalini) throughout the body.

11. Kechari mudra (four stages) – raising the tongue upward in stages to (1) the roof of the mouth, (2) above the soft palate to the spiritually erogenous edge of the nasal septum, (3) to the top of the nasal pharynx cavity, and (4) to the point between the eyebrows through the spiritually sensitive nasal passages. Entering stage 2 kechari is one of the most dramatic transitions in all advanced yoga practices. It is a primary stimulator of kundalini, and a major cause of the rise of permanent ecstatic conductivity in the nervous system.

12. Uddiyana bandha and nauli – stimulating the upward movement of kundalini using the diaphragm and abdominal muscles. Nauli involves twirling the abdominal muscles, and is highly stimulating to kundalini.

13. Dynamic jalandhara (chin pump), with or without kumbhaka (breath retention). This is rotating the head while systematically dropping it toward the chest with each rotation, stimulating ecstatic energies between the heart and head, and throughout the body.

14. Samyama – the process of initiating and releasing particular thoughts (sutras) deep within our inner silence, producing powerful purifying effects throughout the nervous system. The effects can manifest as so-called supernormal powers, which are called siddhis. Samyama is done for spiritual purification.

15. Spinal bastrika – rapid breathing in the spinal nerve between the third eye and root, which dramatically accelerates the purification of the spinal nerve, and the entire nervous system.

16. Targeted bastrika – for the third eye, throat, heart, abdomen, or pelvic/root area. This rapid breathing method is for focusing on and clearing out stubborn karmic obstructions lodged in particular areas of our spiritual anatomy, as needed.

17. Crown to root bastrika – This is also rapid breathing in the spinal nerve, going between the crown flower cup and root. It is best undertaken only after extensive purification of the nervous system has been achieved through third eye to root spinal breathing, deep meditation, and other methods that cleanse the nervous system of karmic obstructions in a smooth and progressive manner. Premature opening of the crown can lead to much difficulty, discomfort, and distraction on the path, so this advanced practice is best undertaken only when tests of stability have been successfully conducted at the crown.

18. Loving service to others – a conscious practice, and a natural result of the increasing outward flow of divine love resulting from the purification and opening of the nervous system produced by advanced yoga practices. This is our natural state of being – an endless overflowing of ecstatic bliss and divine love. Nothing on this earth, or beyond, is more real or more powerful than this great truth that is inherent in every one of us. The reality of divine love is the ultimate truth in us. As we become advanced in yoga, this becomes crystal clear. For some it is known right from the very first sitting in deep meditation.

This lesson has been to summarize all that we have covered so far, including the fundamental principles of human spiritual transformation, the natural abilities we have within us that bring about our transformation, and the key advanced yoga practices that stimulate our natural abilities into action.

With a twice-daily routine of practices, we place ourselves on a "fast track" to enlightenment. It is potentially so fast that it is essential that we develop skill in regulating the practices we are doing each day, measuring each practice by the clock. We adjust practice times as necessary to maintain smooth and steady progress without incurring excessive discomfort due to too many obstructions being released in our nervous system.

This regulation of practices is called "self-pacing," and it too is a practice – one of the most important practices. For, without good self-pacing, we are not likely to get very far on the road to enlightenment.

Another aspect of Advanced Yoga Practices is the prudent handling of experiences, whether they are mundane or extreme. This is a path of enjoyment, and we are entitled to enjoy the "scenery" we encounter on our journey to enlightenment. However, the scenery is not what will advance us on our path, It is our practices that will move us ahead. So, after an admiring look at the passing scenery, no matter how beautiful or attention grabbing it may be, we easily go back to the practice we are doing. If spiritual experiences come while we are in our daily activities, as they certainly shall, we then can continue to enjoy the experiences, or go back to whatever it is we are doing.

We always have a choice. Spiritual life is not something that must be hijacking us from ordinary life. If it is, we have probably engaged in some kind of excess in the past, and a stable routine of practices can correct this. Spiritual life is something that can be cultivated to fulfill our daily activities in everyday life, whatever they may be. We are free to live our rising spiritual experiences in a way that is compatible with our needs. It is our life, our journey and our enlightenment. We have no one to become but our Self.

Enjoy!

The guru is in you.

Addition – After reading this lesson, you might ask yourself, "What is a typical routine of practices that would result from all these principles, abilities and practices?"

It can vary from one person to the next, depending on the condition of the nervous system, bhakti (desire), time available for practices, experiences, and a number of other factors. For some people, meditation will be plenty. Others may go for spinal breathing and meditation. Others may go for the "whole ball of wax." In the case of someone who has built up to a routine involving all of the methods in lessons, the routine could look something like this:

- Asanas – 10 min
- Spinal breathing – 10 min
- Chin pump – 5 min
- Spinal bastrika – 5 min
- Meditation – 20 min

- Samyama – 10 min
- Yoni mudra – 5 minutes
- Targeted or crown bastrika (optional) – 5 min
- Rest – 5 min (or more)

That is about 75 minutes – an hour and fifteen minutes. It is one of many possible routines of practice that could evolve, depending on the preferences and experiences of the yogi or yogini. In lesson #209, we will get into strategies for managing the time associated with keeping up such a routine under varying circumstances in daily life.

Lesson 205 – More on Kechari

Q: Namaste: I want to request you to provide a picture with the different stages of kechari clearly shown. Your verbal description of kechari mudra is very elaborate; still a picture would make it easier to understand. After all, a picture is worth 1,000 words! Someone who underwent the cutting of the frenum told me that he had difficulty speaking clearly when the tongue became very long – is this true in your experience? He also said that elements (the five elements in the body) became unbalanced (not sure what exactly it means other than it does not sound very nice).

Your description of kechari mudra is superb and unparalleled compared to what I have come across so far. I am very grateful for this.

A: Yes, a picture is worth 1,000 words, and for kechari they have been hard to come by. Illustrations for kechari stages 1-5 are provided with lesson #108 in this volume. Additionally, you can find several images by others listed under "Kechari" in the AYP links section on the web site.

Very gradual tiny snipping (I prefer that description to "cutting") does not lengthen the tongue. It only gradually frees it from being tethered to the floor of the mouth, so it is able to go back and up. In the lesson on kechari, I pointed out that the tongue is already long enough to accomplish all the stages of kechari, and how you can measure that for yourself.

Milking, or stretching of the tongue does lengthen it, but I don't regard it as the best means to achieve stage 2 or 3 kechari, and have only engaged in it to a modest degree myself. There are stories about yogis who have lengthened their tongues to the extent that they can touch the point between their eyebrows from the outside. It is not necessary. It is only another version of extremism in yoga, which I am not for.

I first entered stage 2 kechari 20 years ago, and have never found any difficulty with speech, swallowing, or anything else physical because of it. I won't say it was completely easy all the time either. It does rearrange the inner energies substantially, and perhaps that is what your friend is referring to about the elements. But it is a natural rearrangement that leads to much more enlightenment in life, and that is why we are doing yoga, right?

As with all yoga practices, some self-pacing may be required from time to time to keep temporary energy imbalances associated with purification in the nervous system from becoming too extreme. Kechari is no different in that respect. In time, the energies readjust at progressively higher levels of functioning, which correspond with higher levels of spiritual experience. Then we can stay in kechari throughout our sitting practices, and beyond, with nothing but waves of whole-body ecstatic bliss coming from it. Who would avoid kechari when it gets to be like that? Not me!

Kechari is a long journey with many challenges and rewards along the way, and it requires a lot of bhakti to undertake and carry through. It is well worth the effort. It is an important aspect of our journey to enlightenment. Can we do without kechari? Perhaps. I can't really say for sure, as I am one of those who chose to go the way of kechari, and I don't know where I would have ended up without it. Certainly with far less spiritual transformation than I have experienced.

Kechari is one of those natural spiritual abilities we all have. When the time is right, it happens.

The guru is in you.

Lesson 206 – Varieties of Spinal Breathing

Q: What are the different variations of the spinal breath? There are two different kriyas revealed by Norman Paulsen. Also, one of Sri Lahiri Mahasaya's original kriyas is available over the web (this involves breathing up and down the spine with chanting of *OM* at the spinal plexuses). It would be worthwhile to know the different varieties of kriya, as I think that everyone's optimal kriya is different.

A: The number of versions of spinal breathing is limited only by the imagination. The essential ingredient in all of them is the brow to perineum route of attention with slow breathing. 90%-plus of the results come from that. It is that simple. It is easy to make it complicated, and risk watering down the results by adding chakra imagery, sounds, colors, mantras, etc. Any or all of those additions don't contribute much. In fact, all that can distract from the essential function of purifying and opening the spinal nerve between the third eye and the root.

As you know, these lessons put separate attention on deep meditation, and we don't divide the mind by trying to do both spinal breathing and deep meditation at the same time. Of course, anyone is free to do as they wish in spinal breathing, and may have been taught spinal breathing differently elsewhere. In the lessons, we try and keep it to the least common denominator in all practices, so as many as possible can benefit from a straight-forward approach. That is why spinal breathing is taught in the simple way that it is here.

Assuming one is doing deep meditation right after, there is little that can be added to substantially improve the effectiveness of this simple form of spinal breathing. It would be very easy to add a few twists and say, "Here is the best form of spinal breathing." Well, maybe we have done that. What you get in these lessons is spinal breathing without all the bells and whistles, and it works just fine. This is the essential practice that marries the root and third eye. That is what spinal breathing is about. Energetically, everything else in the nervous system flows automatically from that. There is no need to fiddle around much in the middle when we are effectively merging together both ends.

In this approach, instead of bogging ourselves down with a lot of detail in spinal breathing, we stick with the basics, and then take the opportunity to move quickly into many other practices (mulabandha, sambhavi, siddhasana, yoni mudra, kechari, chin pump, spinal bastrika, etc.) that make a huge difference in our spiritual progress. So, instead of "gilding the lily" of spinal breathing, we bring in a lot more lilies. By doing this, we are able to develop a powerful and well-rounded integration of practices in a reasonably short period of time, without a lot of tedious and unnecessary detail.

So, I don't agree that each person needs a different form of spinal breathing. Certainly, each person may have a preference based on tradition, personal whim, etc., and that's okay. Just keep in mind that it is going between the third eye and root that produces the results. In the end, those two divine poles are merged and we are drowned in ecstatic bliss.

The guru is in you.

Lesson 207 – Left or Right Side Imbalances

Q: Three weeks ago I had an intuitive flash while meditating. I was in the attic of a very large and luxurious house. I had been cleaning this house from top to bottom until it was immaculately clean. It sparkled! It was perfect. Then when I reached the attic I found a door. When I opened the door I discovered that there was an entire wing of the house that I had not known about. It was in horrible disarray. Everything was covered with an inch of dust. Wood rot, water damage, mildew, broken windows ... It was bad! I wanted to close the door and forget what I had just seen.

The house is me, and the attic is my third eye. At that moment I realized that the right side of my body is very energetically strong but my left side in thin, weak and blocked. I was floored! The magnitude of this was like looking in the mirror for the first time and realizing that I have been walking around for the past 30 years with an elephant strapped to my back! How could I have missed this? For the next few days I felt as if I was two different people joined together at the center of my body.

With effort I have been able to direct energy to the left side of my body, at first with great physical pain on the left side of my third eye. I can tell that this balance from right to left is going to take some time.

What does this indicate?

A: The obstructions in the nervous system can take nearly any form, and sometimes can be skewed to the left or right side of the body. It is difficult to know how it got that way, but yoga practices can gradually dissolve it all at its source, and bring us back into balance. The fact that you are seeing these things more clearly now is an indicator of purification going on from your practices, particularly in the third eye. The thing to do is continue with your practices as you have been doing them and let the process carry forward naturally.

Generally speaking, it is not a good idea to try and direct the purification process in a specific direction outside the third eye to root spinal nerve, or the well-rounded (global) effects of deep meditation and samyama. We just can't know intellectually what the natural order of purification will be, whereas, inner silence and our ecstatic energies will find the purification channels of least resistance. How the purification happens will depend on so many karmic factors unique to each person. It can all be taken care of in a balanced way by eliciting the natural processes of purification from within with our advanced yoga practices.

If we think we have an imbalance on the left side and focus attention on fixing that, we could cause more imbalances. Better to use meditation, spinal breathing, mudras and bandhas, yoni mudra, spinal bastrika, chin pump and so on. All these work up and down the central nerve and will not lead to left or right side imbalances which can be destabilizing. If you have a left or right side imbalance, the best way to resolve it is to do practices in the middle. That is the focus in the lessons. If you go the middle way with spinal breathing, meditation and the other practices, you will find increasing balance from top to bottom and from left to right. The spinal nerve (sushumna) between the third eye and root is the master key. All is balanced by purifying that.

The practices that have brought you to this level of seeing are the same ones that can safely clear out the obstructions that are becoming more visible.

Remember the guideline on visions – if we see something, we do not try and push it out or become overly attached to it by engaging in it excessively. We just easily go back to the practice we are doing and continue the purification process.

By staying with a twice-daily routine of advanced yoga practices, balanced with an active life in line with our interests, we will be moving steadily toward enlightenment.

The guru is in you.

Lesson 208 – Inner Energy Collisions and Strong Emotions

Q: I have been doing kundalini yoga for about a year now and have recently taken a teacher training program. I have been practicing on my own and in class and have done my first sadhana at home yesterday. I found myself feeling fine until later on at night. I was suddenly enraged in anger and wanted to punch something. This is not my usual tendency and I felt it this morning as well. I was wondering if it had to do with doing too much kundalini or maybe my system is cleansing too much too fast. I'm really not sure and wanted to run this by you to see what you thought. It was as if something took over me, and my emotions were so overwhelmed. This is unusual since I usually take things easier and haven't gotten enraged like that since I was a child.

A: Strong emotions can come when inner energy collides or is having excessive friction with obstructions in the nervous system. Interestingly, ecstatic experience is created in the same way. It is just a matter of degree of energy flow and getting the inner dynamics of purification in the right order.

This is obviously not a static situation. If we increase energy flow without sufficient removal of obstructions first, there can be unpleasant collisions and friction. If we are releasing obstructions too fast, then our ordinary inner energy flow can run into the loosened and lingering obstructions, causing irritability. In the lessons we have a variety of strategies built into and around the practices to avoid the uncomfortable aspects of this situation. For the most part it works, and we can move ahead smoothly and quickly with purification and opening of the nervous system. In the case of kundalini yoga, what I keep running into with people that are having symptoms like what you described is premature crown openings. I don't know what you are doing in the way of practices, but these symptoms are often associated with practices at the crown. You may wish to read the earlier lessons on crown openings.

With a premature crown opening, the energy flow is often too much for the matrix of obstructions still embedded in the nervous system. A prematurely opened crown and a more or less average nervous system are not a good match, and, if pressed, can lead to years of misery. Gopi Krishna is the classic authority on this kind of "doing it the hard way" road to enlightenment.

Traditionally, the smoothest path to enlightenment has been via purification and opening of the third eye to root spinal nerve. This is the approach in the lessons, and we hit it from every angle with an integrated system of practices. By this means, the crown is opened by indirect influence, and the extremes of an energy flow/obstruction matrix mismatch are usually avoided. Instead, the path is filled with steadily rising inner silence and ecstasy, which is what we want from our yoga. So, with the little you have shared, that is my best guess – you may be moving too much energy up with the crown, instead of working it through the third eye to root spinal nerve first. There is much more detail in the lessons on this, particularly in the more recent ones.

If premature crown opening is not the culprit, there is also the possibility that you are doing more practice than your nervous system can comfortably absorb at this time. In that case, the thing to do is back off to a stable level of practice, and ramp back up later when the coast is clear. This is self-pacing. I wish you all success on your chosen path.

The guru is in you.

Lesson 209 – Fitting Daily Practices into a Busy Schedule

Whatever system of spiritual practices we are following, the chances are that we have heard, or figured out on our own, that daily practice is the key to success. The journey of human spiritual transformation takes time, and the inner changes that lead to our enlightenment require daily cultivation. Daily spiritual practices are also needed when we already have spiritual momentum, meaning if we have some degree of dynamic inner opening occurring either through previous practices or a "spontaneous awakening." If we rely only on the energies that are moving in us spontaneously, then we can be prone to imbalances that will make our journey homeward toward unending ecstatic bliss and divine love considerably less comfortable, and potentially longer than necessary.

So, no matter what our approach or level of attainment is, reaching our destination in a reliable fashion depends on having daily spiritual practices firmly in place. This was emphasized in these lessons with the first instructions on deep meditation, and with many reminders since then.

Way back in the lessons on meditation and spinal breathing, some suggestions were given on how to fit these practices into a busy schedule. Wherever we may be, we can close our eyes and meditate – in trains, airplanes, waiting rooms, just about anywhere. The same is true of spinal breathing. In fact, light spinal breathing can be done with eyes open while on the way home from work in the car, without taking our attention off our driving. So, by the time we are home we can go right into meditation. It is not ideal practice, but can be done if the clock is pressing us at home. If we are willing to be flexible and compromise on our practices from time to time, we can keep up the habit under the most adverse circumstances. There is great value in this, for it assures us of a continuation of practices over the long term, which is the key to enlightenment.

We do not live in an ideal world. Even with the best plans for regular practice in our meditation room, it can all go out the window with a family emergency or other intervening events. Does this mean our daily practices have to go out the window too? Not if we have a strategy. That is what we will cover in this lesson. Ways to keep our practices going, no matter what is happening.

As our routine of yoga becomes more sophisticated, involving more practices, keeping it all going in a busy schedule presents both challenges and opportunities. With so many pieces to work with in an advanced routine, we can be pretty creative in compressing our practices when time is short. Where there is a will, there is a way!

Let's talk about the basics of establishing and keeping a habit of doing daily spiritual practices. One of the easiest ways to do it is make a rule for ourselves that we will do our routine before we eat breakfast and dinner – twice a day like that. If the time of one or both of those meals isn't stable, then we can tag it to be done upon awakening in the morning, and as soon as we arrive home in the evening. If we are traveling, it gets a bit more complicated, but practices can be done to some degree in just about any circumstances, as long as we honor our habit.

Keeping the habit is not only about doing a full routine. It does not have to be "all or nothing." The habit is an urge we build into ourselves to do something about spiritual practice at the appointed time that comes twice-daily. Having the habit is having the "urge to practice." This cultivated urge is the seed of all daily practice. It is like getting hungry at meal times. It just happens, and we want to eat. If we have the urge for spiritual practices cultivated like that, then we will do them. Most days we will be doing our whole routine. On other days, we may be doing less.

But we will always be doing something every session. This "always doing something every session" is very important.

To illustrate what we mean by having the "habit," let's suppose we are hurrying down a busy street. We are on our way to a business dinner appointment that will tie us up until bedtime. We are walking quickly, weaving our way through the people we are passing on the sidewalk. The restaurant is just around the corner now. Almost there. But wait! We see a bench, an empty bus stop bench on the sidewalk in the middle of all the people hurrying this way and that way. We have that urge to do practices built into us. It is time. So what do we do? We stop and sit on that bench for a few minutes and meditate. It might be only for two minutes. But why not? Who will miss us for those two minutes? And we have kept our habit to sit. It is amazing how doing something small like that can renew us for an entire evening – centering for just a few minutes, picking up the mantra just a few times. The nervous system says, "Thank you!" And we are calmer for the rest of the evening.

But it is not just about centering for a few minutes. It is also about keeping our habit of twice-daily practices. If we are in a crazy schedule for days or weeks like that, and can just sit for a few minutes before breakfast and dinner, then when we recover control of our schedule we won't be struggling to find our practice routine again. The habit will be there, and then we can indulge it with our full routine, which we know will fill us to overflowing with inner silence and divine ecstasy.

So that is the first thing, you know – keeping the habit, even if it for two minutes on a bus stop bench. It does not matter where it is, or what is going on. We can keep the habit if we are committed. Then it will keep us committed, because it becomes a hunger that comes on its own at the appointed time. Then we will not have to struggle to restore our commitment to yoga once we are free to do twice-daily full routines of practice again.

It is more likely that we will be faced with compromises in our practice time that are not usually as extreme as having to take a few minutes on a bus stop bench. Let's talk about those.

If we are doing spinal breathing and meditation, followed by a few minutes of rest while coming out, it is not difficult to tailor our practice to a time limitation. Say we are doing 10 minutes of spinal breathing, 20 minutes of meditation, and 5 minutes of rest. That is a 35 minute routine. Then one day we may find ourselves with only 15 minutes to work with. We can just do 10 minutes of meditation, rest for a few minutes and get up. We can also put a few minutes of spinal breathing in front. If we know we will be short on time, we can start with some light "walking" spinal breathing before we get to our seat. If we have to choose between spinal breathing and meditation, we always choose meditation. One thing we do not do is combine spinal breathing and deep meditation at the same time. The reasons for that are discussed early in the lessons (#43).

Let's suppose we are doing a "full plate" of practices – everything in these lessons to a moderate degree. So let's lay it out. It is a typical routine. If you are doing more or less of any of the practices, then you can make the necessary adjustments in translating the suggestions on what to do when the schedule crunch hits you. The idea is to develop some strategies that will enable us to keep our routine together when time is short. Think about it in advance – "What will I do if my practice time is cut in half?" There is no absolute right or wrong answer. Beyond a few basics, keeping practices going when time is short is an art. So here is our moderate "full plate" routine:

- Asanas – 10 min
- Spinal breathing – 10 min
- Chin pump – 5 min
- Spinal bastrika – 5 min
- Meditation – 20 min
- Samyama – 10 min
- Yoni mudra – 5 minutes
- Targeted or crown bastrika (optional) – 5 min
- Rest – 5 min (or more)

That is about 75 minutes – an hour and fifteen minutes. There is nothing sacred about the times in this routine. Maybe you are doing 20 minutes of spinal breathing, and no samyama. Or maybe no asanas. Maybe no spinal or targeted bastrika. Whatever the combination is, it is up to you. Just make sure you are not skipping meditation or rest. Those two (cultivation of inner silence, plus a stable transition to daily activity) are the foundation of all spiritual progress. Spinal breathing is right behind meditation and rest in importance. So, spinal breathing, meditation, and ending rest are a powerful and full routine of practices. All the rest of the practices are for enhancing and building on the effects of these.

This "pecking order" is what we use as a guideline when we begin compressing our practices into a tighter schedule.

So, let's say we have this wonderful one-hour-plus practice routine, and all of a sudden due to circumstances beyond our control, we find ourselves with only 30 minutes to do our afternoon routine. Without a plan, the inclination might be to just bag it for the afternoon and try again tomorrow. All or nothing, you know. That is not a good strategy. Not only will we lose the benefit of a skillfully compressed routine, but we will also dilute our habit to practice twice-daily. The urge to practice needs twice-daily reinforcement. Just remember the bus stop bench. If it was good enough to keep the habit going, isn't thirty minutes in a relatively quiet room a luxury? It really is. So here are some suggestions on what we can do.

First, we hang on to meditation. That is always the first priority. But we'd like to do some of the other practices too, so let's trim the meditation to 15 minutes in this 30 minute plan. We know we need up to 5 minutes of rest at the end for a smooth transition back into activity, so that is 20 minutes, leaving us with 10 minutes to work with. Next is spinal breathing. We can do 5 minutes of spinal breathing in front of meditation and then use the last 5 minutes for other things. Which practice should the last five minutes be for?

At this point, it depends on our preference. If we love our samyama, then we can go for five minutes of that and leave asanas, chin pump, spinal bastrika and yoni mudra for tomorrow. Or, if we want chin pump and spinal bastrika, there is a trick we can do. We can marry spinal bastrika and chin pump together for three to five minutes – that is doing spinal bastrika while doing the chin pump at the same time. It is not ideal, but it provides a combined injection of bastrika and chin pump. Two for the price of one, you know. With this scenario, we are giving up the kumbhaka in chin pump, and probably won't have time for yoni mudra either. It is also possible to incorporate chin pump into the last few minutes of spinal breathing. You will recall that this is called "chin pump lite" (lesson #144).

Additionally, in a few minutes before we sit for practices, we can do a short standing asana routine that includes twisting left and right, bending back, and bending forward and touching toes. A little uddiyana or nauli can be done also. All of the elements of an asana routine can be touched on in this way in a few minutes. It is far from optimal, but it is something in the asanas department we can do before we sit. (See the addition to lesson # 71 for instructions on basic asanas and the abbreviated standing routine just mentioned.)

So, in this way, we can do a pretty good routine in 30 minutes if we are faced with a time limit like that. It can be done in less time too. Of course, then we are dropping more practices off. But we can always do something, even if it is sitting on a bus stop bench for a few minutes, picking up the mantra and dipping into pure bliss consciousness.

Is should be mentioned that we don't have to give up any of the "parallel" practices we do while sitting. These are siddhasana, mulabandha/asvini, sambhavi, uddiyana/nauli and kechari. To the extent we are practicing these and they are habits, they can be present with our core sitting practices in every session, no matter how short the time is. Indeed, they will be found creeping into our everyday activity naturally as ecstatic conductivity is coming up in our nervous system. By then, mudras and bandhas have become part of our normal neuro-biological functioning, and we will never lose them.

Of course, we have to be mindful about practices we are doing in public view. Doing full-blown chin pump in a busy airport waiting room could lead to a call for the rescue squad. Either that, or an exorcist! A vigorous bastrika session might lead to a similar call. But most of our practices can be done discreetly. That certainly applies to light spinal breathing, meditation, samyama, mulabandha, mild uddiyana/nauli and kechari. Sambhavi is not noticeable if done with eyes fully closed, which is recommended anyway. Even siddhasana can be done discreetly in a public place if one shoe is removed and our heel is slipped up under our perineum. Sometimes where we happen to be will determine what practices we will do. As the old saying goes – "Discretion is the better part of valor."

There are many ways to piece together practices if we are faced with a short schedule, or less than ideal location. After spinal breathing, meditation and ending rest are taken care of, it is up to our personal preferences. Give it some thought. When the need arises, we can find interesting and creative ways to keep our practices going. With bhakti, we will find a way.

In this busy world, we will all be faced with the challenge of having limited time for our practices. As we continue with yoga, our spiritual desire (bhakti) will become stronger, and we will find ways to keep the necessary time available. Even so, there will be things that come up occasionally that will limit our time, so it is wise to develop an attitude of flexibility and a willingness to compromise when necessary to make sure that we are always honoring our habit to practice twice each day. If we do that, there won't be much in this world that can keep us from reaching our divine destination.

The guru is in you.

Lesson 210 – Handling Automatic Yoga and Siddhis

Q: I need a small clarification. While doing deep meditation I automatically go into jalandhara (chin lock). If I try correcting the posture the feeling of "being-in" which gets built since the start of meditation goes away. If I don't come out of jalandhara I don't get distracted but I am concerned that I will not stick to the "just meditation" routine while meditating. Please advise.

A: Automatic yoga of the physical variety is common during meditation, and also in samyama. The reason is because we are deep into our pure bliss consciousness and then the nervous system gets urges to facilitate the purification process. You have the right approach favoring your meditation practice with your attention. If our body is going in a certain direction, we don't fight against it, nor do we cling to it. It is the same way that we treat thoughts or anything thing else that comes up in our meditation. So, we don't have to be concerned about the jalandhara (chin lock) being there or not. It will take care of itself as we take care of our meditation.

I can tell you with certainly that the automatic yoga will change as we continue our practices day in and day out. We just are easy with whatever is happening. It is purification. The jalandhara will give way to some other energy event. Others have written in about the head going back, the torso going forward, shakes, fast breathing (automatic bastrika), sobbing, and you name it.

With samyama it can get even more dramatic – like hopping around on the bed, or roaring like a lion. We always treat it the same, just easily favoring the practice we are doing. Early stage siddhis (powers), which are inevitable with samyama practice, should be handled in the same way – when they come up we just easily go back to the practice we are doing. It's purification happening in the nervous system.

Automatic yoga is a symptom of practice, not the practice itself. We will do best to stick with the primary causes, which are our meditation, pranayama, samyama and other practices. Automatic yoga is an indicator of progress on the road to enlightenment, and will ease up as our nervous system becomes increasingly purified. The less friction (obstruction) there is in the nervous system, the fewer the physical movements will be, and the more pleasurable it will be inside.

Eventually we will be sitting there looking pretty ordinary, filled with oceanic waves of ecstatic bliss. Only the glow of divine love will give us away.

The guru is in you.

Lesson 212 – Whole Body Mudra

Q: I wanted to let you know that the sambhavi you have described is very powerful. It is a lot more powerful than mulabandha. Is this really true or does it vary from person to person?

A: I'm glad sambhavi is working well for you. It is a very important mudra, because the ajna (third eye end of the spinal nerve) is the master controller of the entire nervous system from the standpoint of ecstatic conductivity, both in cultivating it and in advancing it after it starts to comes up. Then, with the nervous system wired together ecstatically like that, it is all one whole body mudra led by sambhavi. Mulabandha/asvini is then part of sambhavi, as are uddiyana/nauli, kechari and many other visible and invisible movements occurring in the body. All the mudras are part of a whole body ecstatic stimulus/response, with sambhavi leading. In this situation, when the eyes go up as the brow furrows slightly, everything goes up.

When the eyes move devotionally, all the mudras will subtly move by automatic reflex. Ahhh... That is why we nudge all of these mudras along in practices until ecstatic conductivity comes up, building the habits, setting up for further evolution in the nervous system. Then, with ecstatic conductivity, there is only one mudra – the whole body mudra, made up of all the parts. Sambhavi is the leader of it. That's why we see pictures of the sages with their eyes raised. They are in whole body ecstatic bliss just from that, with divine energy radiating out in all directions.

The rise of the whole body mudra reflex is further evidence of the connectedness of yoga throughout our nervous system. It also demonstrates that human spiritual transformation is a neuro-biological process, not ruled by any particular philosophy or belief system. Anyone can do this!

The guru is in you.

Lesson 213 – Conscious Sleeping

Q: I find sometimes less sleep in the night because of the consciousness. I try to sleep but my mind is so fresh. It leads up till to morning. Can you please explain this!

A: A luminous sort of restlessness can happen at night when energy is moving through our purifying nervous system. That kind of interruption in sleep will not last. Make sure you do your practices in the early evening before dinner, and then have some good activity (physical, mental or social) in the evening before bed. This will help smooth it out – it helps integrate the inner energies before bedtime. If we meditate right before bed, it can lead to that kind of restlessness, like a "buzz" going on inside, because meditation is a preparation for activity. Activity after meditation is an essential part of integrating and stabilizing pure bliss consciousness in our nervous system.

Another kind of wakefulness that can happen during sleep is "witnessing," which is the normal rise of inner silence from practices. This is part of the first stage of enlightenment, introduced early in the lessons (#35, "Enlightenment Milestones"), and is a permanent condition that will not disrupt our sleep, even though we may feel awake inside. This kind of conscious sleeping is called "yoga nidra." The first stage of enlightenment is the rise of uninterrupted inner silence, which we find to be our unshakable inner silent self, present throughout waking, dreaming and deep sleep. It is the proverbial "rock" of pure bliss consciousness in us that cannot be washed away by any storm. Continuous inner silence is a good thing. It is the quiet foundation of all the glamorous later stages of enlightenment. It is also the source of our increasing peace and stability in daily life.

The way to tell if it is the first or second experience occurring during sleep is in how rested we feel the next day. If we are a bit tired, then it is likely the first experience of excess energy running around inside, and that will pass as we regulate our practices to keep balance between the cultivation of inner silence and our daily activities. On the other hand, if we feel rested after a night of conscious sleep, then we will know it is the rise of inner silence, which is our normal enlightenment coming up.

It can also be a mixture of both of these experiences, in which case we just do our practices in the early evening to keep our sleep time smooth, and then enjoy being peacefully aware while we are sleeping. That's life on the road to enlightenment. Good things are happening!

The guru is in you.

Lesson 214 – Finding Your Spiritual "Hook"

Q: I have a question. It has to do with a general sense I have of feeling unguided and needing a guru or teacher for my meditation, but unable to find anything that sparks a sense that I have found that. There are many teachers, but no "hook," no staying power. There are many out there willing to tell me that they will be my guru, or master, and I have even been told that I cannot know if someone is my guru, that I just have to obey. But somehow this feels wrong. Meanwhile, my practice is erratic because I don't really trust myself to know what would be my best routine. I've been practicing yoga for over 20 years...

A: I think relying on an outer "hook" is unreliable. Even the best physical gurus have a few failings, and that is okay. No one is perfect. But they are expected to be perfect, and that is a guarantee of failure. Spiritually speaking, the real shortcoming is always in the practitioner who is looking outside for primary inspiration, where the only place it can truly be found is inside.

So the approach in the lessons is for everyone to find their own inner inspiration through solid daily practices, and the resulting experiences that do not deceive us. Inner silence is inner silence. Ecstatic conductivity is just that. Purification and opening of our nervous system is an objective phenomenon, at least from our inner view. The cause and effect of practice and experience belongs to the practitioner. There is no mistake about that. Personal spiritual experience is the best hook. Spiritual practices, done daily, can cultivate it in the yogi/yogini with a high degree of reliability.

The practices in the lessons are not unique, but their integration, combined power and relative safety are rare. Few have dared to cross the rigid traditional lines and integrate these esoteric methods into a workable system before. It has been done here, and the results have been very good. So the practices are offered openly for wise seekers to explore for themselves. It is an inter-traditional scientific investigation that has been done, and everyone can carry the work forward in their own self-paced application of the methods. Such an approach has been much needed. However, it is not for everyone. If someone needs a lot of hand-holding, ritual, etc., then a physical guru may be necessary. That is not me. I am happy to help with questions on practice, but I am not here to be anyone's physical guru. I am making some good tools available. Everyone has to take up their own journey, using the best tools they can find. Even with a physical guru this is the case, though few emotionally dependent disciples like to hear that.

I view yoga as neuro-biological science. No mumbo jumbo. Just cause and effect. That is what we'd like to have in our yoga – good methods that work, that we can be confident using year in and year out. Then we know we will find more and more ecstatic bliss and divine love welling up within us over time, and the world will be changed for the better by our unfoldment. What else matters?

Good yoga operates like clockwork. We can see steadily expanding results over time.

So, try the lessons and see for yourself. Start at the beginning. 20 years is a long time on the path. Even so, everyone should start at the beginning, because correct deep meditation is the key to everything in yoga – at least in this kind of yoga it is. Inner silence is the foundation of all spiritual progress, and that is what deep meditation is about. Then we add very effective spinal breathing pranayama. These two are the core practices, and everything else builds on these. So, starting at the beginning is very important. The lessons can be used as a stand-alone teaching, or to supplement any other path as "food for thought."

No allegiance is necessary here. It is your journey. You are in charge. In time you will come in tune with the primordial guru inside, your inner pure bliss consciousness, and then you will have the real hook. Your bhakti will fly high, and knowledge will come to you from all directions. Then you will know what this game is about. It is not about anything but your own inner purification, opening and divine union. This is the approach throughout the lessons. Here there are no promises of deliverance by someone outside you. Just practical information on practices, and how to apply them within yourself for the best results.

I wish you all success on your chosen path. Enjoy!

The guru is in you.

Lesson 216 – Kundalini Jolts and Self-Pacing in Practices

Q: Thanks for sharing your knowledge and insights. I had an experience last night that slightly concerns me. While sleeping, I felt something like electricity coursing through my body from the head to root. There was pain and soreness, throbbing as well. It got more intense as I relaxed and surrendered to it. After about two minutes of this, which felt like massive amounts of electricity jolting through me, I woke up. I noticed only two hours had passed since I went to bed, but felt alert and fully rested.

I felt giddy and started giggling for a few minutes. I went back to sleep, and felt tired and groggy for most of today. I do 10 minutes of pranayama with sambhavi and mulabandha, then 20 minutes of the *I AM* meditation. I added the sambhavi and mulabandha about one week ago. I skipped my evening practice on the night this happened, prior to sleep.

Am I going too quickly? My only concern is the pain. I've experienced this "painful electricity" twice in the past month or so, and it tires me out for the day. Otherwise, I feel great and the practices are of great benefit to me. The pain is bearable, but I wonder if it's telling me to alter my practice. And what exactly is the electrical sensation? It causes me to laugh uncontrollably afterwards. Please advise.

Thank you for listening. You are providing a great service to people seeking a true spirituality.

A: Thank you for writing and sharing. Something is going on there for sure. The feeling of electricity is energy creating friction in not yet fully purified nerves. The giddiness is from this also, as is the let down later on. It is a bit too much going on during those short episodes – it is a classic kundalini overload, albeit a small and short-lived one.

It is surely not an experience we want to have happening on an ongoing basis, even though it does have the pleasant short-term aftermath. What we want is a smooth and pleasant long-term aftermath, always. Perhaps you should lighten up a bit until things stay steady for a month or so. The spinal breathing generally has a stabilizing effect on inner energies, if not taken to excess. Likewise with deep meditation. Even so, if you step back from 10 and 20 minutes to 5 and 15 minutes, that would be an appropriate lightening up. As for mulabandha and sambhavi, it should be okay to use them for the lesser time of spinal breathing. They are shortened in time by proxy. Try that for a month, and see if the jolts become less frequent. If not, then consider trimming a bit more, or at least not increasing anything significantly until you have a level of stability settling in that satisfies you.

Make sure you take plenty of rest coming out of your sitting practices. And make sure you have good activity during the day and evening after practices – mental, physical, social, a good blend of these over the weeks and months. If we don't stabilize what we gain in practices with good activity, it can sometimes lurch through during sleep like that. Activity is an important part of the process of purification and the stabilization of inner silence and ecstatic energies.

A set of light asanas before sitting practices can help with stabilization also, as can a diet that is neither too light or too heavy. Moderation is valuable in all aspects of life, including yoga.

One thing I suggest you not do is forge ahead with more new sitting practices until you find the necessary balance and smoothness that is just right for your nervous system. Only you can do that. Good self-pacing is an art – balancing the speed of purification with stability in daily life, including sleep time. I suggest you look for at least a month or two of good stability before stepping up to the next level.

Except for the electric wrinkle, yoga looks to be going very well for you.

I think if you work with the elements mentioned, you should be able to smooth things out. It is up to you. Use your best judgment, and with a little trial and error you will get the feel for your own process of unfoldment. Then nothing can stop you from forging ahead safely and surely toward your goal. It's kind of like learning to drive a fast car, only there can be a delayed reaction as we put our foot on the gas pedal, or take it off. Keep that in mind as you move forward, and make your adjustments accordingly.

I'm honored to be able to help out, and wish you all success on your chosen spiritual path.

The guru is in you.

Lesson 217 – Responsibility

Note: This is a follow-up on the previous lesson called, "Kundalini Jolts and Self-Pacing in Practices."

Q: Thank you for the advice. I'll tone it down, per your suggestions, and see how it goes for a month or two.

From this experience, I really get your message about not going too fast. I no longer feel the intense need to burn through all the practices. My desire to keep it up and experience the divine is still strong, but I now feel that the later practices can wait. I realize this process is actually quite fast enough without me charging ahead.

This experience and your advice have really helped me to see this.

A: Yes, now you have it. It is a journey that requires prudent regulation of practices. Only the practitioner can do that.

I have been very impressed with the level of responsibility nearly everyone has shown in taking on these powerful advanced yoga practices. There have been perennial predictions that open knowledge of spiritual practices would lead to disastrous results. It is not true, at least not here and now. Self-pacing is a concept and a practice that is easy to understand. The "learning to drive the fast car" analogy is one we can all relate to.

It seems that the tendency toward desperation and overdoing in practices is driven more by the lack of practices than by the open availability of them. What is withheld we tend become desperate for, and we often overcompensate with the practices we do have. What is freely available, we must develop the skill to use responsibly, and we will. It is that simple.

So, my hat is off to you (and everyone) taking up the challenge of Advanced Yoga Practices and developing good self-pacing skills at the center of your approach.

It means you are well on the way to self-sufficiency in your spiritual endeavors. That is a very important part of the enlightenment process. It means you can do it yourself. Once you know that, then there is no stopping you. Bravo!

The guru is in you.

Lesson 218 – Meditation Sensitivity and Head Movements

Q: I am new to this group and have some problems I would like to discuss with you. When I start to meditate the first thing that happens is my head starts to move from side to side. As the mantra begins to become subtler this movement will increase until it is uncomfortable. I consciously stop this, and then ticks start in my face followed by jerks in my arms, which become more and more violent until I have to stop meditating. Have you ever come across a problem like this before? And do you know the answer to it?

A: Thank you for writing, and welcome. Movements during yoga are not uncommon, though they are not usually as strong as you describe. It means your nervous system is spiritually sensitive, and a lot of deep purification is going on. It is energy moving inside, and what is happening is your body's natural response to accommodate that. It is a good thing, and it will smooth out in time. In the meantime, practices should be managed in such a way so you will have comfort on your path. Otherwise, you might not be inspired to carry on.

It is suggested you look up "automatic yoga," "connectedness of yoga," and "self-pacing" in the topic index. These topics will bring up most of the discussion on movements in yoga (and other energy/kundalini symptoms) and various ways to deal with them. See lessons #160 and #200 for some immediate help on extreme sensitivity to meditation. Not the same symptoms, but a similar degree of sensitivity. The measures suggested there may be appropriate in your case.

Also, if you read through the lessons from start to finish, you will find other aspects of practice that tie in with your experience. For example, there is an advanced practice called "chin pump" that involves vigorous, yet systematic and safe, rotational movement of the head. It would appear that your body is attempting to move in that direction in the experience you describe. When these tendencies become organized they are called "automatic yoga," and there are quite a few manifestations of this discussed in the lessons. However, before trying chin pump, it is suggested you start at the beginning of the lessons and work your way through. There is a lot of groundwork that should be covered before chin pump is undertaken. If you read through the lessons you will see that the steps of practice are logical and take into account the many kinds of experience that can come up.

Keep in mind that these sometimes crazy purification stages do pass with good self-pacing, and wonderful openings often follow. Your experience fits right in with all we have been discussing. You came to the right place.

I wish you all success on your chosen spiritual path ... Enjoy!

The guru is in you.

Lesson 219 – Irritability in Activity

Q: I have been meditating for many years and have tried many methods. The problem that I have is as follows:

I will do spinal breathing, bastrika and alternate nostril breathing all with proper mudras and bandhas. Then I will do mantra practice as described in your lesson. This is my favorite. When I am done my mind is very clear and calm. Very pleasant. However, while my core of silence is still more or less intact, I find that I am very intolerant and pretty unloving. I think my mind is preferring the inner quiet over the normal irritation that is found at work or at home. This has actually caused conflicts at work. However, I have found that if my meditation is a mindfulness practice based on observation of the rise and fall of the belly with breathing; that the effect is that I am calm and tolerant. I would prefer to do the teachings that you are offering instead of the above-mentioned Buddhist practice. I think the problem is that when I get too much energy in my head, that I get intolerant. My belly as the focus of the mindfulness practice is a larger and lower focus and the energy accumulated seems to be more generalized and more balanced. Of course that will never progress to kundalini, etc. Any suggestions?

A: Thank you for writing and sharing. Too much energy running around in the upper centers (from the heart up) is probably a good assessment of why you are having irritability in daily activity. But why?

There is probably too much practice happening too fast, so you are left with more purification than can be comfortably integrated during activity. Even with long experience in meditation and yoga, anyone can overdo when adding or rearranging practices too often and/or suddenly increasing overall practice times. If there is some inherent sensitivity in the nervous system (as discussed in the last lesson, #218), this can compound the discomfort afterward. Inner silence can be there while discomfort is going on. The peacefulness of inner silence (witnessing) is a good thing, of course. In the formative stages of the rise of inner silence there will be a contrast with outer activity, and there can be the impression of conflict between our inner peace and the roughness we may be experiencing on the outside, as you point out. But it is only an impression. There really is no conflict, only the uncomfortable friction of too much energy bubbling to the surface through our nervous system that is not yet purified enough to accommodate the amount of flow coming through. That is not caused by the inner silence or any conflict with it. It is caused by too much energy moving, which is on the Shakti side. As you know, inner silence is the Shiva side. The solution to this is to regulate practices so our inner energies can be comfortably integrated and balanced in everyday activity. If we take the view that our salvation is to be found in our inner silence alone, and not outside in the ebb and flow of the world, then we will be missing the opportunity for the higher stages of enlightenment. These involve a complete integration of inner silence with the flow of energy in all avenues of life. When this is accomplished through a balanced blend of practices and activity, then we come to know the complete marriage of silent bliss consciousness and ecstatic energy flowing everywhere, and this is liberation in this world. All becomes the One, and that is who we are.

What then can upset us? Then we will be in the best position to stand firm in the world on the things that are important to us, smiling all the while.

The practice of mindfulness of breath in the belly you mentioned may be bringing some relief, but I don't know how progressive that practice would be over the long term. It has its inherent limitations, as you point out. It could also be causing some "doubling up" of practice time in pranayama and meditation if you are also doing deep meditation and spinal breathing on the same days you are doing the breath awareness practice. Doubling up means more purification from doing similar practices on the same day, which can stimulate excess energy flows inside. It may not be obvious this is being set up while we are doing the practices themselves.

So, what is the solution? First of all, it is suggested you get a handle on what is doing what, beginning with the core practice of deep meditation. If you have not already, try going back to a simple practice of meditation only for 15-20 minutes twice a day with nothing else added, and see if that brings more stability in daily activity. Make sure you take at least 5 minutes of rest coming out of meditation. Coming out too fast alone can lead to a lot of irritability during the day. If that simple routine is smooth during the day, then you will know that you were doing too much somewhere in your previous routine. Then it becomes a matter of maintaining that stability and, if desired, gradually adding things on one by one, stabilizing each new level of practice in activity before adding more. Keep in mind that with most practices there will be a time delay in energy effects, so it takes a good month or two at least to stabilize any single practice before taking on more will be appropriate.

If 15-20 minutes of meditation alone with good rest coming out still leaves you with irritability during the day, then you will know you are dealing with either a temporary or ongoing sensitivity in your nervous system. Then you can try decreasing the time of meditation (and increase rest afterward) until the daily activity smoothes out. Adding 5-10 minutes of spinal breathing in front of meditation can help stabilize the internal flows. A light set of asanas (5-10 minutes) in front of sitting practices can help stabilize things afterward also. You may have to try several combinations before you find what works for you (lessons #160 and #200 cover this process). Hold off on adding things like mudras, bandhas, siddhasana, kumbhaka, etc. until you find a stable platform of practice that gives you smoothness in daily activity. All those additional practices turn up the heat, you know. Once you know you have a stable platform of practice, then you can add things on one at a time, stabilizing each one before adding the next one.

I know all this sounds very tedious and time consuming, especially if you are advanced already and wanting to get on with it. But there really isn't any other way to build a stable practice that will give us the ecstatic bliss in activity that we certainly deserve. If we are experiencing instability, we have to go back to a stable level of practice. It can happen with advanced practitioners as often as with beginners. In fact, it is very common for adjustments to be necessary as we move up into the more refined realms of advanced practice and experience. We can be moving along doing just fine, and all of a sudden hit a big release (or a series of them) deep inside that sends us back to a reduced level of practice for a few days, weeks, or months. It can happen to anyone. It is part of the journey. It is important to recognize that we will go into sharp curves in the road from time to time, and that we must take our foot off the gas pedal temporarily at those times, or risk a wild ride, or even a wreck. That's how it is. Once we know the advanced practices, how smoothly we travel home to enlightenment is all in the self-pacing.

I wish you success on your chosen spiritual path.

The guru is in you.

Lesson 220 – Opening the Heart Chakra

Q: I have developed heart and kidney problems over the last few years. I had a heart attack at the age of 39 for which I was forced to slow down tremendously.

Recently I saw a very great practitioner of Shanti and Reiki healing due to my distress over this situation. I have been in meditation on the Holy Names of both the Maha-Mantra and the Mantra Rajas for over 25 years. (Unfortunately, we are not taught the science of meditation)

I was told by this healer, and by a couple of other practitioners, that my heart chakra is "clogged" and that it must be opened and cleared. That this is the cause of my physical distresses. Forgive me, but I am most ignorant of this technique. I know what the chakra centers are from the Vedas, but not the techniques on how to open them.

I live a very simple life, but being a teacher and guru in our tradition, I do have stress at times. I have a strict sastric diet, follow my dosha recommendations and chant over 100,000 Holy Names daily, which means I am in active meditation over 10 hours a day. This is not the problem, since it has been daily routine for many years.

If you could please recommend some reading, or explain this technique, I would be most grateful. My healer says that this would greatly enhance my health, preaching and ministry, and also allow more of the Light of Nityananda-Gauranga to flow from me to those around me.

Thank you for your time in this.

A: Thank you for writing and sharing. The practices in the lessons are geared toward overall spiritual awakening, and not so much on individual chakras – except the ajna to root connection, which is especially important for enlightenment. Of course, the heart is opened also by this overall purification in the spiritual anatomy. While meditation and spinal breathing are global and open the heart "by proxy," other techniques like uddiyana/nauli, chin pump and targeted bastrika can work more directly in the heart area as part of the overall process of purification and opening.

In general, I am not for focusing on individual chakra openings, because how can we know what is the right order? Unfathomable karma sets each of us on a somewhat different path, and that is why the broad approach in the lessons is offered, rather than a specific chakra by chakra approach. In this way we allow pure bliss consciousness to cultivate natural opening of the nervous system from within, relying on intellectual decisions very little. Through the practices in the lessons, we are systematically surrendering to the process of spiritual transformation that is inherent within us. Of course, pure bhakti is the greatest of all practices, and you know that already. If human desire is raised to the level of bhakti (intense desire for God/Truth), then all the methods of yoga are stimulated automatically. We only need hear of them once (if at all), and we are off into practice!

Having said all that, here are a couple of additional suggestions on opening the heart chakra that are holistic in their effects:

There is a pranayama technique that works directly in the heart that has not been mentioned in the lessons so far. It is like spinal breathing, but in reverse direction. We can call it "heart breathing." It provides the opportunity to bring our ishta (chosen ideal) directly into our heart using the breath with profound effect. What we do is inhale from the third eye (point between the eyebrows) back to the center of the head and down the spinal nerve into the heart, and then exhale back out the same route through the third eye. On the inhalation we bring our ishta in, and on the exhalation we send out impurities. If we slow down the breathing (comfortably), the effects will be enhanced. Breathing through the nose is preferable, but not mandatory. This method has great benefit for the heart, purifying and opening it. During this practice, our heart is filled with our Beloved and impurities are expelled. It can be done for 5-10 minutes before or after sitting practices, or anytime. Be careful not to overdo it in the beginning, as it can bring excessive karmic releases in the heart if overdone. It is suggested you start off slow and work up gradually according to comfort and effect. This practice has not been offered in the lessons so far because of the reverse direction aspect and possible confusion to beginners in the traditional spinal breathing that is given beginning in lesson #41, which purifies the heart in a more general way. Also, many people do not have a clear ishta to use, which can be confusing to those coming to yoga with a non-worship orientation. This is clearly not the case with you, so perhaps you can use this practice with good effect. It may even combine nicely with your other practices. It is in your hands.

For those who wish to try this practice without a specific ishta (deity, avatar or guru), the purifying and healing power of universal truth can be brought in through the third eye and down into the heart during inhalation, and impurities sent out on exhalation.

A second suggestion is on the physical/lifestyle level. Much of the contraction in areas of our nervous system can be reinforced in our daily habits – how we interact and carry on our daily routine of activities. Sometimes just bringing in a new behavior, changing the routine, can reduce the contraction. In the case of a heart problem, the solution is straight forward, coming from modern medicine. Daily aerobic exercise is one of the first prescriptions to build a healthier heart. No doubt you know this already. Daily exercise (20+ minute brisk walk, or equivalent), and a low fat, low salt, vegetarian diet are good for both the heart and the blood pressure. It is not unusual for a sattvic (pure) diet to have a lot of fat and salt in it, so being sattvic in diet alone may not be adequate. I found this out many years ago when I had a tendency toward high blood pressure in spite of a pure vegetarian diet, which was easily resolved by the measures just mentioned. Doing these things will also change the way we carry on our daily routine, including our relationships with other people. So, putting some emphasis on these physical health measures will affect our life in nonphysical ways, which is good for the heart also. Some letting go is necessary to make these changes, and that can reduce the contraction in our heart. An opening heart is one that knows how to let go. An opening heart laughs a lot too!

Cultivating the habit of letting go deep in the nervous system is at the root of deep meditation, samyama and many of the other practices in the lessons. As inner silence comes up in our life, we are able to let go of the daily stresses more easily, even as we are engaged in activity. Letting go while remaining active in life is, of course, the essence of karma yoga, so it all ties together.

If you want to take a more focused "spiritual energy work" approach to opening the heart chakra, I am probably not the best person to ask. Perhaps an energy healer you are already seeing (Reiki or other) can help with that. I am not much for focusing too much on particular chakras for the reasons mentioned. I try and keep the chakras "under the hood" as much as possible so as not to distract from the overall task of "driving the car" home to enlightenment. My role is to stay focused on that.

I wish you balanced health, and continuing success in your important spiritual work.

The guru is in you.

Lesson 221 – Expanding Heart Space

Q: I really enjoyed your write-up on heart breathing (lesson #220). I've been having good experiences with spinal breathing since beginning about 6 months ago, and this adds a new dimension. With regular spinal breathing I often feel like I am opening up inside into a boundless space. Sometimes it is just a joyous emptiness. Other times there are very pleasant sounds, like a trickling mountain stream, church bells, or music like I have never heard though my physical ears. Sometimes there are golden or multicolored lights. Sometimes no light at all. I don't know where it all comes from, but it is usually expansive and very, very pleasant. This space seems to be in my heart, but infinitely bigger than my physical body. I tried the heart breathing at the end of my practices the last couple of days. Though I don't consider myself to be very religious, I come from a Christian background, and imagined breathing Christ into my heart through my third eye, and letting whatever impurities that are in there go up and out the eye with the out breath. Well, the inner space is coming alive with huge waves of love and compassion and a sense of indescribable strength and purpose. It is amazing. I have been walking around like this after practices too. Is this Jesus Christ inside me? Or is it something else? Whatever it is, I want more.

A: What a beautiful experience. It is a wonderful example of how spinal breathing combined with deep meditation and other practices will open the heart as part of the overall purification of the nervous system.

This is the "heart space" we enter as our nervous system opens and our inner sensuality begins to rise. The Sanskrit word for the heart chakra is "anahata," which means "unstruck sound." Sensory experiences come up in the heart space out of nowhere, and can be experienced simultaneously everywhere inside. The sounds are "unstruck," and the inner lights are "unlit." What is in the heart space just is, as if there is no cause and effect operating there, just a radiation of the qualities of pure bliss consciousness coming endlessly from within, and playing on our refined perception – an eternal fountain of bliss inside us.

By inviting an influence into our heart space in heart breathing, such as our ishta (chosen ideal), there will be a filling that occurs corresponding to our openness and intention to receive truth and harmony. We all know in everyday life that positive intentions (and habits) expand our heart space and enliven us, and negative intentions (and habits) contract our heart space and deaden us. With advanced yoga practices, we are working on the opening on much deeper levels in our nervous system. So deep that our experience moves into the celestial realms – all contained within us. There, the negative intentions (and habits) are melted by the pure love of our divine qualities coming up from within, so the experiences of heart contraction becomes less and less, even as we navigate through this physical world where nothing lasts for very long. We continue to expand as we naturally identify ourselves more with that inside us which is all bliss and does not whither away.

If we have a religious background and are inclined to use an ishta from our tradition, it can work very well for us in the heart breathing. It will work equally well for any person sincerely longing for truth through any tradition or belief, because it is the devotion we have for our ideal that stimulates the purification and opening in our heart. So too does our devotion/bhakti stimulate all of our practices through the connectedness of yoga, as has been discussed in previous lessons.

There is an interesting connection here with the practice of samyama, which was first given in lesson #150. Our expanding heart space is analogous with our expanding inner silence. We know that inner silence (cultivated in meditation) is the vast reservoir of divine power we let go into with our sutras during samyama practice. In doing so, we cultivate the expansion of inner silence in many directions according to the range of sutras we are using. This is expanding our heart space. We stimulate the expansion of our heart space in many ways during our routine of practices. The heart, while not often mentioned in the lessons, lies at the center of all we are doing in Advanced Yoga Practices. This local spiritual energy center we call "the heart" eventually becomes everything.

The opening heart is the means by which our inner silence, inner sensuality and ecstatic bliss expand gradually to encompass all of our surroundings in the physical world. Then do we experience the entire world through our senses in the same way we experience the heart space in these early stages of inner expansion, as you have described. Eventually, all the world is contained within our own expanding heart. Our outside becomes inside, and our inside becomes outside – a divine paradox. That is unity – Oneness. Then when we breathe out from our heart space, all the world is purified.

This experience may seem to be very mystical. Yet, it is rooted in the neuro-biological transformation of our nervous system that we cultivate through our daily practices. We are wired for it. We are all mystics in the making.

The guru is in you.

Lesson 222 – Chimes in Inner Space?

Q: I've been doing spinal breathing and yoni mudra for a few months straight now and I'm having some strange things happen. They usually happen late at night or in the morning upon waking. Upon waking, I've been getting a rapid vibration in my chest area and inside my jaw sockets. It was strange but not uncomfortable. I also hear strange, mystical "chime like" sounds after I do my nighttime meditation. Sometimes I am awakened by them as I dose off in corpse pose after meditation. The sounds are hard to describe and it's hard to tell where they are coming from. I think they are coming from outside my house but a lot of the time there is no wind and I never hear them any other time. I've practiced yoga and meditation for several years and have come across lots of strange things but these sounds are really different. I am wondering if they are somehow linked to the practice and if so what might they be? I know it can be just a coincidence I hear them when I do, but I think there may be something else happening here. Thank you so much for the lessons and your time!

A: Thank you for writing and sharing. If it is not the wind chimes outside, then it is likely the expansion of your heart space and inner sensuality, as was discussed in the last lesson (#221). When this happens (common with spinal breathing, especially with yoni mudra kumbhaka added) inner sounds that are "celestial" in nature may seem to be somewhere outside. This is because our inner dimension has expanded out into our surroundings. So, it can seem like we are experiencing something outside our body while it is inside us and "out there" at the same time. The uncertainty you feel about where the sound is coming from is common in this situation. Don't be concerned about it. Good things are happening. So, if it isn't the outside chimes, it is probably the inside ones that are "anahata" – unstruck sound.

If any of these experiences become uncomfortable or excessively distracting (the vibrations or the sounds), be sure and apply prudent self-pacing in your practices. Otherwise, enjoy!

I wish you all success on your chosen spiritual path.

The guru is in you.

Lesson 223 – Kechari Stage 1 and-a-half? (a dialog)

Q1: Thanks to your instructions (lesson #108) I have made some progress from stage 1 kechari, but did not find exactly what I expected yet.

After some experimentation and feeling my way about, I am thinking I am in a sort of stage 1 and-a-half, with my tongue longer than needed for stage 1, but not quite long enough for stage 2 yet. I don't know if perhaps the existence of this intermediate stage is a feature of my own particular anatomy, which other people would not experience because of a slightly different layout. Here is what I experienced:

By stretching the tongue upwards and to the right I was able to find what seemed like a hole through which I was just about able to push the tongue. I tried using a finger, but I seemed to be unable to make use of it since the tongue was already at the limits of its stretch.

However, through that hole I sensed tissue of a type that I had not felt before. I could sense this because it was salty! Salty probably because of a thin layer of salty mucous on it.

I kept the tip of my tongue on that special tissue and moved it towards the center. (The experience was dramatic and ecstatic.) In the earlier days (it's been over a week now) it always slipped away before I got near the center but with practice I was able to get it to the center.

However, there are no nostril-openings to be found at this point, and no septum between them. The organ I am resting my tongue on is relatively flat, with a hint of a ridge in the middle. It is normally covered by the uvula but I have gotten my tongue under that covering. When I turn my head to the right, the right side of that organ bulges towards my tongue, and correspondingly when I turn my head to the left.

I believe the nostril-openings and septum are just "above" where my tongue is currently able to reach on that organ. Therefore I think I am in a sort of transitional stage between 1 and 2.

Do you think this is right?

A1: Yes, I think your description of what is happening is pretty accurate. Congratulations on getting behind the soft palate! It is the beginning of a new world of progress and advanced experiences.

Maybe I can add a few clarifications that will be helpful. It sounds like you are feeling the back edge of the hard palate from behind the soft palate (behind uvula). The septum comes down to the center of the edge of the hard palate. That would be the "hint of a ridge" you feel in the middle. So, yes, you are still shy of the septum, eustachian tubes, inner nostrils, etc. But you'll get there.

To go higher, it might be helpful to think not only about length, but also about releasing the tongue from the floor of the mouth bit by bit. Most people have the length already, but are limited by the tether (frenum) tying the tongue to the floor of the mouth. By focusing on length only we are, in effect, taking a detour back and around the soft palate with length to compensate for the tongue being tied down toward the front. If we untie the tongue, it goes up much further much faster. That, combined with lengthening (milking) yields the optimum progress in kechari. All of this is covered in detail in lesson #108.

I'll not tell you what to do on this, as it is a very personal journey, dependent on each person's bhakti and preferences. I'll point out the mechanics. The rest is up to you.

Q2: Thank you very much again for your response.

I used to pull the tongue but I found that a lot of pulling seemed to be required to make even a little progress. I've been quickly converted already by your posting to the idea of nicking the frenum with a cuticle scissors. So when I say "length" I really mean "length as allowed by the frenum."

The only thing I'd like to mention is that I do make a number of tiny nicks rather than only one (I make about 10) and I make them at separate spots along the frenum surface). I expect that this greater number speeds up the process. Actually, it seems to; after one nicking session I can already feel a greater extension.

This larger number of nicks heals just as quickly as a single nick, that is, in about three days.

Making more than one nick might be inappropriate in maybe the most typical case because of the effect of the extra speed. But I feel ready. Behind me I have twenty years of yoga and meditation, including about 14 of kechari. If you had any comments on that I'd be interested.

I agree with you that nicking is ultimately less traumatic on the tongue. The frenum is only a tendon, relatively insensitive tissue with a simple task, while the tongue itself is muscles and nerves largely.

A2: You are on your way, knowing what you have to do. Bravo! Regarding snipping, I don't think simultaneous multiple snips along the edge of the frenum will speed up the process much. The reason I say that is because the strings of tendon are piled up on top of each other in the frenum by the thousands, and snipping in multiple places at the same time may be snipping mostly the same string multiple times, which will not produce additional new freedom for the tongue once the string is snipped in one place. Except for a slight increased risk of infection, It certainly doesn't hurt to try though.

It takes some time for new strings of tendon to come up and present themselves once a string has been snipped. It is an interesting phenomenon that occurs with snipping which is mentioned in lesson #108. Once a snip is taken, then there is healing for a few days. At the same time, kechari practice stretches it out. Then the unsnipped tendons underneath are stretched to the surface, presenting a clear target for the next snip. The more days that pass, the more prominent the edge of the new tendon string becomes. Taking this snipping, healing and stretching new strings to the surface approach results in steady progress over time, and with little to no pain or bleeding, because the stretched tendon strings come up to the surface with an edge like a callous that can be snipped easily. It is as though the frenum was designed to be trimmed in this way.

All the while we are going higher, and soon ravishing the secret spot!

Q3: Ah, is that the way it works?

I had imagined that the pieces of the broken strings separate but join again with scar tissue, the scar tissue producing extra length. For that reason, I had thought that multiple snippings along the length would help. Do you know that idea to be wrong? (You know, it might be. I think I heard that tendon never heals...)

Your description of how it works is very helpful. This tells me that whereas there may be little to be gained by snipping "along" a tendon, if I were to do a series of snips in a line "across" the tendon, in that way snipping distinct fibers, it would probably speed it up ...

To help avoid infection, I use antiseptic mouthwash before and after the snipping, and I position the snipping between meals so I don't eat for a few hours after. This way I have not experienced even the mildest infection, even in the early days when I made a mistake and snipped a larger piece than I should have. When the snips are small enough I find that the surface is never even sore, it is just slightly more sensitive.

" ...All the while we are going higher, and soon ravishing the secret spot!"

Oh yes! I'm looking forward to that!

A3: Without kechari practice for weeks or months, there can be a tightening up of fleshy tissue under the tongue. This is easily stretched out again once kechari resumes. Once a tendon string is snipped, it won't reconnect to itself or anything else that presents a strong limitation. Once a tendon string is snipped there will not be much there to hold the tongue down that can't be easily stretched at any time in the future.

Make sure you stay in the middle when snipping. It is recommended that you not venture far from the center edge. The path of least resistance in the stretched tendon is there. If you go too far to either side, you run the risk of getting into the arteries in the tongue. It is not very likely, but that is obviously not the direction we want to be going in.

Someone wrote a few months ago suggesting that there is risk of cutting an artery when snipping any part of the frenum. It is not so, as long as we stay on the stretched edge of the tendon string in the center with our tiny step by step snipping.

Q4: That makes it really clear to my engineer's mind. I'll make a few snips across the tendon. I'd never go near the blood vessels, don't worry.

I only snip what shows up as taught when I pull out the tongue. In fact, I've taken to pulling it out, drying the underside and marking the taught, hard high-tension spot with a non-toxic laundry marker! Then only the marked spot is eligible for snipping. I find the actual snipping is easier when the tongue is not pulled out. I use a hand-held cosmetic mirror in strong light, turn the tip of the tongue to the roof of my mouth and put the cuticle scissors in and snip the marked spot.

A4: Sounds good (except you probably don't need the laundry marker). Carry on at your own safe speed.

The guru is in you.

Lesson 224 – Automatic Kechari and Visions

Q: I just came out of a 10 day silent retreat in India. A most incredible experience. I tried to apply self-pacing and meditate as lightly as I could (most of the time staying away from mantra or any advanced practices), but it was overwhelmingly intense. Inner silence and meditation invaded every moment. One of the remarkable experiences I had was a realization of a new level of kechari. I rolled my tongue deeper into the soft palate, and suddenly hit an inconceivably ecstatic spot. A feeling I could never imagine. However, after pushing it for some time, I stopped as I realized this puts my tongue in a very problematic position, perhaps "milking it backwards." I still have nasty marks on it, and it feels a bit loosened. Are you familiar with such spot? Is it a taste of stage 2 kechari?

Also, some remarkable experiences having to do with the third eye: One night, while lying on my bed (definitely wide-awake) a shining spot appeared at the edge of my field of vision. It slowly moved to the centre, stabilizing in the middle of it, and suddenly got a heart-like shape and grew a misty, dark colorful aura, greatly concentrated in color and resolution. I turned my head, and there it appeared again. Once again I looked the other way – and again it showed up. I closed my eyes – yet it lingered in its place for some time, Until finally gone. A similar incident happened yesterday night as well.

Do you have any idea about the meaning of such occurrences? Does it have anything to do with the third eye? Next time it appears – what should I do with it. Can I apply it for further experience in any sort of way?

A: Welcome back. Sounds like you made some wonderful progress on your India trip.

On kechari, the automatic yoga inclination was strong enough to pull your tongue back maybe further than it has been so far. If the tip got to the place where hard and soft palates meet, this is right below the bottom of the septum, and is very sensitive. There can also be sensitivity further back in the soft palate itself, and even in the throat. But the septum (higher up) is the focal point of ecstatic experience. Once you get behind the soft palate (stage 2 – see previous main lesson #223 and tantra lesson #T34) the tongue will be free to go up and you will find incredible sensitivity up there, and you will never be the same. I look forward to hearing from you when that happens! In the meantime, don't force things too much. Where have we heard that before?

Visions through the third eye can occur as the sushumna (spinal nerve) is purifying. Some people start having them as soon as they learn spinal breathing. The common one is a tunnel with a star at the end, out in front of the brow. This is often first seen as a circle with a bright light in the center. Other visions (variations) can occur there too, as you have seen. You may want to check the lessons on this (#92 and #179). There is advice in these on how to regard visions – not doing much with them at all. If you look in the topic index under "scenery" you will find a group of lessons on having and dealing with visions, etc.

The more advanced we get, the more visions can happen. Fortunately, by then we are much more grounded in inner silence, so can resist getting off on the tangents where visions can sometimes take us. Visions are symptoms of progress, not transforming causes, nor the enlightenment itself. Enjoy them, be inspired, and regard them as scenery along the road to enlightenment. Then you will be able to keep focused on the practices that promote the ongoing transformation in your nervous system. Carry on!

The guru is in you.

Lesson 225 – Clearing the Clouds

Q: I am impressed with your simplicity in explaining complicated subjects like yoga and meditation. I started practicing the pranayama – spinal breathing for approximately 10 minutes followed by 15 to 20 minutes of meditation using mantra and about 10 minutes rest, twice a day from August 9, 2004. On August 11th evening, I had wonderful feelings, free mind with lot of creativity and energy for the first time in my life. I am very sorry to say this incident never repeated till today even though there is no change in my routine. What could be wrong?

A: It is wonderful that you have had such a clear experience in your early days of meditation. The variation in experience does not mean anything is wrong. It is not unusual for experiences to change over time as we proceed with long term daily meditation. As impurities become gradually less in our nervous system, the experience will become gradually clearer.

Think of if as a slowly clearing cloudy sky. Even on a cloudy day we might see the sun shining through occasionally. Then, over time, as the clouds become less and less, the sun is visible more of the time. Eventually it is all sun. That is how pure bliss consciousness comes up in a purifying nervous system.

Remember to keep your attention on regular daily practices, rather than on the ups and downs of experiences. The practices will keep our journey going steadily forward. Experiences will vary according to how purification is progressing in our nervous system at any given time.

Also keep in mind that we get used to rising pure bliss consciousness very fast, and the contrast will not be noticed as much after a few days of more clarity. Then we become eager for the next level of clarity. The ups and downs and the plateaus in experience are a normal part of the journey – the scenery, if you will. This is also true when ecstatic experiences arise. There is always more. Once we have glimpsed the divine coming from within we are hungrier for God.

Keep up practices over the long term, and your experiences will become gradually clearer as your nervous system becomes pure, eventually giving you the experience of ecstatic bliss all the time.

I wish you all success on your chosen spiritual path.

The guru is in you.

Lesson 226 – Expansion on Our Mind

Q: I am practising meditation and pranayama for the past two and half months. The effects I got are:

First of all, I got the ability to concentrate on one thing in my life for the first time. I have tried a lot of methods before, but there is an inner satisfaction only now. After each meditation session for the next hour my mind gets filled with peace and happiness. In my last two meditation sessions one or two times I lost the ability of watching myself whether I am thinking the mantra or not.

Now my questions:

Can I meditate more than twice a day? Can I meditate one hour after meals and before bed? In this stage can I go to next step of siddhasana? (I have not yet experienced any special colors and sounds as you mentioned.)

Can mantras like Gayatri mantra when repeated large number of times help me for my development?

Guide me please.

A: Thank you for writing and sharing. I am very happy to hear your meditation and pranayama are going well.

Meditating more than twice a day in our regular routine is not recommended. It is easy to have too much of a good thing in yoga, and that can lead to excessive purification, discomfort, and less progress. In a retreat situation more than two meditations can be undertaken if there are no responsibilities and the routine is designed to accommodate it. If you go to the topic index and look up "retreats," you will find a couple of lessons covering this. At home in our regular work schedule we should stay with the measured twice-daily approach. With experiences like you describe, we all would like to expand it for sure. The way to do that is to gradually add practices into our twice-daily routine. The lessons are for that.

Meditating before eating is preferred, so meditation will not be competing with digestion. An hour or more after eating is okay too. But close to bedtime is not recommended, as it can lead to restless nights. Meditation is preparation for activity, not sleep. Daily activity helps stabilize the inner silence and ecstatic energy brought up during meditation, pranayama and other practices. That is why we meditate before the morning meal and before the evening meal. Then we have some good activity afterward, which is the right dual cycle of meditation and activity each day, producing the most efficient progress.

Siddhasana is after spinal breathing, mulabandha and sambhavi in the lessons. If you have already stabilized these, one at a time, then you may be ready for siddhasana. Try not to take on too much all at once, as it can lead to an unwieldy routine that is hard to stabilize. Step by step, you know. Rome was not built in a day. You are the one in charge.

If you undertake other mantras during the day, like Gayatri, it will certainly speed up purification, but maybe excessively. With all the good techniques available these days, the challenge is not in achieving the purification. It is in digesting it in a way that facilitates stable progress and the rise of ecstatic bliss over the long term. The lessons take a particular approach to the task. There are other approaches too. Mixing them together may not bring the best results.

In the approach here, daily activity is used to stabilize the effects of practices. The best way to do this is to go out and engage in worthwhile activities of our choice. Then our activities, inner silence and ecstatic energy are naturally blended to bring about higher functioning in our nervous system. The end result is life lived in ecstatic bliss with divine love flowing out into everything we do. Our life naturally becomes joyful service, wherever we may be.

There are many things you can do that will hasten purification in your nervous system. But there is only so much purification the nervous system can assimilate in a given period of time. The order in which practices are done is important too. Think of it as being like athletic conditioning. It takes time, particular exercises, and a gradual build-up. That is the approach here. The practices in the lessons, combined with prudent self-pacing (very important), provide a means to go gradually faster without risking excessive instability. Then we can keep up our daily practices indefinitely without overloading and burning out.

Stable long-term daily practice is the key to enlightenment. The journey is more like a marathon than a sprint. With right practices and good self-pacing it can be a pretty fast marathon!

You are doing great. Keep up the good work. I wish you all success on your chosen spiritual path.

The guru is in you.

Lesson 227 – Meditation, Activity and Sleep

Q: I'm wondering about activity after sadhana (practices). First of all, the lessons have mentioned interpersonal interaction as well as physical activity. Is the main point to become re-engaged with the external world/re-grounded? Is vigorous physical activity the best for promoting integration after meditation practice (after the rest period)?

I also find that frequently I want to (feel compelled to) sleep after meditation and have sometimes slept for an hour or more. Am I better off going with the flow and taking the sleep that my body and psyche seem to want, or would it be better to ignore the sleep and move purposefully into some kind of activity? Is there a drawback to sleeping after meditation practice?

A: Yes, activity "grounds" the inner silence and ecstatic energies we cultivate during meditation, pranayama and other practices. Actually, the word "integrates" is a better description. Over time, as we do practices daily and are active in normal life according to our inclinations (no special conduct or activity required), we come to naturally sustain the qualities of inner silence and ecstasy all the time, no matter what we are doing. That is the fruit of all this – being out in the world, living our life as we choose, becoming a self-contained bundle of unbounded ecstatic bliss, and radiating that wherever we go.

Meditation will always give us what we need, because we are bringing up pure bliss consciousness from within, the source and sustainer of all that we are. If there is some accumulation of fatigue in the nervous system, meditation can bring us into a sleep-like state during or right after practice. This sleep associated with meditation is of a much deeper variety than ordinary sleep. Deep-rooted impurities are being dissolved. So, we don't force against sleep if it comes during or right after meditation. Of course, if we have to get up and go to work, then we do that. If we have the time to honor a need for more rest, we should allow it. There are cycles that come and go along our journey in practices. We may go through a period of falling asleep during or after meditation. And then one day, we are wide-awake and radiating bliss. Some clouds have been dissolved. As mentioned in a recent lesson, sometimes we can have both the bliss and the clouds. It is all part of the process of purification on the road to enlightenment

The guru is in you.

Lesson 228 – Heart Opening and Service

Q: On the heart chakra matter, as my understanding is (I am a pranic healer, and in our school the first meditation we are taught addresses the heart chakra...), heart chakra difficulties stem from one of man's most primary tendencies – that of receiving and not giving, be it of love, money, emotion, time, what have you.

We are comfortable taking things, but not so much in giving. The best way to open up the heart, our guru tells us, is to serve other sentient beings, be they human, animal or even subtle beings.

We do this by healing. In Western countries I am sure there must be many opportunities of community service. It does not matter whether the receiver is appreciative of our gesture, so long as we are "giving from the heart", so to say.

Of course, the flip side – all giving and no receiving – is not good either. There needs to be a healthy balance.

Aside from that, from my understanding of chakras, it would not be just the heart chakra, which needs a bit of cleansing, but also the accompanying solar plexus chakra, which is where we tend to store our emotions. And bastrika pranayama and nauli are excellent to get the solar plexus chakra going.

In my experience, it is also a good idea to invoke the divine for protection before embarking on the day's practises. A small point, but one that seems to be omitted astonishingly often.

A: Thank you for your feedback on opening the heart chakra. It is a chicken and egg thing – service and heart opening. Which comes first, service or heart opening? Service is both cause and effect of heart opening. Heart opening is both cause and effect of service. I lean toward beginning with the latter, using advanced yoga practices to purify and open the heart (and the entire nervous system), and service comes up naturally with the resulting inner silence and ecstatic conductivity. Service then plays an important role in marrying silence with ecstasy into an endless fountain of divine love pouring out and merging with everything everywhere, and that is enlightenment. Service is encouraged in the lessons to promote this process, i.e., meditate, and then go out and help someone in need.

What I am reluctant to do is beat people over the head with codes of conduct, including the "service imperative." I think everyone will find their service tendency naturally. All it takes is some good yoga and an occasional reminder. Service lives within us all. It is called karma yoga, and comes up naturally through the connectedness of yoga that we have discussed previously in the lessons.

Going inward first is the approach to yama and niyama (codes of conduct) in the lessons – purify and open first, and then let's go share our bubbling bliss with the world. That kind of service never burns out. Enforced service behavior does burn out, because it has a limited spiritual foundation underneath.

That is why the practices come first in the lessons – first build a foundation of inner silence, and then build the house of living generously with our energy in the world. Practices and service go together. One without the other leads to stagnation. A foundation without a house is pretty boring, and a house without a foundation can't last (and can lead to heart problems). So both are needed at the same time, and it really doesn't matter much which one we start with, as long as we end up with both. This is how the heart can be opened with great effectiveness. It is a formula for good health all the way around – spiritual and physical.

I agree that starting our practices and daily activity with remembrance of our chosen ideal is very good. In fact, a continuing hunger for our chosen ideal (ishta) is a blessing. This is bhakti. Cultivating our desire for the divine to a fever pitch is the greatest yoga practice of them all. With that, all of yoga and its fruits come quickly.

The guru is in you.

Lesson 229* – Spinal Breathing in Inner Space

Q: I would also like to ask for clarification about spinal breathing. When we talk about tracing the spine during spinal breathing and bastrika, is it necessary to have an actual visualization? And if so, is it important for the visualization to be either from outside the spinal cord/sushumna nadi looking in or, alternatively, visualizing from within sushumna and travelling along its passage? My usual experience is to notice a slight kinesthetic sensation of pressure moving up the spine during inhalation, and the flowing warmth down the spine during exhalation. (I'm not currently experiencing the coolness rising up.)

And, as long as I'm full of questions today, I'd like to ask your opinion of another version of spinal breathing that I had learned – 12 count inhale, 3 count kumbhaka, 12 count exhale, 3 count kumbhaka. The kumbhakas feel very natural and quieting, but I wonder if you feel that the counting is too much division of attention? With this form of the practice, I have been able to experience the coolness rising, as well as the warmth flowing down.

Thank you for your patience and generosity in answering all of our questions.

A: It is everyone's tendency to begin spinal breathing looking from the outside, imagining the tiny thread of a nerve between the perineum and brow. Over time it internalizes due to the rise of inner sensory experience. The experience of the cool and warm currents is the beginning of that, an excellent "handle" to bring the attention inward during spinal breathing, and that is why it is discussed in the lessons (#63). On our journey from external to internal, we can imagine being inside, but not to the point of strain, as this will detract from the natural flow of spinal breathing. It is like meditation in that sense – we just easily favor the direction we want to go in, not forcing.

There are many forms of spinal breathing (lesson #206). This is acceptable because spinal breathing is not nearly as delicate a procedure as deep meditation due to the physicality of breath, which regulates the overall process. So, there is room for variations while maintaining effectiveness. This is not so with deep meditation, which involves the management of attention only. That is why we are "stingy" with our attention in meditation, always favoring the easy procedure of picking up the mantra and letting it refine naturally to stillness in the mind.

In spinal breathing, as long as we are slowing down (restraining) the breathing and cycling the attention with it going between the brow and the perineum, it will work. Due to this relative sturdiness of spinal breathing, we are able to introduce and stabilize into habit many of the other practices in the lessons. It is relatively easy to incorporate new practices while doing spinal breathing without disrupting our practice excessively. Of course, if we shift to the crown instead of the brow in our attention cycle with breathing, all bets are off. That dramatically increases the risk of instability of our inner energies.

Kumbhaka on either or both ends of the breathing cycle in spinal breathing is a further degree of restraint of breath. If this works for you, that is good practice too. Keep in mind that adding kumbhaka into spinal breathing, and later adding more with yoni mudra and the chin pump will be a lot of kumbhaka, and you should be prudent in your self-pacing of practices if the resulting purification and experiences become excessive. You can use the counting during spinal breathing if you like, though I think you will find later that the cycling of breath, kumbhakas, etc. becomes a natural and organic process. Then the counting will not be necessary. So much the better for letting the attention do what it does best – soar in inner space!

When you get to kechari stage 2, and beyond, all of this will take off, as kechari takes the experience of spinal breathing much deeper. That is why kechari means, "to fly through (inner) space." By the time it gets to that stage we are definitely inside, traveling the infinite expanses of pure bliss consciousness between our third eye and root source. Externally, it is a journey back and forth between sambhavi and mulabandha/asvini with uddiyana/nauli in-between. But we don't even notice that when we are inside our infinitely big little nerve, reveling in ecstatic bliss.

It is a metaphor for all of physical life, really, and an emerging reality for the yogi/yogini. The rise of internal sensory experience does, in fact, gradually become the reality of our outer life too. What seems so limited through our outer senses now is seen to be infinite when we purify and develop our inner senses. We are "That," and everything inside and outside is joyfully dancing in That.

As it says in the Upanishads: "I am That. Thou art That. All this is That." What is That? It is pure bliss consciousness, of course – our own radiant inner silence.

The guru is in you.

Addition – This is a good place to introduce an optional element of pranayama practice called "brahmari," which means "bee sound." It is most effectively used during spinal breathing, once ecstatic conductivity has begun to come up.

You will recall that when we first introduced spinal breathing, a partial closing of the epiglottis was recommended during exhalation. This is called "ujjayi." It creates some pressure in the lungs, and some vibration in the throat in the form of a high hissing sound. These two effects stimulate the circulation of prana in the nervous system, and the awakening of the higher neuro-biology in the upper body and head.

Brahmari has features similar to ujjayi, though it does not occur in exactly the same place anatomically. Brahmari operates in the larynx (voice box), which is just below the epiglottis at the entrance to the windpipe. The escape of air from the lungs can be limited either with the epiglottis (ujjayi) or with the vocal chords in the larynx (brahmari). Brahmari occurs when the escape of air on exhalation is restricted in the larynx by the vocal chords coming together and making a hum like the sound of a bee in flight.

The effects of brahmari are similar to ujjayi. The main difference is the resonant vibration created by brahmari deeper in the throat, which has a more stimulating effect in the upper body and head, particularly in the medulla oblongata (brain stem). The medulla oblongata is where the natural vibration of *OM* emanates as ecstatic conductivity comes up in the nervous system. Brahmari stimulates this natural neuro-biological occurrence of *OM*, so it can be called an "*OM* stimulator." The effects of this stimulation are profound once ecstatic conductivity is present in the nervous system.

For most people, brahmari is a more challenging practice than ujjayi in the beginning, mainly because it requires a balancing of pitch with the rate of exhalation. The higher the pitch, the slower the rate of exhalation. The lower the pitch the faster the rate of exhalation. Therefore, the pitch used in brahmari is related to one's rate of spinal breathing on exhalation. So, doing brahmari is a bit trickier. Ujjayi can be regulated more easily to suit the pace of comfortable spinal breathing. In both ujjayi and brahmari the throat is opened wide during slow inhalation during spinal breathing, without any restriction being applied.

There is a social aspect to brahmari. It makes a noise that can be heard rooms away from where it is being done. Under some circumstances this may not be desirable. Ujjayi makes practically no noise, so can be practiced discreetly almost anywhere that one does spinal breathing.

Although brahmari has extra benefits, ujjayi may be the preferred practice due to its simplicity and quietness. Maybe ujjayi will be preferred at certain times, and brahmari at other times. Just be sure to be doing one or the other during spinal breathing, so there will be some pressure and vibration on exhalation. Which practice to use is up to you. Either one greatly compliments spinal breathing, sambhavi, kechari, siddhasana, and the rest of the mudras and bandhas we are using.

You will know when you are ready for brahmari. It will tend to happen automatically as ecstatic conductivity comes up, because it brings so much pleasure. Then you will be immersed in waves of ecstatic bliss in inner space that will follow you out into daily activity!

Lesson 230* – Crown and Third Eye

Q: It's only been a couple of weeks, if that, that I've been doing mulabandha and have just added sambhavi today (wasn't sure if they were supposed to be together at the start or get comfortable with mulabandha and then add sambhavi – which I did).

My question is that I am getting a lot of activity at the crown though I am not focusing at all there but following your suggestions on focusing from the root to third eye with the spinal breathing.

I am wondering if I should be "taming" this in some way or as it is happening spontaneously, just leave it alone and continue to focus on the root to third eye direction. I have practiced meditation for 20+ years on and off under my own guidance and have enjoyed it immensely.

My concern is that when I first tried meditation, I fell into the silence very, very quickly but after only a few meditations I had a spontaneous kundalini awakening which shot up through the root area quite strongly. It was at a difficult emotional time for me then and led to more difficulties in my life (at least I determined that was the cause of a pathway I followed) for a couple of years.

This was all quite bewildering to me, as I did not have any teacher at the time to advise or explain what was happening. Later, I took some yoga classes and understood a bit more though I never discussed the situation with the teacher, as I just didn't feel comfortable to do so.

Anyway, here I am, years later, so excited to have found your web site and your lessons, eager but definitely not anxious, due to past experience, to push forward but rather would like to move forward easily and naturally. This is a long story to get to the point but wanted to give you the background. The activity at the crown is strong but not unpleasant but as I want to go about this as naturally as possible, do you think I should back off a bit or just let it take the natural course. I do not feel afraid or over-cautious but would love to have your take on this as I am enjoying all of it.

Thank you for the blessings you have bestowed in offering these lessons.

A: Thank you for writing and sharing. Yes, you did right in taking on mulabandha and sambhavi one after the other, adjusting to the first before taking on the second. It is like that with all the practices. Stability is the first priority. Otherwise the whole thing can become too unwieldy, and then we lose our ability to sustain long-term practice, which is the key to our enlightenment.

Speaking of stability, your previous experience with practices in this life (and probably before that) indicates a sensitivity that is manifesting as lots of energy flowing, including the crown experiences you mentioned. It is good stuff. At the same time, the experiences you are having emphasize the importance of sticking with third eye to root spinal breathing. Actually, nearly all of the practices in the lessons (including meditation) are geared toward third eye to root purification. It is suggested you stay with this approach in your practices. In doing so, you will continue to open the crown also, with the elements of safety and control built in. Ajna (third eye) means "command." There are several lessons on crown versus third eye oriented practices. Given the nature of your experiences, you may wish to review them now. You can find them listed in the topic index under "crown opening (avoiding premature)."

Along the way you will come across lots of lessons discussing "self-pacing," which is a skill we must develop having so many powerful spiritual techniques available. As a matter of fact, self-pacing is fundamental to any spiritual path, no matter what level we are at. Everyone responds to practices a little differently, and prudent application of self-pacing is how we customize our routine and expansion of practices to achieve maximum progress with minimum difficulties along the way. It is an ongoing interaction we have involving the relationship between the application of our practices and our resulting experiences, much like driving a car through a constantly changing landscape.

You are wise to take it easy and go step by step according to your capacity. You know what can be accomplished, and what the risks are. You are into some of the best tools available, and are applying them with skill. The possibilities are very exciting. Drive safely, and enjoy the ride!

The guru is in you.

Addition – If there are some sensations at the crown, this is normal as we continue with our regular brow to root advanced yoga practices, because the crown is also being gradually opened in a controlled way. Over time the crown sensations will become stronger in concert with overall purification in the nervous system. If the energies do not become uncomfortable, we can just continue with our daily practices. It is not a danger to notice what is happening at the crown, as it does not constitute focused practice. There will be a time when we can go directly to the crown with nothing but complete absorption in ecstatic bliss being the outcome. This is how it is when the nervous system is adequately purified. So, all we do is let the crown come along naturally with our regular advanced yoga practices. If things get excessive, then we know it is time to apply self-pacing and back off a bit. With this approach the crown is not so much difficulty. It is just like any other kind of self-pacing situation we encounter in the nervous system as we proceed with our practices.

Lesson 231 – Dusty Rooms

Q: I have been meditating for the past five months. Now one bizarre thing is happening in my life nowadays. Previously I used to be a goody-goody kind of person meeting people helping them, happy to be in groups, etc. I had seemingly good relationships with all and used to be known as a nice person. Of late I have become too introverted, sort of disinterested in people, just keeping to myself, avoiding people. In fact, my relationship with my family also is not very good. There is a sort of unsaid sadness hanging around. I am happy to be with myself, but having people around me is not very comfortable. People don't understand me any longer. It sounds queer, but strangely this is what is happening. I really am in a fix. Is it the meditation? Or is it some deep emotion? Kindly help. I want to be the same loving nice person I used to be.

And on the technical part of meditation, as soon as I put the tip of my tongue on the palate a sort of salty taste occurs, and soon I start getting a feeling very strongly that I have to vomit out something and it goes on till I remove the tongue from the palate. Please tell me what to do. May God bless you.

A: Thank you for writing and sharing. You are that same nice loving person, and even more. What is happening is purification in your nervous system from practices – a bit more than is comfortable. It is a temporary disturbance that can be corrected. This indicates a sensitivity to meditation and other practices you are doing. The sensitivity is a good thing. It means your nervous system really wants to open. On the other hand, it also means that you should use good self-pacing in practices to make sure you don't have so much coming out every day. It can cause the kinds of symptoms you mentioned – reclusiveness, irritability, heavy mood, etc. There can be physical symptoms also, as with your kechari.

Think of yourself as living in a big house, and you just discovered several new rooms. They are full of dust and you want to clean them. If you go in there swinging a broom every which way, the dust will fly up in great quantities and you will run out coughing. Better to do a little sweeping at a time, picking up the dust and disposing of it a bit at time. Then the rooms can be cleaned without causing a lot of disruption in the house. The nervous system is like that. When we undertake meditation, we enter into new areas inside that have not been active much before. If our practices are too much, there can be a lot of dust kicking up. And that is what can cause the uncomfortable symptoms, moodiness, etc. It is odd, because our same practices of meditation and pranayama, done in balance with activity, will make us more joyful than we were before.

The solution in your case is to scale practices back to have good cleaning without causing undue disruptions in life.

But first, make sure you are taking plenty of time of rest coming out of each meditation. At least 5-10 minutes. Lying down during this time is good. This enables the "dust" of released impurities during practices to dissipate before we go into activity. If we get up too fast, there can be irritability or moodiness in activity.

If coming out slower does not help, then consider scaling back your time of meditation five minutes. It that doesn't work after a few days, try scaling back another five minutes, and so on. There is a discussion of this process in lessons #160 and #200. Also, if you look in the topic index under "self-pacing," you will find more lessons on this subject. It is a very important skill to develop, especially if a high sensitivity to practices is there. We all have this at one time or another along the way toward enlightenment. No one can make the journey without making adjustments in practices from time to time. The journey of purifying the nervous system with practices is like driving a car across a varying landscape. We have to be sensitive to our changing experiences and make adjustments in our driving accordingly. Comfort is the first measuring rod to use. If there is discomfort, it is a signal to adjust our practices.

Another thing to consider is spinal breathing. You did not mention it. If you are not doing any, you might try doing five minutes of it before meditation each session and see if that helps your emotions during the day. It will often help if there is an energy imbalance in the nervous system. In fact, spinal breathing is one of the best remedies for energy imbalances in our yoga tool kit. So consider that too.

On the discomfort in kechari (tongue going back), this is also a sensitivity to practice, with lots of impurities coming out when you do that. It is a good thing, but, again, we want to do it in a measured way that does not disrupt our life. In time it all clears out and what we have is pure bliss consciousness and divine ecstasy shining up through us in vast quantities. Along the way we will have many glimpses of this as it gradually rises to become a full time reality in our life.

You are that wonderful loving person you have always been. You will be even more like that, because it is your true nature. Just apply some good self-pacing in your practices and I think you will find a much smoother ride. Don't be afraid to experiment with your routine to find the right balance between practices and your experience in daily living. The journey should be both progressive and fun. Aim for that...

I wish you all success on your chosen spiritual path.

The guru is in you.

Lesson 232 – Meditation and Automatic Yoga (a dialog)

Q1: I recorded my experience today with the *I AM* meditation. I am just beginning so this is as far as I have gone. The experience was awesome, as they say. I am keeping a diary of what I experience. I have copied my experience and pasted it here. I wanted to find out if what I experienced is "normal". Thank you.

August 16th, 2004, 8:34-8:55: 2nd attempt at *I AM*. First time I did this was lying in bed. Did it for about 20 minutes and then went to sleep. Did not notice anything spectacular. Probably wasn't a good idea to do it in bed as it is too relaxing and I was sleepy when I did it.

Had coffee, no food prior to beginning: 2nd time, sat in my office chair with doors closed. Palms on thighs. After some time, felt as though I was about to float out of top of head but only very briefly. Felt like a floating sensation. This happened twice.

Then after some more time, an overwhelming tingling sensation washed over my body and became stronger and stronger. I noticed my breathing change with it. It was intense like a wave similar to waves of ecstasy one has in approaching orgasm. It was definitely sexual in nature and ran throughout my entire body, not just one area.

When it first started however it also resembled the feeling one gets when one experiences some excitement of the kind that gives one goose bumps and butterflies. Similar to what may be referred to as an adrenal rush but, but a good one. This tingly sensation of excitement soon led to the waves of ecstasy described above.

After several moments of this it was almost as though I could take no more, and then it backed off for some moments. Then a second wave came like the first. I actually made some verbal sound as a sigh or groan as it continued and my breathing became heavier and deeper. I noticed too I felt like I might be trembling but am not sure now whether my body was actually trembling or it just felt that way.

After this second wave passed, for some reason I was ready, perhaps even anxious, to end the session but was aware that I was supposed to do this for a full twenty minutes. I looked at my clock and saw that I still had a little more than 5 minutes or so to go so resumed it. After some moments, again, the feeling started to come as described above but this time it was more jolting, not as smooth as the first two. I felt this jolt twice. After some moments I ended the session, having gone a total of about 20 minutes. I took several deep breaths and remained sitting and rested as advised and then wrote this so that I forgot nothing.

A1: Thank you for writing and sharing. You are off to a very good start, finding out right away the difference between meditating lying down and sitting up! Keep in mind that your experiences will vary over time, sometimes very deep, sometimes with lots of energy (even sexual – you will read more on that in later lessons), other times dull, and sometimes a bit restless. All experiences are correct as long as we favor the easy procedure of meditation. What is important is long term daily practice. That is what purifies and opens our nervous system. See lesson #180 with a response to someone having strong start like you did.

Our experiences during practices are mostly due to purification going on in our nervous system, and will vary greatly. Even ecstatic experiences are largely purification. It all comes out according to how the impressions of past actions are stacked inside. There is no accounting for it, and all we have to do is our procedure of practice, and purification and opening happens. So, don't become too attached to experiences that occur in meditation. Practice is good if we follow the procedure, no matter what happens experientially in our sitting. Of course we all love blissful and ecstatic experiences. Enjoy them when they happen. But keep in mind that experiences are symptoms, not the practice itself. We don't want to become distracted from our practice by experiences that come up. So when experiences come, we notice them, and go back to the practice we are doing. That is what keeps us going forward toward enlightenment. As you read through, you will encounter many lessons that discuss this from a variety of angles.

Q2: Thank you. I am somewhat relieved to know that I don't necessarily have to expect to repeat that experience. Otherwise I may have thought I was doing something wrong if nothing happened next time.

I just read lesson #39 and #41 on pranayama, which I have not yet tried. I did some deep breathing before starting my meditation on *I AM* that morning. Maybe that was one reason my experience was so dramatic.

I am taking another course that gives the sound *OM* to chant. I haven't been doing it lately but thought I would start again. I saw one of the Q&As where you state the difference between *I AM* and *OM*, that latter being circular. But I am wondering if I should wait a while after the meditation to do my *OM* chanting.

I have several questions:

Can you tell me when I should start trying spinal breathing pranayama? That is, are there a certain number of days that one should do the *I AM* meditation before doing the pranayama exercise? Also is it advisable to set an egg timer so that I will know when my 20 minutes are up? Is it necessary to do it two times per day to achieve optimum results? Do you state somewhere in the Q&As why the lotus position is better than sitting in a chair?

I am really surprised at how powerful that mediation technique is. I still can't believe it. I had always wondered at the significance of the phrase "I AM" in the *Bible*. Now I am even more curious and want to go back through all the places where it is referenced.

My husband is going to try it sitting up now. He too had only tried it lying down before so I am anxious to hear of his results. I didn't tell him about mine because I didn't want him to be expecting a certain result.

A2: Given that you have just started and have lots happening already, it would be wise to stabilize your meditation practice for at least a few weeks before adding pranayama. Then you will have a good platform from which to expand. As you read through the lessons you will see a lot on "self-pacing," which is essential for success in yoga. You already have seen the first lesson on this (#38) called "What is Your Time Line?" A very important subject – more important than any single practice. Without a skilled driver, the car is not likely to reach its destination.

Self-pacing applies to taking on other practices outside AYP too, which is risky to begin with because the effects in combination with AYP practices can be unpredictable. You are in charge of your journey. Be measured in your approach, always stabilizing what you have before moving ahead. Each person is different. Stabilizing could take weeks or months. In some cases (as with mantra enhancements and advanced pranayama-kumbhaka methods given later in the lessons) it could take years. A few days will rarely do it. Even experts in yoga have to apply prudent self-pacing in practices to accommodate the many experiences that come up as the nervous system goes though stages of purification. So, satisfy your thirst for knowledge by reading on, but build your routine very gradually so you can remain consistent in your practices over the long term. That is how enlightenment happens. Rome was not built in a day.

It is okay to use an egg timer for meditation, but don't become too dependent on it. It is best to develop the inner clock for timing practices, with occasional peeking at the watch or clock as necessary. Once we have this "inner clock" skill, then using an egg timer is not our sole means of timing. That way, if you are without your egg timer, you won't be at a loss.

Siddhasana (not lotus) is the way of sitting that the lessons evolve toward. You will see why as you read on. It is a simple and powerful practice for raising ecstatic energy. The cultivation of inner silence and ecstatic energy, and their natural union (inner lovemaking of "Shiva and Shakti" or "Father and Holy Spirit"), is the key to human spiritual transformation.

On the twice a day, check lesson #148. Many of your questions you can find answers to in the topic index. I will be happy to help with anything that you cannot find a satisfactory answer on.

The methods in the lessons are the simplest and most powerful I have encountered over more than three decades on the path, integrated together into this system of practices. So, yes, this is all very powerful stuff. Use good self-pacing, avoid tangents (lots of those will tempt you), and you can go very far with this over the long term. Enjoy!

Q3: Thank you much again. Yesterday I again received the waves washing over me, up and down, which felt, as I can best describe, like an electrical current. I noticed my breathing began to change each time this occurred causing me to take deeper breaths, which I immediately corrected. I soon found that I could control the waves at will. Not sure if I should allow them or discourage them?

I also noticed my head began both times to rock gently back and forth and then to eventually sway side to side in what seemed a figure 8. After the experience, I did a search under "swaying" and found where one of your students also experienced swaying but with his entire body. I read your responses about not letting all these sensations detract from the main purpose.

For the first time today, I did my meditation in the lotus position with my back against my couch. It wasn't as comfortable and was a bit distracting a few times but I managed to keep directing my attention away from the discomfort and concentrate on the mediation. The electrical waves came again, but this time were a lot more subtle. And again when the breathing intensified I immediately stopped it and calmed it and stayed quiet.

I did away with the egg timer and peeked at the clock again. I think I may have been a little more anxious to end the session because of the position I was in. When it was over, my lower leg was asleep. I didn't see any instruction on "when" we should start the lotus position. I did see lesson #33. I will start doing some exercises to limber my joints up a bit which I remember from ballet school many a year ago. I still felt my mediation was good though it wasn't quite as smooth as in the sitting position.

A3: You are having the classic symptoms of what I call "automatic yoga," from just a few days of meditation. It goes without saying that you have come "wired" for this from past lives of work in yoga. We are all wired for it by virtue of our human nervous system. Some have more neural conductivity than others because they have done direct work on the circuitry before. You are one of those, and now you are picking up where you left off. We all have the same journey and destination – purification and opening of our nervous system to unending ecstatic bliss and outflowing divine love.

By automatic yoga, I mean physical, mental and emotional tendencies coming up out of nowhere, seemingly unrelated to the practice we are doing. This happens because there is a connectedness of yoga throughout our nervous system. This is explained in other lessons, particularly in discussing the "eight limbs of yoga" (lesson #149). For now, just know that your rising desire to study, practice, take on more, etc. is all coming from the few dives you have taken into pure bliss consciousness within. So too are the bending legs, breathing symptoms and head movements from this. Pretty amazing, isn't it? The lessons will help you guide all of these tendencies step by step into a safe and effective routine of practices.

When movements or deep breathing come up in meditation, we don't entertain them, or force them out. We just easily go back to the procedure of meditation, picking up the mantra at whatever level of refinement we left it, and let it continue to refine.

Breathing generally becomes very quiet during meditation, as the metabolism slows way down. If it is getting deeper or is speeding up, that could be associated with ecstatic energies beginning to move. Don't dwell on that, as it will take your attention away from the simple process of meditation. When you begin spinal breathing (a separate practice done before meditation), then you will have the opportunity to cultivate the ecstatic energies in a progressive and balanced way. Favor the procedure for using the mantra during meditation over anything that comes up. The same goes for head movements and other symptoms that can occur – just easily let it go in favor of meditation. Much later in the lessons, you will see that head movements also will be part of practices in the form of an advanced method called "chin pump." That is way down the road though. You are just starting out. Take things one step at a time. Gently favor the practice you are doing, no matter what else comes up. If some of these things become so strong that they seem to be dominating your meditation time, then just be easy and let your attention be with the movements or sensations (without encouraging them) for a few minutes without picking up the mantra. That will help stabilize the energy flow. Then after a few minutes you can go back to meditation.

On the folding legs, the lessons do not teach lotus (feet up on thighs). We use siddhasana instead, which is a more direct means for cultivating the ecstatic energies within. Once you get through spinal breathing, mulabandha and sambhavi, you will come to siddhasana. You are doing right to be loosening up the legs now. No need to go up on the thighs with your feet though – just develop some comfort having the legs folded with toes tucked under a bit, as discussed in lesson #33. This builds a foundation for things to come, with a minimum of distraction to meditation. If it becomes too distracting, ease off the folded legs. Try one folded until two works. Try legs folded only one sitting out of two each day. It is a gradual process of adjustment that can take weeks or months to work into. In the meantime, keep as comfortable as possible while meditating. In time, sitting with legs folded will be completely natural and unnoticed during practices. So will siddhasana, except for the fountain of unending ecstasy coming up from it. Well, that is another subject.

Timing for taking on new practices is discussed in the course of the lessons. It has to do with your ability to assimilate things more than anything. That is why specific times are not given. Everyone is different. The main thing is not to get too far ahead of yourself. Even that is not the end of the world in the short term, as long as you know to back off when you get a little too far ahead of your nervous system's ability to digest new practices. It is a process of always testing, stepping forward, and stepping back – gradually learning the ropes of this wonderful transformable spiritual vehicle we are living in – the human nervous system!

Q4: I took a quick skim of the chin pump lesson (#139) and it seems that describes something very similar to what was happening to me.

This is getting quite exciting but I want to take it step by step as you suggested so I didn't read it in detail. There are so many lessons that to do otherwise would be very difficult in any case. Yesterday for the first time, I did the meditation twice. My legs were just crossed. (I haven't even attempted the lotus position and am glad to hear we won't be expected to use it!) Again, sitting cross-legged was very distracting but once I got into the meditation it became smoother.

I am wondering about the meditation on *I AM*. Over the past weeks before I found your group and web site, I had been doing a mental affirmation throughout the day, "I am in harmony with Christ". I even have a pillow speaker under my pillow with me speaking that affirmation. The reason for this was that I had read in one of several books (reading Spalding on the Siddha Masters, Collier, Trine & Hill, so I get them mixed up sometimes) that one of the reasons for sickness, stress, etc. was being out of harmony with Christ. Also they all talk about us as being Divine, that God is within us. I suppose I grew up like a lot of people thinking about Him as being up there somewhere separate from us.

So sometimes in my meditation, while thinking *I AM*, I am thinking of God, then I alternate with just meditating on the words *I AM* without thinking of God. So I suppose I'm uncertain as to how to think/feel when I think *I AM*.

At one point, for just a few seconds last night in my second session, it seemed I stepped out and forward from the meditation on the words, into a circle with some colors and there were no words or thinking. It was just like a complete separation from thought and body. But it was just for seconds and then I was back thinking *I AM*. This occurred a couple of times very briefly. I wanted to explore it more but it didn't happen again. It was as though I was on the very edge of something but couldn't quite get there. Then during this morning's mediation, I felt that same separateness but this time rather than moving up into a circle I felt as though I were falling backwards and floating into that separateness. Again, all thought of thinking *I AM* and my body was forgotten. It was so "still." I wanted it to last longer again but it was only for a few seconds a couple of times. For the first time since beginning the meditation, I wasn't anxious to come out of it. I was content to stay there but went ahead and ended it at 20 minutes since that's what you have advised.

I do have a question that is confusing me even while I meditate: Should I think of God as I meditate with *I AM* or try just to meditate *I AM* without its meaning or thinking of God or my Divine nature? Should I try to divorce the meditation form thoughts of God?

I wanted to check about something new that happened last night.

Yesterday and last night I noticed at times, my breathing was so slight, that once I thought I had stopped breathing. But the newest thing is last night; the area in my solar plexus was pressed inward to such a degree that it felt as though my entire rib cage was exposed with the area in the middle under the breastbone going inward. It must have actually been drawn inward towards my back for I could feel the movement under my breast. It wasn't painful, just really intense. I didn't think I was holding my breath and cannot remember now this morning exactly how my breathing was when this happened. I should have made notes right after this. So naturally again I am wondering about this and if you have ever heard of this happening?

A4: The mantra is used for sound only, not meaning. In the topic index you can find several lessons on this under "mantra – language and meaning." Another way to spell the *I AM* mantra is *AYAM.* Same pronunciation. None of this takes away from the meaning and mystique of the Christian phrase, "I AM." It is just that when we use it as a mantra, it is the vibration that matters, not the English meaning. My background is Christian also.

So, when thoughts come up in meditation regarding the meaning of *I AM,* or God, or whatever, we just treat them like any other thoughts that come up and easily go back to the mantra. The same is true for all experiences we have in meditation, no matter how ecstatic, profound, revelatory, strange, or dramatic – when we realize we are off into something, no matter what, we just easily go back to the mantra. That is the procedure of meditation.

Ah, you noticed the breathing slowing down and nearly stopping. As mentioned before, that is normal.

The diaphragm pulling in and up is another of those automatic yogas. It is called "uddiyana." You can find discussions on it in the practices section (top) of the topic index, under "uddiyana/nauli."

Take it step by step, and enjoy!

Q5: So in other countries, in other languages they also use *I AM* rather than their translation of *I AM?*

I just did a quick read of the article you referred to on uddiyana. This is so incredible that my body is doing all of these things on its own. Though I hadn't mentioned it, my tongue has also been cupping and pressing against the roof of my mouth near the front. I didn't realize it was something that you consciously try to do. I guess whatever my body starts to do from here on, I can safely assume it knows better than I.

I am trying to follow everything step by step. By my body jumping into all of these things on its own, am I at risk in not developing properly since I seem to be doing things out of order? I only start out by thinking to do only the mediation. These things are just happening on their own. I've had some other things happen as well that I may later learn are automatic yoga.

A5: Yes, since we are using the sound of *I AM* (*AYAM*) and not the meaning, translation of meaning into other languages is not advised. The sound has a universal vibratory resonance in the human nervous system. That's why I call it a universal mantra.

Ah, the tongue has gone up? That is called "kechari," a very important one we talk about a lot in the later lessons. You can look it up in the topic index.

With all this coming up, I can see that you are a little concerned about how to manage it going forward. I suggest you don't even try. Just do your practices according to plan, taking on new ones gradually over the coming months and years, with the priority being to establish stable practice each step along the way. Whatever comes up as automatic yoga, regard with equanimity, and stay the course with structured daily practice over the long term. If you do that, then all these things will fit together naturally in due course. Given your fast moving situation, the most important things I recommend you keep in mind are patience and self-pacing in practices. If you try and accommodate all that is going on at the same time, it will be very difficult. You have many gifts of yoga sprouting there. Tend your garden with care, day by day, and you will travel far.

Always remember that the most important practice is deep meditation. This is what cultivates our foundation of inner silence underneath all of the external hub-bub. Without it we will be flailing about in the wind, with no center, no matter how much automatic yoga we have going on. Inner silence (pure bliss consciousness) is the key to all progress in yoga.

As it says in the *Psalms*, "Be still, and know I am God."

Q6: Thank you for your answer to my many questions. I was a little concerned about how to manage these things but that has now been put to rest by your answer. I will proceed methodically as though these things weren't happening.

Yesterday, I only did the meditation (with spinal breathing) once rather than twice. I had been for several days, experiencing a difficulty in putting my mind/energy on the more mundane tasks that my work requires. I had no motivation to do my work and thought that it might be a result of the mediation. I remember that you have stated that it is advisable to rest after the meditation and I never really did that beyond a minute or two at most so perhaps that is what I needed to do.

But I decided yesterday to try doing without the morning session and only did the evening session. I looked in your Q&A for any information on whether you are to do it everyday, 7 days a week or if its desirable to perhaps occasionally skip a day or one of the two sessions once in a while at least at the beginning. It may be there in the postings but I didn't find anything that addressed this question.

One other thing I wanted to ask about: I had written after my second or third mediation that I had found I could control the waves of energy charge that pulsed through my body at will. It started off happening without conscious effort but then I found I could make it happen again with minor effort. But lately, the last couple of days, I have been experiencing this in my daily routine out of mediation as well. At times during the day or night I feel the urge to push this energy current through my body at will. It might be while making a protein shake or working at my computer or while watching the news. It's becoming somewhat addictive I think. It's happening at least once about every hour. If I don't do it willingly, then it comes on its own. I don't feel it's a bad thing. It feels rather pleasant and gives me an unexplainable feeling of empowerment. Is this an enhancement of my spiritual powers or merely a part of the purification process?

A6: Yes, taking it easy, and one day at a time, is the best approach. It is the best approach whenever big changes come into our life – whether it be sudden wealth, fame, or realizing that our nervous system is opening us up to become infinite pure bliss consciousness encompassing the entire universe!

Yes, the experiences are part of purification and will change – expand actually, so there is much more to come. And yes, it can be addictive. That is in the very first lesson – my addiction to yoga and the experiences it brings. To borrow a word from the 12 step program for addicts, maybe we are all "recovering" yogis and yoginis. Recovering what is ours that has been long lost, that is. It is not primarily about the ecstatic experience of the moment. It is about something infinitely bigger than the greatest ecstatic pleasure we can have today. Enjoy your experiences, and incorporate them into your everyday life. The best way to do that is by taking your bliss and sharing it with others in simple ways. Simple living for the benefit of others is the best way I know to keep rising ecstatic experiences from going to our heads. That's part of why I am writing these lessons. What good is rising enlightenment if it is unshared? Not much good at all. Down-right self-indulgent. The truth is, enlightenment can't happen fully until it is shared in service for the benefit of others, because enlightenment is, by nature, all-encompassing.

It is not our fault that the true nature of life is ecstatic bliss. The human nervous system is an ecstasy machine. Should we run from that? I don't think so. As we move into our natural state of ecstasy, we can do so with responsibility. That is how we can make the journey. Ecstatic bliss must flow outward to the world to find its fruition, and so too must we. To do anything less is a form of spiritual hedonism. We may do that for a while, just indulge inwardly in our ecstatic experiences. That's okay. Sooner or later we will go out into the world with our ecstatic bliss. It is inevitable. Along the way in yoga, we unravel one of the greatest of all mysteries through our direct experience – the role of sexuality in human spiritual transformation.

As for daily practices, it is better to stick with two sessions every day, because developing and maintaining the habit is so very important. This was covered in a lesson not long ago (#209) called, "Fitting Daily Practices into a Busy Schedule." I know that lack of time is not the reason you have tried cutting back to one session, but that lesson gets into the reasons why keeping the twice-daily habit is so important. So does lesson #148, "Why Practices Twice a Day?"

If you are feeling a bit over-stimulated in your practices, then the thing to do is cut back on time in the twice-daily sittings. If you are doing 5 minutes spinal breathing and 20 minutes meditation, and are having too much happening, then, rather than doing it once a day, try cutting breathing back to a few minutes and meditation to 15 minutes twice a day. If that is still too much, then try meditation at 10 minutes. It can be ramped back up later as your nervous system adjusts to the energies. This is the all-important topic of "self-pacing" which is discussed extensively in the lessons. The key is to find a balanced and stable twice-daily routine. That way, we can cultivate inner silence and ecstatic energies in our nervous system and stabilize them in activity using a twice-daily cycle, which is much more effective than doing a once daily cycle with longer practice. Of course, there will be times that we are too pressed for time or too exhausted to do much of anything at practice time. Then we just keep the habit by sitting for a few minutes with eyes closed. See how that works? It is about the twice-daily habit. As they say, "use it or lose it." We can be flexible with our times and practices within that twice-daily commitment, as necessary.

Q7: I had a session yesterday that was, well, all I could think afterwards was, Wow! I had had two days of quieter mediation with the usual "automatic" head rocking and circling but the experience was much milder and quieter without all the involuntary surges of energy as before and no new automatic yoga experiences.

So I decided to move on and incorporate lessons #41, #54 and #55 (on spinal breathing, kundalini and mulabandha) in my session yesterday. The experience was the most powerful I have had yet and there were a lot of new things, what you call "automatic yoga" going on, I think.

A7: As you add on new practices, keep in mind that there can be a delayed reaction in effects. So we don't really know all of what a new practice is doing for a few weeks at least. If you have piled on two or three new practices, and things take off, it may be hard to figure out what is doing what – and that's when self-pacing gets tricky – what to back off on when the energy is flying everywhere? Getting a bit ahead of yourself is not the end of the world, as long as you know to back off when necessary for a smoother ride. You'll get the hang of it.

Just remember you have a spiritual Ferrari there (an extra fast one) and you have to learn how to drive the thing without running off the road. You are in the driver's seat.

All the best on your journey. Vrrrooom!

The guru is in you.

Lesson 233 – Yoga and Religious Beliefs

Q: Thank you for all the lessons.

I already completed the lessons, and am progressing with two times daily practise. But if I have a shortage of time, then I only do pranayama and meditation.

I have a question. Is it OK to practice AYP without interfering with our faith? Practicing AYP is like practicing tennis or playing chess. It is only a matter of physical body including brain and nervous system.

A: Your practice sounds very good. Yes, that is right, yoga is a matter of purifying and opening the nervous system to its natural higher functioning, which will not interfere with any religious belief system. AYP is non-sectarian, meaning, not tied to any particular belief system.

Interestingly, as our nervous system purifies and opens we become much more attuned to inner truth, and that can strengthen our spiritual life in whatever religious tradition we are. Each religious tradition has its own terminology and metaphorical language to describe the process of human spiritual transformation, which is the same neuro-biological process in everyone.

And if we are not involved in any religious belief system, that is okay too. Yoga will work just as well in the nervous system, as long as we have a strong desire to practice and progress toward greater inner peace and happiness.

The guru is in you.

Lesson 234 – Inner Wisdom Shining Through

Q: It's a month now since I have followed meticulously the meditation technique using mantra. Earlier it was difficult to sit at one place for 20-25 minutes and now, I would like to remain in the meditation posture with my mantra as long as possible, If I continue for more than 30 minutes, my mood becomes very dull later. Hence I restrict the meditation only to 20-25 minutes and feel relaxed and fresh some time. However, I am not getting any telltale marks in doing meditation. Kindly tell me, am I not cheating myself that I am meditating?

A: Thank you for writing and sharing. Your meditation practice sounds very good. You have found the importance of regulating the time so as not to overdo. This gives you the maximum rate of inner purification with minimum discomfort. That is perfect. Your feelings of peace and relaxation are just right. As you continue with practice, it will expand and progress over time, gradually illuminating your daily activity.

As you move through the lessons, you will learn additional practices that will begin to enliven the ecstatic side of the enlightenment equation. Spinal breathing is next, and, step by step, many other means. The formula is for a blending of inner silence and ecstasy. Meditation is for cultivating inner silence. Many of the other practices are for cultivating ecstatic conductivity in the nervous system.

It is normal to have a few doubts now and then. It is some dust kicking up in the purification process. You can be sure you are on the right track. Just keep going at your own pace. Your inner wisdom is clear and shining through.

The guru is in you.

Lesson 235 – Blending Inner Silence and Ecstasy

Note: This is a continuation of the discussion with the same practitioner in lesson #232.

Q1: I was wondering about something: After about the second week, I stopped having all that sexual energy raging through me when I meditated which I first wrote you about. (This is day 24 for me)

I recently started using a rolled up sock to sit on since I can't get my foot under me. And I haven't noticed any difference in my experience during the spinal breathing or meditation as a result of adding the sock. My meditation is more peaceful now and, as I said, all that surging energy has stopped. My head feels lighter when I meditate and I think it's deeper now. But is the decline of energy rushes something to be expected?

After I read lesson #75 (on siddhasana), I expected that "bucking bronco" which is what I experienced the first week or two to repeat itself but it didn't. I'm not complaining. Believe me, I'm glad that has stopped. It was somewhat overwhelming. But I just wanted to check on this. Do most people who first experience the "bucking bronco" also have it calm down and stop after a while?

My other question is that sometimes my meditation gets so still and quiet, that I realize after some moments that I have forgotten to repeat the *I AM* mantra. There are no thoughts coming in. I am just blank and enjoying the stillness. Should I not worry about it when this happens and just allow myself to be blank and enjoy that stillness or go back to the mantra?

And lastly, sometimes when I go to bed, if I don't take something to help me sleep, my body, mainly in my head, seems to be vibrating. It's like a low energy current going through my head. Sometimes I see flashes of color (eyes closed) but mainly it's just a feeling like I'm buzzing. Is this one of the chakras trying to open?

A1: So many energy experiences are due to what I call "friction" in the nervous system – energy passing through partially loosened obstructions. This can give the impression of a lot happening (erotic feelings, heat, vibration, physical movements, mood swings, etc.). Once the obstructions have been cleared out somewhat, then the experience can be much smoother and blissful. Same energy – less friction. I mentioned early on that experiences would change. That is the reason – changing patterns of obstructions in the nervous system as they are loosened and dissolved. This does not mean you are on the verge of total purification (though we'd all welcome it) – just that there is more clarity at the moment. You are seeing between the slowly dissolving clouds. It will change again.

As for siddhasana, if there is no bucking bronco, that is okay. Look for pleasant sexual stimulation in the way you do siddhasana. Not to overdo or anything. But it is a tantric practice, you know, the essence of which is preorgasmic stimulation. That, combined with inner silence, is the enlightenment formula. It takes time to cultivate the appropriate blend. Make sure to check out tantra lessons #T16 and #T28. Both provide additional perspective on siddhasana. It is pretty advanced stuff, so don't expect to have it all pulled together in a month. It will take time. You will get there. Everyone will. It is written in our genes.

Quiet meditations are nice. When you realize you have been off the mantra, just ease back to it in a very refined way at whatever level of thinking (or non-thinking) you are in. Don't pull it all the way back out to a clear pronunciation. It can be a very faint feeling of the mantra, and then you are gone into blissful silent awareness again. That is right practice. It is correct use of the mantra that got us there, and it is continued correct use of the mantra that takes us even deeper. Then our whole nervous system is infused with blissful inner silence when we go out into activity. That is why we meditate.

On sleep, make sure you are meditating before dinner and having some good mental and/or physical activity between dinner and bedtime. That way, releases in meditation will be least likely to interfere with sleep. If you were inclined toward those energy experiences in sleep anyway, before beginning meditation, then some other measures may be necessary, like the pills. If you work the energy out before bed with more activity, that could help. Over time in yoga, there will be less inner "friction" in sleep also, and in all of life.

If the inner energy movements become excessive in sleep, or at any other time, and seem related to practices, then it is time to think about self-pacing – scaling back in practices a bit until things calm down.

Q2: Before reading the lessons (tantra #T16 and #T28) you referred me to, in my next meditation, I sat on my rolled up sock during my breathing and meditation again. During my meditation, I felt the need to move one of my crossed legs and not finding a comfortable position for it, I put it up on top of my crossed thigh near my body. This resulted in more weight going down on the ball, pressing it harder against that area. Soon my body started to gently rock back and forth, forward and back, a little. This created a preorgasmic sensation. I found it pleasurable and a little frustrating because of wanting to achieve orgasm. But the main thing is even though I was thinking *I AM* my attention was more on the sexual stimulation than on the mantra. It was almost laughable. My body is thinking of satisfying this sexual pleasure and my mind is shouting *I AM*.

So now my question: Should I encourage the rocking to stimulate the sexual feelings? I had the impression that just sitting still it should happen.

A2: Ah, the bucking bronco!

It is suggested you keep it at a level of stimulation that does not disrupt your meditation too much. That means staying pretty still with moderate pressure. Later on the energy can be increased as conductivity rises in the nervous system, so it will not be so frustrating. It is an evolution that takes months, or even years. In the meantime, just keep it near simmering without too much distraction.

If it is too much of a distraction in meditation, you can use siddhasana more in spinal breathing where energy distractions are not so critical, and then leave (or reduce) siddhasana during meditation. You will find your balance, as long as you remain clear about the principle involved – inner silence balanced and blending with ecstatic energy.

Once you get to be an old hand at siddhasana, you will be able to sit is total stimulation with no sexual frustration at all. Just a fountain of ecstasy flowing upward through your nervous system, cascading through endless realms of unbounded inner silence! That is the fruit of siddhasana, and why it is such an important tantric practice. It enables us to transform sexual energy to unending divine ecstasy. All of the tantric practices are for this. Siddhasana happens to be one that can be done daily in our scheduled practices. That kind of consistency in practice is not possible in sexual relations, though plenty can be done with tantric methods when sexual relations do occur. See the rest of the tantra lessons on that.

Over time, as we cultivate the transformation in sitting practices, we find the experience of ecstatic bliss coming up naturally from within throughout the day. Our view of life expands infinitely as this happens, and we find ourselves in a position to joyously give much to those around us. This is what we mean by "ecstatic living."

The guru is in you.

Note: Over time, our daily life becomes an undulating sea of shimmering ecstatic stillness. That is what we are, and that is what we share… Enjoy!

The Tantra Lessons

Lesson T1 – What is Tantra Yoga?

It is funny, you know, how a perception has crystallized as tantra yoga has crept toward the mainstream of our modern society. The common perception for most these days is that tantra is about sex – better sex, more ecstatic sex, more "spiritual sex." So the call of tantra has become, "Sex, sex, sex!" Do we have one-track minds, or what? It is natural enough. For most of us, the peak experience of our life is found in the sex act, particularly in the overwhelming pleasure of orgasm. So it is no surprise that we are a culture obsessed with sex – usually for it, sometimes against it, and always in awe of it. We all know that sex somehow connects us with a greater dimension of what we are. It is a fact that sex binds us together in love, family, and ultimately our spiritual life. So, of course we are obsessed with sex. It lies at the root of everything we are. It defines us. A deep desire we all have is to merge permanently with the ecstasy contained in this thing called "sex."

To unravel the ultimate mystery of sex, we will be wise to take a broad view of it. This is where tantra comes in.

What if I told you that tantra is mainly about meditation, pranayama, bandhas, mudras and asanas? All the things we have been talking about in Advanced Yoga Practices. It is true that tantra is mainly about those things. Yes, it is about sex too, as we have been facing up to in the main lessons since early on. We have not skirted the issue of sex as it relates to the overall enlightenment process. Indeed, enlightenment is not possible if our sexuality is not brought into the process of yoga – the process of union between our inner divine self and the outer world. In cultivating our nervous system toward that, the role of sexual energy must be addressed.

Tantra means "woven together," or "two fullnesses as one." It means the same as yoga really, with some intimacy added. Tantra recognizes from the start that there are two poles to be ecstatically merged for enlightenment to occur – Father heaven and Mother earth, masculine and feminine energies, Shiva and Shakti, yin and yang – and that these two poles are contained in us, in our nervous system. We have already discussed this from various practical angles in the main lessons.

Tantra yoga is the broadest of all the yoga systems that approach life as two realities to be joined in the human nervous system. Included within tantra yoga are mantra yoga, kundalini yoga, hatha yoga, ashtanga (eight-limbed) yoga, and others. The practices contained in these traditional yoga systems comprise what is called the "right-handed" side of tantra yoga. Then there is the "left-handed" side of tantra yoga, which is concerned with infusing pure bliss consciousness into the indulgences of sensual life in the material world. The left-handed side is not opposed to sensual indulgences. In fact, it takes advantage of them for spiritual purposes. The left-handed side is sort of the underbelly of yoga, the part that upstanding citizens are supposed to stay away from. That is the traditional view anyway. That was before the "hip generation" got a hold of tantra. Now it is respectable to practice left-handed tantra. At least in the West it is. Maybe Westerners don't have anything to lose, being so immersed in material living to begin with. Why not bring the spiritual side into material living? Let's have our cake and eat it too. It's got left-handed tantra written all over it.

So, in the tantra lessons we will take a closer look at left-handed tantra as it pertains to sexual methods. What you will find is that we will be connecting with things we have already discussed in the main lessons. We have done a full work-up on kundalini ("a code word for sex") over there, and begun stimulating sexual energy upward into the nervous system with important advanced yoga practices such as mulabandha, sambhavi, siddhasana, yoni mudra kumbhaka, nauli, kechari and bastrika. All of these have been worked into the twice-daily routine of practices to be undertaken in steps according to our capacity.

Everything we have done so far as been from the root on up, above siddhasana, which is systematic stimulation at the perineum. Now, we are going to go below siddhasana, so to speak. It is necessary. For if we do not get a handle on the huge flows of prana involved in the sex act, we may find that we are limited in what we can accomplish spiritually in our nervous system. This does not mean we have to entertain the dreaded "C" word (celibacy). It does mean we will consider some intelligent methods to bring our sexual activities more in line with our spiritual aspirations. In fact, you may be surprised to find that intelligent spiritual sex can be far more enjoyable than the run-of-the-mill kind of sex which is sometimes characterized by the words, "Wham, bam, thank you Ma'am."

So, let's get into it.

The guru is in you.

Lesson T2 – Meditation, Bhakti and Tantric Sex

It was not an arbitrary choice that way back in the beginning of the main lessons we started out discussing desire and meditation. We got our desire focused enough to get started meditating. The process of diving deep into pure bliss consciousness in meditation brings up silent awareness and an instinctive recognition in our nervous system. This recognition resonates with more yogic knowledge we encounter, and then we have more desire for the divine, which leads us to more practices. This rising desire for divine experience is called "bhakti." Bhakti is a product of our desire, combined with purification occurring in our nervous system. And it is intentional on our part – we enter into the divine desire by our own choice. With daily practices, bhakti goes up like a spiral, spurring us onward into ever-higher levels of yoga practice and divine experience.

What has this got to do with considering tantric sex?

For starters, if we approach so-called tantric sex looking just for better sex, under the best of circumstances that is about all we will get, some better sex. A short-lived victory. If we come to tantric sex on waves of bhakti spawned by our daily routine of advanced yoga practices, then it will be a completely different ball game. Then we will become filled with permanent divine ecstasy. So, the first recommendation regarding tantric sex is to put a strong foundation of daily meditation, pranayama and other advanced yoga practices underneath. Then tantric sex will come naturally, and have real spiritual potential, even before we start doing it.

It was the same thing when we started taking on advanced yoga practices such as mulabandha and siddhasana, both for the purpose of stimulating sexual energy upward into our nervous system. Had we done mulabandha and siddhasana first, before meditation and pranayama, we'd be trying to send energy up through mostly clogged pipes, so to speak, with limited potential for a successful outcome. Better to do some house cleaning first, and continue it daily as we begin to move sexual energy upward into the higher realms of our nervous system. The same thing applies in beginning tantric sex.

How will we know if we are ready for tantric sexual techniques? It is easy enough. We will want to do something regenerative with our sex life. It will become important to us. The more we want it the better it will be. The level of bhakti in us is easy to feel, and easy for others to notice as well. It comes as the nervous system purifies itself as a result of advanced yoga practices. It is a kind of magnetism that rises calling us toward more. It takes a strong call to get us into a new spiritually oriented mode of sexual activity, because we have to do something radical. It takes a radical desire to undertake tantric sex. We are embarking on a journey to alter the course of a mighty river. In tantric sex, we are learning to engage in sex for the purpose of cultivating sexual energy upward, and putting our deeply ingrained obsession for orgasm second. Spiritual cultivation of sexual energy first, orgasm second. A big shift in our aspirations. If our bhakti is strong, we will be able to expand our sexual functioning to a cultivating mode, just as we train our arousal brought up in siddhasana to a much higher function over time. It is like that in tantric sex – a gradual training over a long period of time. Tantric sex is not an overnight accomplishment. It is an evolution over time – over many months and years. As our bhakti strengthens it will happen, because it must to fulfill our journey to enlightenment.

The sexual journey through yoga will not be the same for everyone. It will be as different for each of us as our sexual inclinations are.

For those who are light to moderate in their sex life, there is not a great necessity to introduce yogic methods into sexual relations, though learning tantric sex certainly will enhance lovemaking, and the rest of advanced yoga practices as well. Occasional sex is not much of a deterrent to enlightenment. The traditional methods of yoga (right-handed tantra) discussed in the main lessons will be more than enough to get the job done.

For those who are very active in sex, it is a different story. Though the storehouse of prana in the pelvis is huge, there is a limit to how much one can expel and still be spiritually vibrant. This is especially true for men, where large quantities of prana are released during orgasm with the ejaculation of semen. It is somewhat true for women also, but not anywhere near to the same degree. It is the man who holds the keys to tantric sex, for it is he who experiences the greatest loss of prana during orgasm. Because of this, it is also he who determines the duration of the sexual joining, and, therefore, the extent of cultivation of sexual energy that can occur during lovemaking. While a woman may be filled with bhakti to bring sexual energy higher and higher in herself and her partner, it is the man's bhakti that will determine to what extent this can be accomplished in sexual union. So the roles of a man and woman in tantric sex are somewhat different. Yet, in another way, their roles are the same. For tantric sex to occur, both the man and the woman must be involved in the intelligent management of the man's ejaculation. This is true in the beginning stages of learning tantric sex, and remains true for some time.

In time, and with practice, the man becomes the master of his semen and is no longer dependent on help from his partner to control his ejaculation. When this level of proficiency has been reached, both partners are free to cultivate sexual energy virtually indefinitely – the equivalent of an ongoing super siddhasana, if you will. We have all seen Asian visual art of tantric lovers in union playing musical instruments, reading poetry, meditating, or joined in long loving conversation. This is not usually what we think of in the West as sex, or even tantric sex. Nevertheless, this is what real tantric sex is – long preorgasmic cultivation of sexual energy in lovemaking.

It is important to mention a couple of things.

First, tantric sex does not make a good end in itself. It does not stand alone as yoga practice. By itself, tantric sex is a weak practice for globally purifying the nervous system. Meditation and pranayama are the primary tools for this. Once some purification is coming up, traditional bandhas and mudras, siddhasana and kumbhaka are very useful for stimulating sexual energy upward. This leads to a rise of ecstatic conductivity in the sushumna (spinal nerve) and the thousands of nerves in the body. Tantric sex can play a role in this, especially for sexually active yogis and yoginis. Tantric sex is not something we do to get ourselves to be more sexually active. It is something we can do to improve our yoga if we are already sexually active. So, this discussion is not for the purpose of calling everyone to have more sex in a tantric mode. If you are light to moderate in sex and happy in your advanced yoga practices, you are in very good shape. Don't dive into sexual escapades for the sake of these lessons. These lessons on tantric sex are for people who are sexually active already and are seeking ways to bring their sexual activity into the overall spectrum of their yoga practice.

Second, it may seem like a bad idea to some that we are leaving orgasm somewhat on the back shelf while we develop the ability to cultivate sexual energy endlessly upward. It might seem like we are throwing the baby out with the bath water here. After all, orgasm is the deepest pleasure we have known in our life. This is a normal and valid concern, and we are right to ask,

"What about orgasm? What happens to it?"

These lessons are not anti-orgasm. In fact, the path of Advanced Yoga Practices is a path of pleasure, a path of ecstasy. Orgasm is an ecstatic response in the body that is elicited by a particular type of stimulation – sexual stimulation that is biologically oriented toward reproduction. The condition in the nervous system that we call "enlightenment" is also an ecstatic response in the body that is elicited by a particular type of stimulation – stimulation by advanced yoga practices that is biologically oriented toward the birth of our awareness in unending pure bliss consciousness and divine ecstasy.

Is enlightenment at the expense of orgasm? No, enlightenment is a flowering of orgasm, an expansion of orgasm into endless full bloom in the whole body.

Ramakrishna said that divine ecstasy is like innumerable yonis (female sex organs) in continual orgasm in every atom and pore of our body.

So, while in the beginning it might seem like we are putting something important on the back shelf, what we are really doing in Advanced Yoga Practices is gradually expanding our orgasmic response into the cosmic realms through our purifying and opening nervous system. There we find ecstasy to be unbounded in magnitude and duration. It is only a matter of cultivating our nervous system to reveal what is already there inside us.

It is through our desire that all this is accomplished. Each day we choose our path anew.

Okay, let's get into the specifics of the practices of tantric sex.

The guru is in you.

Lesson T4 – The Holdback Method – A Stairway to Heaven

What is perfect lovemaking? Is there such a thing? It is like asking, "What is enlightenment?" Maybe they are the same thing. Whatever they may be in the end, we have to begin from where we are. There is a process we can undertake, a journey. If we believe there is something more, we can begin from where we are and move forward. It takes a continuous desire to make the journey.

There are so many factors in sexual relations. Compatibility is a big one. Do we get along? Are we "good in bed" together? There are many nuances of personal preference and style that we are seeking to match up to our liking. Am I attractive? Is he/she attractive? Is the flirting right? Is the foreplay good? Is the place of lovemaking suitable – the bedroom, the basement, the kitchen table?

In these lessons we will not focus much on these things. They are important for sure. But what we want to focus on here is the act itself. Specifically, how prana (sexual energy) is affected during sexual stimulation, and what we can do to bring that stimulation into the realm of yoga practice. Obviously, an important part of this is answering the question, "What do I want from sex?" If the answer is, "Something more than genital orgasm," then we are ready to begin experimenting with tantric sex methods.

The methods are pretty simple. It is about managing sexual stimulation and orgasm. And it is about male plumbing (piping). Very mundane stuff when you think about it. But we bring so much baggage to bed with us, you know – our obsessions about sex. And that can make it a bit complicated. But it doesn't have to be complicated.

We have obsessions, strong emotional attachments relating to sex. Let's remind ourselves that we are coming to the bed for a higher purpose in lovemaking, and let's use bhakti to direct our sexual obsessions to that. A little bhakti can go a long way.

An important part of this higher purpose is to remember that tantric sex is about our partner's needs. If both partners take this to heart, then there will be great success in tantric sex, or any sex, or any relationship. It is like a Buddhist koan, an unsolvable riddle. If both partners are looking to serve the other, who is being served? If personal need has been transcended, whose need is being filled?

Of course, serving our partner 100% is an ideal, a goal to be gradually fulfilled over a long time. Let your attention come to it easily from time to time as you are making love. It will make a difference. If you are coming to tantric sex sincerely, you probably had this in mind already – that it is about honoring and filling your partner with divine ecstasy. So, take this as a confirmation of what you already instinctively know. Tantric sex is about your partner. Of course, both partners will not always have equal concern for each other. That is okay. Giving does not require a response in kind. Lovemaking is not a business transaction. Lovemaking is making "love." We make love by giving, by doing for someone other than ourselves, not expecting a return for it. This is what love is. It is not necessarily about making a lifetime commitment. It is not about the future or the past. It is just about serving in this very moment.

Sometimes making love means saying, "no." Loving is not rolling over for every desire our partner may have, particularly a desire that is destructive. Under these circumstances, saying, "no" is loving too. Love isn't a pushover. Love is wise. Love is strong. Love radiates peace and light to all of life. This is an important part of what we want to cultivate in tantric sex. It will happen naturally as we progress.

So these are the foundation blocks: Understanding that tantric sex is about cultivating sexual energy upward in our nervous system, that advanced yoga practices provide the prerequisite purification in our nervous system, that we are looking for more than genital orgasm, and that we are there for our partner.

Now let's talk about the holdback method.

In these lessons, we will refer to the male organ as the "lingam" and the female organ as the "yoni." These are the traditional Sanskrit names used in tantra for the masculine and feminine organs of regeneration, covering the full scope of ecstatic union from the physical to the highest spiritual.

The holdback method is most easily done with the man on top and the woman on the bottom. It can be done in other positions also once the partners become familiar with the principles. It is the most difficult to do with the woman on top, as will be come evident.

When a man and woman are in lovemaking, the holdback method involves just what it says — holding back. It is done by the man. It is done before his orgasm, preferably not too close to his orgasm. The idea is not to get to the edge of orgasm and then hold back. It can be too late then, and then the man is out of business until next time. No doubt it will happen that way sometimes, and that is okay. We will discuss another method in the next lesson to help with that. For now, let's continue with the holdback method.

Intercourse is simulative stroking, yes? This is the natural way it goes until the man has orgasm. Maybe the woman has orgasm first, maybe not. But when the man has orgasm it is over, at least for a while. He may come back soon in a semi-recovered state to try and satisfy his lover, and then maybe lose more semen. She may find some satisfaction, but he has paid a high price, pranically speaking. If this goes on daily for a long time, the man's progress in yoga practices will suffer. The woman's progress in yoga won't be helped much either. If it happens only once a week, or less often, it is not such a big deal. But even those who have sex only occasionally can find their yoga progress improved by knowing the methods of tantric sex.

Mastery of the holdback method changes the dynamic of this old style of sex, introducing a new dynamic with many benefits.

In the holdback method, the lingam enters the yoni for a number of strokes and then pulls out and lingers around the opening of the yoni. How many strokes is up to the man, but well short of orgasm is recommended. This is supposed to be a long lovemaking, so holding back sooner rather than later is best in the beginning, as this is when the staying power will be least in most men. A few things are going on when the lingam is in holdback mode. First, the staying power of the man in front of orgasm is being strengthened, recharging to a higher level of staying power than before the previous entry into the yoni. Second, the woman is in anticipation, and this is sexually exciting for her. She does not know when the lingam is coming back into her, and this anticipation will increase her arousal. To add to the woman's anticipation and excitement, the man may do a little teasing with the tip of his lingam, without risking his own orgasm. He may enter the yoni just a little bit and then pull back out. Or he may not touch the yoni at all with his lingam, and then all of a sudden when she least expects it ... Well, use your imagination. An accomplished tantric man won't use the same pattern of stroking and lingering twice in a row. There are lots of ways to play the game.

I won't tell you how to play the game. It is the principles of practice we are after that tap into the natural ability of the nervous system to bring ecstatic energy ever higher in the body.

The important thing in using the holdback method is for the man to pull out in time and give himself adequate time to recharge and increase his staying power. In the beginning this means relaxing outside the yoni for a while and not rushing back in as soon as the lingam has been out for a few seconds. In the beginning, it is all about building up staying power in the man, and this is done by stroking inside preorgasmically and stopping outside, over and over again. This practice can immediately level the playing field between the man and woman in sexual relations.

Everyone knows that the woman is superior to the man in the sex act, and in other things as well. Nature has built her to be biologically superior in sexual relations. The survival of the human race depends on it. She will have the semen no matter what. She does not even have to try. Her beauty calls the semen from the man on sight. Her curves, her lips, her eyes, all call the semen out.

Hundreds of years ago the great reviver of yoga in India, Shankara, said, "Even the greatest yogi cannot gaze into the eyes of a beautiful woman without having his seed jump."

With a knowledge of the holdback method we can balance sexual relations to the benefit of both the man and the woman. Over time, the man's staying power becomes very great, even from the beginning of a lovemaking session. A change occurs gradually in his sexual biology as a result of using the holdback method. This brings freedom to both partners in lovemaking, and solves the challenge of sex that Shankara pointed out.

As we progress with the holdback method we discover that we are on a new path in our sexual relations. It involves longer sex, which is a boon to both the man and the woman. But with the holdback method we get much more then length. We get height, which is the greatest payoff.

What do we mean by height? As the man goes through the cycles of stroking and holding back, a stairway of rising ecstasy is being climbed. Of course, the woman is not inert in this process. She is active every step of the way – coaxing her man when he is in her, and becoming more aroused with anticipation each time he lingers near her entrance. There is stimulation, and then pause, more stimulation and then pause, and so on. With each cycle the pleasure rises. The essences of love, sexual energy, rise to permeate the bodies of the two in lovemaking. Together they go up the stairs of ecstasy being created by the repeating cycles of stimulation and pauses. It is a stairway to heaven.

The holdback method is also called the "valley orgasm" method. The partners go up the side of the mountain of stimulation toward genital orgasm. Then they pause before they get there and slowly dip into a valley of pleasure higher than where they started. Then they go up with stimulation toward genital orgasm again, stopping before they get there, and dip back into a valley of pleasure again, this one higher than the first. And then they do it again, and again, and again. The mountains and valleys get higher and higher. In the end, the lovers are permeated with sexual essences, gone into a bliss state akin to deep meditation.

This is how sexual relations are turned into yoga practice.

So, that is an overview of the holdback method. This is not a practice you are supposed to do for so many minutes twice a day. It is for doing in your normal love life, whatever that may be. Maybe sex is not of much interest to you. Then you won't need any of this. It is here for those who need it, and not here to promote more sex. What we want to promote is more advanced yoga practices. Tantric sex is only one aspect of a growing array of tools we have to purify and open our nervous system to higher experiences of the divine within us.

Next we will talk about getting a better handle on male orgasm. It is not likely that knowing the holdback method alone will be enough for all men to stay in front of orgasm right from the beginning, even with a great desire to do it. It is not an easy thing to master. It takes some special self-training.

So, more help is on the way for that.

The guru is in you.

Lesson T5 – Blocking Male Ejaculation – Putting on the Training Wheels

In the last lesson we talked about the holdback method. It is pretty straightforward. There is only one catch to it. Many men have little or no control over their orgasm. And in the heat of the moment they don't want any control. The semen wants to go, and that is it. Sex is a mad dash for that, and everything else tends to fall by the wayside.

So, how do we get around this? The key is in altering the habit of the inner neurology of orgasm. We do this by giving the male neurology a familiarity with a different way of traveling the road of stimulation. In doing so, we find a different experience of pleasure, and the experience of divine ecstasy coming up through the nervous system. In time, divine ecstasy becomes more charming than the jerking and lurching of genital orgasm, and we become motivated to spend more time in the habit of preorgasmic stimulation. We then have the choice – preorgasmic tantric sex or genital orgasm. Maybe in a single session we'd like to have both, beginning with a long session of the former and finally ending with the latter. Once in a while, why not? That is having the cake and eating it too. Of course, be doing that too often (like more than every week or two) and the cake will be eating up your yoga.

In principle, the holdback method alone can provide the necessary training for the man. We will talk about the woman's evolving role in tantric sex in the next lesson. She is very important, obviously. But first, we have to deliver her a motivated tantric man. Without that, there won't be much tantric sex going on. That is why we are focusing on the man first.

Is the holdback method enough for training the man's orgasmic response? Maybe for some it is, especially if they are experienced and have been working seriously on extending their orgasm already. But for many, the holdback method will not be enough.

We will now talk about blocking male ejaculation. It is an ancient tantric method with a long history of success. It is simple enough to do.

When orgasm is about to come on, the man puts one or two fingers (usually index and/or middle finger) at the perineum, presses inward and forward against the back of the pubic bone, and blocks the urethra channel that the semen is about to come through. The orgasm still occurs, but the semen is blocked from leaving the body. If the man lets go too soon, the semen can still escape. If he holds the block for a minute or two and then let's go, the semen will be reabsorbed and none will escape.

Blocking can be done by reaching to the perineum from either the front or the back. In tantric lovemaking with a partner, the man can reach from the back and block his ejaculation if he has slipped and gone too far with stimulation. He still has orgasm and will be done with sex for a while, but he has blocked the loss of semen from his orgasm.

Beyond the mechanics of stopping the exit of semen from the body, the blocking method has several other aspects related to training the orgasmic response of the man.

First, having an orgasm with the ejaculation blocked is initially not nearly as pleasurable as having one with a free flow of semen. If a man's bhakti brings him to engage in blocking most of his ejaculations, then there will also be a gradual shift in his motivation from wanting to go to orgasm to wanting to stay in front of it. So, blocking, besides stopping semen from leaving, provides an incentive for a man to stay in front of orgasm. Why go there if it is going to be less pleasurable than continuing in preorgasmic sex and climbing that stairway to heaven with our lover?

Second, given what has just been said, blocking is not something that will be needed forever. It is a voluntary, temporary measure, like having training wheels on a bicycle. Aren't you glad to hear that? Bicycles with training wheels are not much fun at all. We want to get them off as soon as possible. So, we have an additional incentive to train our orgasmic response, and reduce our reliance on the training wheels. Once we learn to stay in preorgasmic in sex for long periods, we won't need blocking very often. By the time we get to that stage, having genital orgasm may be part of sex only after an hour or two in union, or maybe we will forget about it completely.

Forget about orgasm? Yes, the experiences in long tantric sex can become so profound that we can forget about orgasm completely. Hard to believe, but it is true. Tantric sex can be that good. And it is good advanced yoga practice too! Over time, the importance of the genital orgasm will fade to the background. We can still have it if we want it, but it will become less attractive as our divine ecstasy expands beyond it. Sex will still be good, but in a different way. Sex will become an expression of our overall rising enlightenment, rather than the obsessive needful thing it has been in the past.

Now we should talk about male masturbation.

It was mentioned that blocking can be done from the front or the back. If a man is masturbating, the blocking can come in from the front. Given the fact that the total semen expelled in masturbation in the lifetime of an average man exceeds the amount expelled in lovemaking many-fold, we should really talk about it.

Masturbation is the greatest expeller of semen for many men. Masturbation also happens to be an advantageous time to be training the male orgasm. It is a good time to practice the equivalent of the holdback method, holding back before orgasm over and over again, and permanently building the staying power to a high level. It is also a good time to practice blocking when orgasm comes. So, all the elements are there. Stimulation, pauses, and blocking as necessary. Only the partner is missing. Interestingly, this is not far from what we are doing in the traditional methods of mulabandha, siddhasana and other advanced yoga practices – stimulating our sexual energy systematically up through our nervous system.

So, is tantric masturbation a kind of yoga practice? Yes, it can be as long as it remains preorgasmic. It is also an ideal self-training ground for a man to prepare for tantric sex with a partner.

None of this is to promote excessive sexual activity, or more masturbation than is already going on. It is just to add an awareness of tantric methods that can be incorporated into what we are already doing in our sex life. If we do so intelligently, dramatic changes in our experience of sex can be achieved, and our overall advanced yoga practices will be enhanced significantly.

The guru is in you.

Lesson T7 – The Woman's Role – Nothing Less Than "Divine Goddess"

Now that we have given the man the primary tools that will enable him to work toward having a strong role in tantric sexual relations, let's talk about the role of the woman.

The woman is everything in tantric sex, and in all of life. She is the divine goddess. Everything we see and everything we do is born of the divine feminine. That is why, in this world, she is called "Mother Nature." It is the divine feminine that attracts the masculine seed of pure bliss consciousness and manifests all. The cosmos and everything in it is born from Her.

When a man and woman engage in sexual relations, it is a microcosm of this great divine process. In tantric sex involving accomplished partners, it begins as a microcosm and rises toward the cosmic joining of the masculine seed and feminine womb. This joining occurs in both the man and the woman. This expanding ecstatic event fulfills itself inside each of the partners as they engage in tantric sex together, and also as each does their sitting advanced yoga practices in their meditation room. This joining of masculine and feminine energies occurs in many ways. It threads its way through all of our advanced yoga practices – meditation, spinal breathing, bandhas, mudras, asanas and so on. Everything in yoga is about this spiritual joining that occurs on every level in the nervous system.

So, when a man and woman come together in tantric sex, this is the beginning of something much bigger in both of them, reaching far beyond the bodies present on the bed. The man's role is seed, whether he is giving it physically or not. If he does not give it physically, it is cultivated up in both partners spiritually.

The woman's role is divine goddess, the flower garden of bliss. She calls the seed from the man. If it does not come physically, it comes up and fertilizes from within both partners spiritually. The more she calls, the more the fertilizing will happen. If not physically, then spiritually. She is the inspiration of both physical and spiritual fertilization. This is the essence of the woman's role in tantric sex. She is the temptress of the physical seed, and the temptress of the spiritual seed. If the physical seed does not come, the spiritual seed will. Her lovely divine bliss and waves of beauty will bring the seed out. If the man is able to hold the physical seed back, then the spiritual seed rises in both the man and the woman, and this is the internal joining of masculine and feminine energies in both tantric partners.

Tantric sex is about that – about stimulating the internal divine union in both partners. It is the same purpose that is found in all advanced yoga practices. If both partners in tantric sex have been doing advanced yoga practices daily on their own, then there will be much purification in their nervous systems already, and tantric sex will be much more effective. The sexual essences will rise and penetrate their nervous systems deeply, and the experience will be like the deepest meditation, rich in pure silence, ecstatic bliss and overflowing with love. This will carry over into daily activity and the regular routine of spiritual practices. So tantric sex can have this very positive and profound effect in life. For people who are sexually active, this is the beautiful silver lining in the dark cloud that sex can sometimes hang over spiritual life.

It takes discipline to get to such a wonderful stage of lovemaking. We talked about the challenges the man faces in learning to become the master of his semen, and what methods he can use. What can the woman do to help this evolution toward tantric sexual relations?

Obviously, her first responsibility is to understand the process of transformation to tantric sexual relations – understanding that it involves cultivating a change in the man's orgasmic response, and that this is not an overnight change. Her partner may not understand this at the start. She has the ability to educate him. Before a divine goddess will be able to engage in tantric sexual relations she may find herself becoming a teacher, a tantric priestess, if you will. This can be very helpful to a man trying to understand his sexuality. But she can only do so much, for it is he who must take up the challenge. A tantric woman cannot do the holdback method for a man. It won't work if he is not committed to take the lead for the benefit of both partners. If the woman takes the lead in the holdback method, it produces the same kind of escalating arousal in the man that occurs in the woman when the man is in the lead. The holdback method with the woman in the lead is not going to give the man the recharging of his staying power. Just the opposite. But, if a man chooses to take the lead in the holdback method, the woman can help by assisting him in taking the pauses necessary to recharge his staying power. She can refrain from egging him on too much in the sensitive early stages of tantric sex. She can remind him about what they are doing in tantric sex if he is wavering. This requires self-discipline in the woman, because instinctively she wants the semen inside her yoni, just as instinctively he wants to release it in her. If the man is consciously trying to practice the holdback method, the woman can help. In the beginning it will be challenging for both partners, like tiptoeing through a minefield. With persistence and practice by both the man and the woman, the sexual relations can be gradually changed to something much more.

In intimate relations where the woman is present while the man is masturbating, or if she is stimulating his lingam by means other than intercourse, she can help as he cultivates his staying power through cycles of stimulation and pauses. She can also learn to perform the ejaculation blocking method on her partner in such situations, though, if it gets to that point very often, her presence may be providing more stimulation than is necessary for his training purposes. So, there a question whether having the woman present while the man is doing self-training is a good idea. Nevertheless, if it is the nature of the relations between a man and woman to be together intimately like that, then it is certainly good for the woman to know the methods the man is working with, and to help him apply them as much as possible. It is in the best interest of both partners, and yoga, that the man continue improving his staying power, whatever the sexual situation may be. If she is aware of the process, there will always be opportunities for her to help him. This could be as simple as giving him the time necessary to do self-training alone.

So, just as it is a challenging period of adjustment for the man in the beginning stages of tantric sexual relations, it can be challenging for the woman too. While he is working to build staying power in front of orgasm, she may be curbing her natural abilities to draw the semen from him. It is a transition period that both the man and woman will go through – a time of training and readjustment.

As the man gradually comes into his own as the master of his seed, things will change. This is when the woman, our divine goddess, can really shine in all her beauty and glory. Then she can fully bloom as the beautiful lovemaker she is by nature. For when the man can manage his semen, lovemaking becomes an act of sexual equals, rather than the one-way flow of semen from man to woman that was the case before the transition to tantric sexual relations. Once the stage of self-sufficiency of staying power in the man is reached, then cultivation of sexual energy can proceed much more actively, creatively and blissfully.

It should be mentioned that as a man becomes proficient in using the holdback method, it becomes possible for the woman to be stimulated to "multiple orgasms." Having multiple orgasms is a natural capability in the woman. It assures that no matter what happens, she will still be soliciting the semen from her partner, and enjoying every minute of it. Is feminine orgasm a regenerative process, a yogic process, and are multiple orgasms spiritually healthy for women? There is some loss of prana in feminine orgasm, and some loss of ability to climb to successively higher levels of divine ecstasy as a woman has multiple orgasms in tantric sex. Clearly, feminine orgasm is much less of a pranic drain than masculine orgasm is. But are multiple orgasms in the woman part of tantric sex? Perhaps many feminine orgasms will eventually add up to the same pranic loss as one masculine orgasm. Maybe it is a stage the woman must go through when she finds herself with access to unlimited orgasms through the holdback method. Then, perhaps after a period of time, she will settle into preorgasmic sex with her partner with his cooperation and loving help. It is in her best interest spiritually to do so, just as it is the man's best interest to stay in front of his orgasm. So the pendulum can swing back and tantric lovemaking can evolve to become a means for both partners to stay in front of their orgasm, climbing the stairway to heaven together – higher, higher, higher ...

In advanced tantric sex, the woman's role can flower fully to the natural and powerful coaxing of the seed that is her gift in sexual relations. No longer does she have to be so concerned about her partner developing his staying power. He has done it already. Of course, she remains mindful of the principles of tantra, making sure they are being applied. If her partner is in principle, preserving and cultivating sexual energy, the woman can use every means she has to draw the seed out. He will know how to dance with her while preserving the semen within himself. This balance enables the two lovers to dance the night away, climbing the stairway of ecstasy in a delightful and natural fashion. It is all about lovemaking then – tantric lovemaking that leads them higher and higher as the cultivation of sexual essences goes upward within them.

Under these circumstances, the woman may find herself becoming motivated to strengthen her sexual charms with kegal exercises and other means that will enhance her abilities to stimulate her partner in tantric sexual relations. So, for the sexually active woman, enhancing her already formidable sexual capabilities may become more important as she enters into more advanced tantric sexual relations.

On the other hand, for tantric lovers who have been at it a long time, it can take another course. As progress in advanced yoga practices and tantric sexual relations reach maturity, the lovemaking never stops inside the two partners. Then, a glance, a smile, a touch, a kiss, a hug, is all it takes to keep the divine lovemaking moving inside. Then the partners may join in tantric sex only occasionally. Or maybe never. Ramakrishna was a married man, but it is believed he never made love physically to his wife. Instead, they worshipped each other as incarnations of the divine masculine and the divine feminine.

Whatever the style of lovemaking turns out to be in the end, advanced tantric sex is a very free state of relationship that is consistent with the spiritual goals of Advanced Yoga Practices.

Before the state of advanced tantric sexual relations is achieved, there is an imbalance between the man and the woman that exists for the purpose of reproduction and the survival of the species. Before tantra comes in, sex is primordial, concerned only with assuring reproduction. After tantra comes in, sex becomes spiritualized to a higher state that is concerned with both reproduction, and the joining of pure bliss consciousness (the seed) and divine ecstasy (the womb).

The inherent imbalance in non-tantric sexual relations is at the root of the difficulties that have existed in the relationship between men and women for thousands of years. When men feel inferior sexually to woman (which they are before learning tantric methods) they tend to try and compensate by dominating women in other ways – trying to control their huge feminine sexual power. This is one reason why women have been held down in many societies over the centuries. Men harbor a deep subconscious fear of women. Men are not fundamentally to blame for this, and neither are women. It is a phenomenon that has its roots in immature biological and neurological processes. As the processes of the nervous system evolve to a higher level of functioning, more equality in sexual relations arises, and the subconscious fears and aggressions gradually disappear. This will be one of the fringe benefits of this new age of enlightenment – a balancing of the sexual energies that flow between men and women. There will be more honor, more integrity, more respect and much more love. Women will receive much more of the deep reverence they deserve. It is happening already.

Shiva and Shakti are neither superior nor inferior to each other. Both are equal polarities joining everywhere in the great expanse of life reaching from unmanifest pure bliss consciousness to the heights of divine ecstasy throughout creation. Through the union of these two polar energies, the birth of Oneness is occurring in us, and everywhere. When we directly experience the polarity of every atom as an ecstatic union of the omnipresent divine lovers, then we know the truth about life. We know that it is all bliss, all love, all Oneness.

The woman's role in this is on every level of existence – from the beautiful feminine being sitting in front of her man, to the dynamic force of creation constantly coaxing every atom in the cosmos outward in its ongoing existence.

What we see everywhere is the divine goddess at play, and that is the woman's role in tantra.

The guru is in you.

Lesson T9 – The Relationship of Brahmacharya, Tantric Sex and Celibacy

Now we are going to touch on a really taboo subject, and tie it in with the tantra discussion. These days, it is a more taboo subject than sex. It is called, "celibacy."

Don't run screaming for the door yet. Celibacy is not going to be a suggested practice here. It will not be pooh-poohed either. We only want to understand how it fits in, because some people are naturally drawn to it. Others may be forced into it either by self-will or the will of others.

But before we get into celibacy, we should talk about "brahmacharya," because it is the key to understanding the spiritual implications of both tantric sex and celibacy, and what they have in common. They have more in common than is generally believed.

Brahmacharya means to walk or abide in the creative force of God, which is the sexual energy in each of us. What do we mean by walking or abiding in sexual energy? Two things: First, to preserve it. And, second, to cultivate it. This is the essence of brahmacharya – to preserve and cultivate sexual energy.

So far in these lessons on tantra we have introduced the primary methods necessary to undertake a process of transformation in sexual relations to do just that – preserve and cultivate sexual energy. We talked about the prerequisite bhakti (desire for something more) necessary to pursue it, the various challenges involved, and the divine consequences of making the journey of tantric sexual relations. Pretty far reaching stuff.

We mentioned the tie-in between tantric sexual relations and the advanced yoga practices we have been discussing in depth in the main lessons, how both kinds of practices have the same aims, and how tantric sex can compliment meditation, pranayama, and our other daily yoga practices.

Where does celibacy fit in? It is a matter of choice, a matter of inclination, a matter of lifestyle. It happens. Maybe we surrender to a guru or organization and they choose it for us. Maybe we do it on our own. Maybe we are never attracted to it at all. Any of these are okay. It is up to each of us to follow our own feelings about it.

What is celibacy? Technically, it is abstention from marriage and sexual relations, including masturbation. It is defacto preservation of sexual energy, though "preservation" may not be what the celibate has in mind. There are other reasons for celibacy that are more oriented toward going away from something negative about sex (obsession, excess, injury) than going toward something positive about it (inner expansion, divine ecstasy, enlightenment).

Celibacy is the first half of brahmacharya, but not necessarily all of it, because without prerequisite purification of the nervous system and then encouraging sexual energy to move to a higher manifestation, there is no cultivation, which is the second half of brahmacharya. This concept of celibacy being one half of brahmacharya is an important point. Without the second half of brahmacharya, celibacy can lead to stagnation and to the emergence of unbalanced obsessive behaviors, particularly if it is an "enforced" celibacy.

So, while celibacy (preservation) is in the direction of brahmacharya, it is incomplete as a spiritual practice without activating (cultivating) sexual energy for a higher purpose. That, of course, is the purpose of tantric sex. Ironically, those who are diligent in their tantric sexual practices can have better spiritual prospects than celibates who are not diligent in their sitting yoga practices and ongoing loving service to others to cultivate sexual energy to a higher manifestation in their nervous system.

Is celibacy a better path to enlightenment than tantric sexual relations? Who can say? It depends on how motivated a practitioner is in one or the other lifestyle. It is the level of bhakti in the practitioner that determines the outcome more than any particular approach. If bhakti is abundant, the nervous system will continue to open, one way or the other.

For either the tantric lover or the celibate, the core practices of meditation and pranayama will have the greatest influence on the degree of bhakti rising in the nervous system. It is the global purification going on daily in the nervous system that determines how much inner silence will be available. This is pure bliss consciousness, our source, our deepest divine quality rising in us. If we have that, then whether we are inclined to be a tantric lover or a celibate, we will hunger constantly for the same destination, divine union. Whatever our chosen lifestyle may be, we will naturally incorporate the elements of brahmacharya – preserving and cultivating our sexual energy as we travel our inner highway to heaven.

The guru is in you.

Lesson T10 – Sexual Healing

Q: The spiritual aspirations of tantric sex are noble as you describe them, but I find it hard to tackle the problem of developing male "staying power" without more down to earth rewards. If I go through all this will it help my marriage? Specifically, will my wife become more interested in having intimate relations with me?

A: The human race is in quite a fix when it comes to sex. We are the custodians of this great power that has been given to us by God, yet we are still to find the maturity to manage it responsibly. Hence, sex is at the heart of much of the debilitating karma we carry around with us through life after life.

Sex isn't really the problem though. It is the immaturity of our human nervous system. We are an in-between species on the evolutionary scale. In-between the animal kingdoms and the divine being kingdoms. We are a species in transition. This transition is intimately tied in with the knowledge of yoga, the knowledge of human spiritual transformation.

The primordial force of sex rules the planet for the purpose of perpetuating the many species. In the plant and animal kingdoms, it functions with impressive harmony. In the human kingdom, where mind and free will reign along with sex, it is not so harmonious.

What does all this have to do with attracting a member of the opposite sex to the love chamber? Everything!

Sexually speaking, we are a race of the "walking wounded," injured over and over again by the immature processes of interaction between the pleasure-seeking mind and sex. Our sense of self is wrapped up in it, and 99% of it is lodged beneath the surface of our conscious awareness in the so-called subconscious mind. Many of the obstructions we talk about in the main lessons are related to these sexual dislocations that have occurred over the course of many lives. There are other kinds of obstructions, but the obstructions created by sexual misappropriation are a huge influence in all of us, as folks like Sigmund Freud have pointed out.

So we need healing, sexual healing. It comes with daily practice of yoga disciplines for sure. We barely have to think about sex as the housecleaning is going on while doing the "right-handed" disciplines of advanced yoga practices discussed in the main lessons. It is a pretty luxurious approach to cleaning up all the subconscious mess. If you don't need sex, and you have right-handed practices, then you have it made.

For those who need sex, we have the "left-handed" disciplines. That is a different story. It is for couples only, you know. Only the brave need enter here.

How do you tell your wife you are sorry for 100,000 years of abuse? Not that you are directly responsible. But someone has to say, "I'm sorry." It may as well be you. And you need the apology as much as she does. We have all been men and women over innumerable lifetimes. We all have the divine masculine and feminine inside us right now, wounded, divided, asleep, and not comfortable to come to the divine bedchamber everywhere inside us. We are as blocked and dysfunctional in our internal lovemaking as we are in our external lovemaking. The two lovemakings are parallel. If one is healthy, the other will be healthy. Everyone needs an apology for past wrongs. Millions and millions of past wrongs spawned by our rising mental power and immature nervous system. No one is to blame, but we all should be sorry for it, and comfort each other. The hurting will end. We are growing up.

So, begin with soft touching, not for sex, but for consoling eons of hurt, for love. That is a good place to start. Dare to trust your sincere tantric lover. It takes a lot of courage. That can only happen with benign sharing, and caring for the other more than the sexual obsession we have. This is where the tantric methods come in. If a man has become the master of his seed, he will not be nearly so obsessed. He will have time to care about the goddess who loves him and who needs his unconditional love.

Most often it will seem to be she who needs the nurturing. But she is not alone in her need. Men are wounded too. They cover it up, you know. Men are not allowed to feel vulnerable in our society. Any sign of vulnerability is taken as weakness, and then the instinctive protector role of the man is compromised. So both the man and the woman need nurturing. You can count on it. Both need gentle touching. Both need to sleep with someone who has no expectations. Can you do that with your lover – sleep with them with no expectations in the gentle spoon pose? Progress in the tantric sexual methods in these lessons will enable you to do this, and not after draining your vitality first. Rather, you can be together intimately with full sexual vitality, unspent sexually, not expecting anything from your lover. This is the power of tantric sex, the power to be vital with prana, without expectations, able to nurture. It is a higher functioning of the nervous system, and how we will travel beyond the immature expressions of sex.

If we work with the methods and principles, we can get on the road to sexual healing. What is sexual healing? First, it is not creating more injury. That happens as our behaviors toward the opposite sex become more mature – more nurturing. Second, it is releasing the obstructions built up over ages past, and in this lifetime. It all can be let go using the right-handed and left-handed methods of tantra. Once we are underway, and it is clear to both partners what the journey is, it is a new world. Then who will not be attracted to the love chamber?

So you see, there is a down to earth benefit in learning male staying power. It is the first step on a journey of healing – sexual healing. It can dramatically change the quality of a relationship in a short time. Just agreeing to work on it together will be a huge leap forward in the relationship. That is the initial payoff. The long-term payoff is even bigger – unending ecstatic bliss!

An American movie came out a few years ago that is recommended for more perspective on the subject of sexual healing. It is called, "Bliss," with actors Craig Sheffer, Sheryl Lee and Terence Stamp. It is a contemporary story about the relationship of a young married couple. It is entertaining, erotic, and also a serious study of relationships, sexual healing and healing of the psyche. You can probably find it at your local video rental store. It is not everything that we discuss here in Advanced Yoga Practices, but it illustrates very well some of the key points about sexual relations we have covered.

The guru is in you.

Lesson T11 – Blocking and the Evolution of Spiritual Biology

Q: I just have a question on this technique that you posted – blocked ejaculation with the finger will result in a retro-grade ejaculation; the semen goes into the bladder; on urinating it will be found that the urine is whitish, cloudy having mixed with the semen. So if the semen is going to be lost eventually (when one urinates), would this technique preferably be not practised at all, other than as a last resort.

A: Thank you. It is a very good question. The answer has a few parts because the expansion of male (and also female) sexuality upward is an evolutionary process and has different functioning at different stages along the way.

Yes, you are correct, in the beginning much of the semen goes into the bladder during blocking and this can be readily observed during urination, as you mention. But this is only the beginning, at an early stage of the change in sexual functioning.

When added to bhakti (hunger for the divine), blocking produces an incentive to work toward staying in front of orgasm. As things progress, blocking will become less and less needed, like training wheels. It naturally reduces over time. In contrast to training wheels, which we throw away, blocking will always be a good measure of last resort, so we will always have it in our tool kit once it is learned and refined.

By "refined," I am referring to more advanced stages of sexual functioning, where much if not all semen is retained without blocking, even during genital orgasm. So, when we block in this situation, not as much semen will go into the bladder. Much of it will be retained in the seminal vesicles, going upward through other routes in the body. But our goal is not to have genital orgasm without ejaculation. This is extremely difficult to attain, and aiming for it will lead to much loss of semen along the way. It does not help our spiritual evolution anyway. Long preorgasmic cultivation does, and this is what we want. We want to be climbing that stairway to heaven in sexual relations, not seeing how many genital orgasms we can have without ejaculating.

Now, here is the kicker. One of the routes that semen naturally takes going upward in the body is through the bladder. This does not mean we do blocking to put semen in our bladder on purpose. This will not help us, as the bladder has to rise in its higher spiritual functioning first. As it does, gradually over time, the semen goes up into the bladder automatically, with no blocking, and even without deliberate cultivation of sexual energy. See how tricky the biological change is? Advanced yogis are always having semen rising up through their body, and they always have it coming up through their bladder, though not in the quantities you are referring to that occur in the beginning blocking stage.

Fortunately, all this is not so tricky for us to worry about in practices, because the biology will change automatically as we do advanced yoga practices, including tantric sex if we are in sexual relations.

So, blocking starts out pretty clunky (you've heard me say that before about other practices, right?), and refines over time. The refinement is in two areas: First, as we find ourselves increasing in ability to stay in front of orgasm, the need for blocking becomes less and less. Second, when we do block, there will be less and less to block over time because there is more control over ejaculation as our sexual functioning evolves.

Interestingly, there is an analogous process that goes on in a woman, though till now it has not been nearly so obvious as in a man. A woman has the equivalent of a prostate located just in front of the inside of her yoni. It is stimulated though the so-called "G-spot." This gland releases a milky substance similar to semen during extreme arousal, and it can be ejaculated through the urethra. "Female ejaculation" has become a hot topic in recent years, a rite of passage for many women as sexual freedom is being claimed. What its role is in reproduction is hard to say. The reason it is mentioned here is because it appears that a woman has similar spiritual biology going on in the bladder that a man does. And, though it is unlikely that a woman will need to engage in blocking like a man does, the same biological components are there. Of course, the woman also has other sexual components that are part of the spiritual functioning of sex, so we can't carry the comparison too far. Vive la difference!

In both the sexes, an accelerated spiritual evolution comes with advanced yoga practices, with various stages along the way.

The guru is in you.

Lesson T12 – Wet Dreams and Premature Ejaculation

Q: I was reading through the messages and I've a question. This is regarding how one can control the sub-conscious mind into not having "wet-dreams." Most of my friends admit to having experienced such incidents. But some of my friends – whom I consider to be spiritually more "pure" – seem to never have experienced this. I personally see this as a lack of control of emotions and thoughts. Can you comment on this please?

A: Wet dreams are usually the product of immature erotic sensitivities, and are a cousin of premature ejaculation. These tendencies are both mental and physical, with mind and body being closely connected.

On the mental side, if we meditate daily we will find inner silence coming up and we will find gradually more awareness in waking, dreaming and deep sleep states. We will "witness" them more from deep within our silent Self. In time, we will know we are dreaming and be less inclined to occurrences like wet dreams. Perhaps this is what you notice in your more spiritually attuned friends. They are more aware and not so prone to the flights of their dreams.

Developing inner silence is the key from the mental point of view, and this comes from more purification deep in the nervous system, primarily through meditation. Some people are born with more inner purification than others, having done spiritual practices in previous lives. We can all become more pure and aware by doing them in this life.

On the physical side, we can develop more staying power in front of orgasm using the tools in these lessons. This can be done either alone or with a partner. As we develop more control of our sexual functioning this will improve the situation of both wet dreams and premature ejaculation. Of course, accomplishing this will give us rising confidence and benefit us mentally and emotionally as well.

It is just a matter of conscious development, moving beyond natural immaturity in our nervous system to natural maturity. A combination of advanced yoga practices from the main lessons and these tantric sexual methods can bring many benefits.

The guru is in you.

Lesson T13* – Energy Rushing up the Spine During Urination

Q: Whenever I urinate I get a strong energy rush up my spine and into my head. Is this something that you are familiar with? Why is this related to urinating? It's been going on for months. It doesn't bother me in any way. It is kind of amusing. Just wondering if you have heard of such a thing.

A: It is a good thing. The energy going up the spine during urination is the beginning of kundalini sensitivity – ecstatic conductivity. As spiritual sensitivity rises, this can be experienced by both men and women, though having it during urination is not an absolute prerequisite for the rise of broad-based ecstatic kundalini experiences.

When the time is ripe, the energy going up the spine may be felt during other kinds of activity too, including sexual relations. The emotions can stimulate it as well – the bhakti connection in our spiritual anatomy. The experiences will gradually expand in your neuro-biology as you continue with yoga practices.

At this stage, as the urine passes through the changing sensitivity in the prostate, the energy goes up the spinal nerve. It is an indication of an opening occurring in your nervous system. In time, the stimulation will be there without urination, and you will be filled with ecstatic energy all the time. It is intimately involved with the evolution of our sexual function, which is the same as the awakening of kundalini.

All of the advanced yoga practices are for stimulating this transformation to higher functioning on every level in us.

The guru is in you.

Addition – As ecstatic conductivity (kundalini) awakens deep in the urinary neuro-biology, there can be periods of sensitivity that bring a need for more frequent urination. It is a situation that comes and goes during the beginning and intermediate stages of awakening, and gradually diminishes as the spiritual transformation in the nervous system advances toward fruition. This can be experienced by both women and men.

Lesson T14 – A Happy Woman

Q: Thank you for the simplicity and power of the lessons. My hubby and me have worked on the holdback and blocking for about a month and we are getting the hang of it. He sure is. Last night we stayed in intercourse without orgasm for over an hour. I got lost after a while. I didn't know where. It was beautiful. I was filled with the deepest peace and sweet loving pleasure all over inside. Time and space disappeared. It is beyond description, beyond anything sex has ever been. I want to stay there forever, move into that place and never leave. It is still with me today, but fading away. I can't wait for him to get home from work so we can go deep again. He loves it too. I'm a happy woman. Can tantric sex replace the other yoga practices? It feels like it could. We are doing the other lessons too and started meditating in January. But we're a bit distracted from that lately, ya know.

A: It is wonderful that you and your husband are having good success with the tantra methods. It makes this old heart feel good.

As you continue, it will go deeper, and the experience will be more present in your daily activity. That is the purification and opening of your nervous system to divine experience. Preservation and cultivation of sexual energy is an important part of that.

Is tantric sex a replacement for sitting practices such as meditation, spinal breathing, mudras, etc? No, it is not, for a couple of reasons.

First, tantric sex is in a similar category with mulabandha/asvini and siddhasana, and success with these sexual energy-stimulating practices is dependent on continuing global purification through spinal breathing and deep meditation. You can go only so far with tantric sex without the prerequisite practices. Then progress slows down because you are using sexual energy alone for purification that requires broader and deeper measures in the nervous system. The same is true of the sitting practices that stimulate sexual/kundalini energy alone. Without spinal breathing and meditation, things will bog down. There can also be imbalances, kundalini symptoms, etc. So, sitting practices are very important, spinal breathing and meditation in particular, to complete the journey with a minimum of slowdowns and detours.

Second, purifying and opening the nervous system to divine experience is very dependent on daily practice – stimulating the nervous system to open like clockwork twice a day, every day. This twice-daily practice is not very practical with sexual relations, though many would love to try for it. It is better to enjoy sex when it comes to us naturally, using the tantric sex methods to preserve and cultivate for higher experiences at those times. Tantric sex will be enjoyable whenever we happen to do it, and a big help to our yoga. Then, the rest of the time, we will be doing our regular daily sitting practices, which assure us that we will be moving right along with our spiritual progress.

So, whether we are having sexual relations or not, advanced yoga practices will be there every day at the same times, morning and evening. If tantric sex is there too, then our yoga will be even better, and all of life will be beautifully illuminated.

The guru is in you.

Lesson T15 – Lustful Pleasures

Q: I have always been very easily corrupted and have allowed my form to be used in ways that are damaging to my inner growth. Before I began reading your posts I had no reference, nor a concept of how to go about solving my dilemma. I've awakened the inner teacher in myself, and so many questions are readily answered for me. Yet, this area has been the most difficult because in the past I have enjoyed my sexual exploits and basically ignored the inner voice in these kinds of situations, because weakness was greater than my desire to move ahead. I understand that there is no condemnation, that I have the free will, and that I willingly chose lustful pleasures over the Higher Love pleasures. Having said all that, thank you again. Since I've begun with the exercises you've shared, I've been able to see a change in my expression. There has begun to be a true devotional loving, and I think you call it ecstatic energy in my body, from the base of my spine up to my heart and throat centers.

A: We know that lustful pleasures are intense but short-lived. As we move to a more spiritual orientation with our sex, then we are cultivating long term changes in our nervous system.

It may be difficult with a partner if you are used to having his seed and your satisfaction right away. There could be factors relating to relationships with members of the opposite sex – a subconscious need to sexually exploit or be exploited. Yoga practices will eventually get to the bottom of these karmic influences and release them. That is sexual healing, as discussed in an earlier lesson (#T10).

In cases where working with a partner in tantric sexual relations is difficult due to strong lustful habits, it might be beneficial to work alone for a while, establishing a good routine of "right-handed" practices – meditation, spinal breathing, mulabandha, siddhasana and so on. There can be good stimulation of sexual energy for yoga in sitting practices. Solo masturbation could also be explored in tantric mode, if you are already inclined toward it. In that case, when you masturbate, see if you can develop a habit of staying in front of orgasm using the solo version of the holdback method. With all this, in time, your desire for lustful pleasure will lose some of its luster. That is because the inner spiritual pleasure will be coming up more and more, and it is very satisfying, not just for the moment, but ongoing day and night.

A strong libido is actually a great advantage in spiritual practices, assuming you can bring some discipline to your stimulative practices. That is really the key. Passion with a purpose, you know. You will know you are making progress when you can just be aroused without having to go to climax. It takes time. Siddhasana is a great practice for cultivating that mode of constant stimulation without expectations. The "bucking bronco" of siddhasana will settle down eventually. Then you will find ecstatic bliss trickling up and down all through you. Lustful pleasures will seem a small thing then, and will slip from consciousness during yogic sexual stimulation, and in regular daily activity as well.

Gradually, you will begin to view men differently. Then you will be able to engage with a partner, if you choose, without it being in exploiter or exploited mode. If it is still either one of these, then consider working some more on your own until you can invite someone into your bed with enough divine love to be there for him more than yourself. It will happen if you persist in your practices. You will attract men of higher spiritual quality too. Or maybe you will move beyond sex with a partner altogether. It all depends on your inclinations. It all depends on where your bhakti (divine desire) leads you.

The guru is in you.

Lesson T16 – What is the Best Tantric Practice?

Q: I have read many books on tantra, and I'm still not sure what it is. Is it about sex, or is it about yoga? What is tantric practice, and is there a "best" tantric practice?

A: Tantra is very misunderstood in the West due to over-embracing of the sexual aspect, and in the East due to under-embracing of the sexual aspect.

In both cases the sexual aspect is an obsession, either for or against. It is because sex is about deeply personal pleasure. We are all fascinated by deep pleasure, especially our own. It is a preoccupation, a fixation, which makes it a hazard to yoga. But without sex, there can be no higher yoga, so it has to be addressed.

What is tantra? Of course, from the first lesson here, you know it is everything in yoga from top to bottom, and from left to right.

If you are asking, "What is the definition of tantric sexual practice?" Then I have to say it is one word – "Brahmacharya." By that, I do not mean celibacy, though it can be that. What I mean is preservation and cultivation of sexual energy as part of the whole of yoga practices. Genital orgasm is not part of that. We go for orgasm because we need it to satisfy our reproductive urge. Genital orgasm has little to do with spiritual progress, except as it is expanded (preorgasmically) to unending whole body ecstasy. The rise of whole body ecstasy is nature's way of calling us to the spiritual realms, just as orgasm is her way of calling us to reproduction.

Hence, any teaching that claims to give a bigger, longer, or better orgasm is not really tantric. It is only about having better sex, which is what most people are looking for. Not that there is anything wrong with that. But let's be clear about our yoga.

Are these lessons anti-orgasm? No. We cannot deny our humanity. We just do our best to nudge ourselves toward the divine using the best means we can find. We will slip off this way or that way every day. It doesn't matter. What matters is our continued favoring of the principles and practices that purify and open the nervous system. Life can become an easy sort of meditation, like that. Just favoring natural principles that enable our nervous system to purify and open itself. Nothing is accomplished by negative judgments. So, when we slip, we just pick up and keep going in the direction we know leads home. That is part of tantric sex too, part of the process of brahmacharya – gently favoring preservation and cultivation of sexual energy through thick and thin, without judgment.

What is the best tantric practice? In terms of consistently preserving and cultivating sexual energy, the hands-down winner is siddhasana.

"But that isn't having sex!" you cry.

That is correct. We have the methods discussed here in the tantra lessons for working towards staying in principle (preservation and cultivation) during sexual relations. But how often do we have sex every day? And for how long in front of orgasm? And how about without orgasm? Taken as daily spiritual practice, tantric sex is hit or miss at best. Certainly, tantric sex is wonderful, and a definite aid on the path. It can be taken to great heights by skilled partners. Even so, over the long run, it doesn't hold a candle to a steady disciplined diet of siddhasana during our regular sitting practices twice every day. This is why siddhasana wins. It is twice-daily for 30 minutes or more. It is stimulative and always preorgasmic, once stabilized as a regular part of our practices. Doing it simultaneously with pranayama and meditation has the powerful benefit of cultivating sexual energy while our nervous system is engaged in deep spiritual processes, so the effects of siddhasana and all concurrent practices are amplified.

If siddhasana becomes orgasmic (perhaps in the learning stage), it can also be used by a man for blocking ejaculation, simply by leaning forward on the heel. The heel then does what the fingers do in blocking at the perineum. Siddhasana is an all-purpose tantric practice.

If you want to review, the particulars of siddhasana are covered in main lessons #33 and #75. Does this mean everyone has to forget about sexual relations and just sit in siddhasana every day? Of course not. Siddhasana is a foundation tantric practice for serious yogis and yoginis. Siddhasana means, "seat of the perfected ones" for a reason. If siddhasana is there during pranayama, meditation and other sitting practices, the foundation for tantric practice is there, no matter what else may happen with sex. Beyond that, do whatever comes naturally in your sex life. If you are devoted to your yoga, you will find yourself naturally drawn to the principles of preservation and cultivation in your sexual relations. The methods given in these lessons (holdback and blocking) are easy to learn, and are very effective. There are more complex methods one can use. Whatever tantric practices you choose, the underlying principles of brahmacharya remain the same – preservation and cultivation of sexual energy.

In the end, what matters in yoga is the permeation of our body and surroundings with ecstatic bliss. If we have accomplished that, then exactly how we handled sexual energy is a mute point.

If we apply the underlying principles, we will get the results.

The guru is in you.

Lesson T17 – Reclaiming the Body-Soul Connection

Q: Hello. I have a question. I have been baffled by it for a while. Why is it that the idea of the reduction of the self to a material object in sex is appealing? Sometimes I feel that sexual energies would be better transmitted if my mind did not have a part in them, just my body and soul. Perhaps I think my mind would just be a deterrent and that pure and intentional will comes from the soul. I know this is somewhat of an odd question and maybe I'm the only one who feels this way. Any clarification on this thought would be helpful.

A: It is a good question. You have pinpointed a feeling that many have, I think. The question itself is an opening. That is how bhakti (desire for truth) works.

It is a question of self-awareness, and where that is manifesting. The mind will go where self seems to be. It is determined by the amount of obstruction lodged in our nervous system. If our main identity is with the body, the mind will tend to indulge in that experience. With sex it can be very strong because it is the peak of externalized sensory experience. The mind being identified like this is the essence of sense attachment and lust.

The senses are not bad because of this relationship of mind with body. Making that judgment is like "shooting the messenger." If we undertake meditation and other practices that purify and open the nervous system, the sense of self gradually expands inside to silent pure bliss consciousness. The senses also expand gradually inward to more enjoyable levels of ecstatic experience. Then the mind finds something more than the physical body to be fascinated with – pure bliss consciousness, which is the mind's essential nature, and also refinement of sensory experience to levels of divine ecstasy. So, the mind is naturally drawn to an expanding reality within, and a more stable and satisfying sense of self.

It is not a matter of shutting off or excluding the mind. It is about expanding the experience of self and senses inward, and mind will go there. Indeed, the mind is a primary vehicle for cultivating that. The mind has the inherent ability to go to stillness, and this is what we capitalize on when we go systematically inward in daily meditation.

So, we don't want to shut off the mind. We want to expand it to embrace more and more peace and enjoyment inside. Then we expand beyond narrow attachments to external sensory experiences of the body, and all that. The mind becomes a bridge between the body and the soul. The heart is opened by this process, so divine love emerges, which expands our sense of self beyond our body. Then we see our lover, and everyone, as an expression of our self. We come to live and love for the other.

All of this has a profound effect on sexual relations, producing the effect you describe – body and soul merged as one. Everyone longs for this in sex, and in all of life. It is our natural state. We instinctively want to reclaim it. And we can.

The guru is in you.

Lesson T18 – Enlightenment with and without Orgasm?

Q: Your Q&A section is very educative. Thanks for the same. I have a question. For a woman who has never had a sexual experience, I mean if she does not know what is orgasm, is it possible to raise kundalini? If so, what will be best way? Please answer my question. Thank you

A: Thank you for writing and sharing. Orgasm is not a prerequisite for raising kundalini, or for enlightenment. On the contrary, it can be an obstacle due to the obsession many people develop about it, and the resulting loss of vitality that comes from too much non-tantric sexual activity. So, maybe you have an advantage. This is assuming you are not seriously repressed about your sexual energy, because it must come up into the nervous system for enlightenment stages 2 (ecstasy) and 3 (unity) to be reached. You will recall from the main lessons that stage 1 is permanent inner silence ("the witness").

So, an opening for sexual (kundalini) energy needs to happen at some point – not down, but up. This has its own kind of ecstatic reverie that fills the whole body. How can this be accomplished? It can be done with meditation alone, but it will take a long time. Meditation is best for establishing enlightenment stage 1 – unshakable silent pure bliss consciousness. If spinal breathing is added, the entire sushumna (spinal nerve) will be enlivened with prana from root to third eye, and this stimulates the awakening of kundalini much more than meditation alone. By definition, kundalini is prana awakening in the spinal nerve and then throughout the nervous system, coming up from the vast storehouse of prana in the pelvic region. To speed it up more, targeted physical practices (and kumbhaka – breath retention) can be added as discussed extensively in the main lessons. As mentioned two lessons ago here, siddhasana is the most directly stimulative sitting tantric practice.

So, all this you can do without external sexual activity or orgasm, though you will probably have some strange new sensations in your pelvic area and upward as your yoga advances. It is inevitable. When strong love feelings come, you can direct them to your spiritual ideal, rather than into a sexual channel, and redouble your bhakti for doing practices. You can have a wildly passionate love affair with God, and remain celibate all the way though, if this is your preference. Many great yoginis and yogis in history have gone this route.

How far you go in taking on practices is a function of your inclinations. Maybe the direct stimulation of siddhasana is not for you. Maybe you are not inclined to do some of the other targeted practices either. If that is the case, it is okay. With meditation and spinal breathing alone, the whole job can be done. Even meditation alone can take us very far over the long run. It is up to you – how fast you want to go, and how much ecstatic energy you want to get moving in your nervous system. It can be a pretty crazy life having a fast rising kundalini, and it is not for everyone. Slow and easy may be better for some. We don't always have a choice. Kundalini can develop a mind of her own. When she takes over, we end up in a partnership.

No matter what the inner experiences may be, everyone is free to go at their own speed with advanced yoga practices. That goes for everything, including tantric sexual methods. The most important thing is that we understand the natural abilities inherent in our nervous system, and then choose whatever methods for stimulating these abilities we feel are appropriate for us. Even another path altogether is okay. In that case, just regard all these lessons as "food for thought."

Don't worry, not being sexually active is not a disadvantage. You can do it your own way. It is your choice how you will travel home. As you explore the various methods that stimulate your nervous system to purify and open, you will find your balance in practices.

The guru is in you.

Lesson T19 – Sex, Love and Bhakti

Everyone knows that sex is about hormones. There is the old joke that, "Teenagers are all hormones." Maybe that applies to many of us adults too. The more hormonal vitality we have, the greater our sexual status, and self image. When the juices are flowing we feel more alive.

It is all about prana, you know. Prana is vitality, the life force that flows inside us. It is what is behind all those hormones. Through yoga we influence our prana by influencing our body chemistry, and vise versa. We think according to a certain procedure and we become physically and mentally still inside, and inner silence expands. We become empty self-contained awareness. That is meditation. We breathe a certain way and the energies flowing in our body are enlivened in noticeable ways. That is pranayama. We make love a certain way, or engage in certain types of solo stimulation of sexual energy, and our inner experiences are dramatically expanded into vast inner flights of ecstatic euphoria. Then we are both empty and euphoric at the same time. The joining of these two makes divine love – a self-fulfilling flow that needs no object. It just is.

The great kriya yogi, Lahiri Mahasaya, said, "My worship is of a very strange kind. Holy water is not required. No special utensils are necessary. Even flowers are redundant. In this worship all gods have disappeared, and emptiness has merged with euphoria."

So, ultimately, human spiritual transformation is not about external objects or rituals. It is about our inner processes, our inner awareness (emptiness) and our ecstasy (euphoria). When these two merge, all that is left is divine love flowing out from an endless inner reservoir. It is its own source. It exists for no object, yet serves all. It is its own fulfillment, which is the common good. Divine love is hormones taken to their highest level of functioning in the human being.

But what of ordinary love, the kind most of us feel at some point in our life? The kind we feel in our hearts and in our loins. How do we expand from that to divine love? It is in choosing a higher manifestation of our energy, choosing a higher level of functioning of hormones, and making the journey of transformation using yogic knowledge.

When we become sexually aroused, our hormones are stimulated into high gear. We feel euphoric. We feel attracted. Attracted to what? Something. Someone. This powerful euphoric attraction needs an object. We lose our mind when this happens. The emotions take over. Only the object matters.

"Love knows no reason."

What is this ordinary love? It is an extreme flow of hormones. We are drugged from within. It fills us with devotion for the object of our affection, at least for a time. At least until the hormones settle down. Then what? Then "the honeymoon is over," and we move into a different phase of the process, a less intense one.

The difference between ordinary love and divine love is that the intensity in divine love never stops. The honeymoon never ends. It never goes away. It becomes more, and more, and more. Divine romance is like falling into an endless abyss of love. As we fall, it flows out of us to everyone around us. In divine love we become a channel between the infinite and the world.

Divine love, divine romance, is as much about sex as ordinary human romance is. Divine love is about internal sex, and it never ends. Ordinary love is about external sex, and loses its intensity in time. Ordinary lovers cry and moan in ecstasy for a few minutes or hours. Lovers of the divine cry and moan in ecstasy for decades.

If you read the poems of Rumi and St. John of the Cross (see AYP links section on the web site), you will see that these sages had passionate relationships with the divine. Intensely romantic relationships in terms of their own "ishta," their chosen ideal. As Lahiri Mahasaya points out, even the ideals are eventually overshadowed by the reality of the inner transformation, which is the merging of inner silence with inner ecstasy, a neuro-biological process occurring inside us.

Ah, the divine romance! We have to put it in some sort of language. We describe it with metaphors, deities, the language of our culture. After all the analysis and all the yoga, when divine love bubbles up there can only be poetry, and maybe not even that.

It's like that in tantric sexual relations also. The hormones are cultivated higher and higher. Our lover is the divine before us, inside us, enveloping us. If we have used the method of bhakti, we know all our desire, all our passion, all our hormones are going for that high purpose in us. Nothing matters but that. Our ordinary love will be morphing to divine love in every minute. Love objects become spiritual objects, and then melt inside us. Our body, our lover, and everyone we see are expressions of God, and for that divine lovemaking that dissolves separations. We may seem crazy to ordinary people when we are in this state of divine passion.

Crazy or not, if we are prudent we will keep our love going higher with sitting practices when we are not in tantric sexual relations. This we can do every day. Then the romance never stops. It creeps into our everyday living, flowing out of us in waves of beautiful bliss. Daily practices are important for this. Eventually it becomes self-sustaining. The nervous system wants to rise to this divine state. It asks us to do yoga by calling us quietly from deep inside our heart. As the nervous system opens in yoga it takes over, and there is no stopping. Then we are along for the ride.

So, if you are in love, in lovemaking, or even just contemplating love, keep something in mind. Your love has a great destiny far beyond the attachments and pleasures of the moment. You don't have to go anywhere to find your destiny. You don't have to renounce your family, your career, or anything. You only have to realize that your desire and your passion can be pointed higher.

How?

The intention alone sets things in motion. Can you feel it moving inside you now? A quickening of devotion. A magical expectancy stirring deep inside. Favor that. Favor it as you feel your love flowing. Favor it as you join with your beloved in the bed. Feel it as you use the methods that will cultivate the divine energies higher in your lover and yourself. Feel it as you do your daily sitting practices. Rise high in divine love. You have the means.

The guru is in you.

Lesson T21 – Ancient Advice on Tantric Sex

Back in 1957, a little book was published in Japan called *Zen Flesh, Zen Bones: A Collection of Zen and Pre-Zen Writings*, compiled and transcribed by Paul Reps and Nyogen Senzaki. It includes writings from some ancient Indian scriptures. Several of these; the 4,000 year old *Vigyan Bhairava* and *Sochanda Tantra*, plus another, were combined to form the 112 techniques called "Centering Practices." This is an all-encompassing survey of the techniques of tantra yoga, covering both right-handed and left-handed methods.

The 112 techniques are a few lines each, and, all together, fill up a few pages. You can find them in the AYP links section on the web site under "Centering Practices."

As was discussed in the first lesson here, tantra is the broadest of all the yoga systems, leaving nothing unattended as a tool of spiritual transformation. Virtually all of the lessons of Advanced Yoga Practices are touched on in one way or another in the 112 techniques, which is amazing, because they were not used as a guide for writing the lessons. What is true in yoga today was just as true, and was documented, 4,000 years ago.

You will recall that the principle of brahmacharya is at the heart of managing sexual energy for spiritual purposes. Brahmacharya is preservation and cultivation of sexual energy. This is accomplished in particular ways in sitting practices, and in other ways during tantric sexual relations.

Technique #43 of the 112 techniques captures the essence of tantric sex, and contains within it all of the sexual practices discussed in the lessons:

"At the start of sexual union, keep attention on the fire in the beginning, and, so continuing, avoid the embers in the end."

From this one sentence, all of tantric sexual methods can be derived. In fact, volumes have been written to expound upon it. The late Osho/Rajneesh, the famed tantra guru, wrote a 1,000-page book expounding on the 112 techniques. It is called *The Book of Secrets*, published in 1974.

Nothing is new in yoga. The human nervous system functions the same today as it did thousands of years ago. It is just a matter of understanding the underlying principles involved in human spiritual transformation. Once we know those, it is easy to evaluate the efficacy of spiritual practices, and integrate them into a simple, powerful routine that can alter our lives, opening us up to unending ecstatic bliss.

The guru is in you.

Lesson T22 – Kundalini and Sexual Attraction for Guru and God

Q: I have not felt sexually attracted to anyone in years, which is odd because even as a small child I was attracted to men. I had an active kundalini, even back then. Now I can see men and think they are attractive, but there is no libidinal flow/response to them within me. Men find me attractive, but it's like I see their energy and have absolutely no desire to be with them. The only one who comes close to being what I want is my guru, and I don't want a physical union with him. Is this all just part of the process? Or is it something to do with not grounding enough?

A: It is a normal process of transformation having many stages. Sex is an important part of yoga, particularly in relation to the evolution of kundalini energy. Since your kundalini has been active since way back, this is drawing your energy and attention up and away from external sex. It is not absolutely necessary that it all go up. The energy can go both ways. It depends on background and inclinations. For those with energy wanting to go for sexual relations, we have these tantra lessons to give methods for use in sexual relations in support of yoga. As discussed previously, celibacy is not a prerequisite for success. Preservation and cultivation of sexual energy are, and there are multiple means through which that can be accomplished.

In successful yoga, the range can be anything from tantric sex, to non-tantric sex in moderation, to celibacy. It is really up to you. If the energy is going up and you want to go with it, that is okay. If it is going up and you want come back down for sex, that is okay too. Just understand the tantra yoga aspects of sex and you will be fine. Some people are inclined to sexual excess, and that is not very good for yoga, and it has to be addressed in some fashion for spiritual progress to occur. It seems everyone is in a different place with sex. There is no need for judgement about it. Be who you are, and, however sex may be manifesting in you, favor the corresponding means to bring sex into support of your yoga.

Another thing – the spiritual path becomes very sexy as ecstasy rises with kundalini. You probably know this already. The whole body can be in an ongoing quasi-orgasmic state any time once the nervous system is purified to a certain level. One devotional thought can set it off. We are living ecstatically then, and running to our meditation seat (siddhasana!) every day. It is a divine romance between the yogi/yogini and God, with lots of juicy sex going on up and down inside. Enlightened celibates have extremely active sex lives with God. For them, the passion never stops.

Martin Buber's *Ecstatic Confessions* is a good anthology of diary testimonials throughout history on the subject of ecstatic relationships with God. Ecstatic bliss flowing profusely in the cloistered convents of medieval Europe!

It is also good to read Rumi, Saint John of the Cross and Saint Francis of Assisi for personal descriptions of what hot romance with God is like. Blistering bhakti! Links for those are in the AYP links section on the web site.

None of this means you have to give up sex for a so-called divine romance. It evolves more or less naturally in all of us. Sex and passion have a broad spectrum in us, and it is easy to be doing one thing and wondering why we are not doing something else. The options are endless. It is a matter of what we want. If we want God, and keep on with that desire (bhakti), we will keep moving higher somehow.

Maybe the "man" you want is "God." If a person symbolizes that, then you may be drawn to him. It is normal enough for someone in a kundalini transition (even a very long term one) to be attracted to a guru. Gurus in-the-flesh are affected by that, and many have taken liberties with their disciples, often at great cost to their credibility. It doesn't really do the disciple(s) any good either. I think you understand that. God is in you, and men are always going to be men.

On the other hand, you may find someone you love, get married and raise a family. Then yoga will be carried on within the framework of a busy family life. That's the route I took. It is a common outcome on the spectrum of romance. Love can carry us forward in so many ways, if we will but let it.

When the nervous system is open, it is all love, and there is not so much preoccupation with sex and personal romance anymore. Then it is about divine romance – with love flowing out all the time, not needing anything in return.

The guru is in you.

Lesson T23 – The Count Method – How to Stay in Front of Orgasm

Q: Thank you for your great lessons here and over in the main yoga lessons too. You have made a believer out of me. Well I'm trying. I am one of those who is hooked on orgasm. I don't know if hooked is the right word. I just get going, you know, and don't know how to stop in front of orgasm even though I want to and know it is the way. I got my boyfriend reading the lessons so maybe he will give me some help. Even in masturbation (I do a lot) I can't stop either. It is like I am a runaway train and can't stop till I have gone over the cliff. I go and go and how do I stop that? Also, I like to use a vibrator sometimes, and I don't know how to stop that before orgasm either. Should I give up the vibrator? I started using siddhasana recently and am having some success staying aroused and in front orgasm in meditation, but I'm masturbating sometimes in it too and I feel guilty. It seems like the only time my body wants to stop is after the big thrill and then it's too late. Help!

A: You have the essential ingredient for success – desire. And I don't mean only sexual desire, which you have plenty of. You can use that to your advantage. All desire (including sexual desire) can be transformed to high spiritual purpose, which you are beginning to do now. It is bhakti.

You are finding in your passion that all-important desire to do what is necessary to go higher inside with your sexual energy. That means being aroused in front of orgasm for extended periods. That is when the preservation and cultivation of sexual energy occurs. That is brahmacharya.

You know from previous writing here that even the ecstatic nuns kept themselves aroused for God for months and years on end.

For we ordinary mortals who have not forsaken reproductive sex, the question is, how do we stay in front of orgasm when the gods of reproduction are hurling us mercilessly toward it? By now we know the principle of preservation and cultivation of sexual energy. But how do we do a better job of turning principle into practice? There is another technique we can apply that will stop us before orgasm, guaranteed. And I don't mean setting off a stick of dynamite next to the bed just before we go over the edge. That may not help.

We can all count, right? This is called the counting method. How unsexy can you get? Just mention of counting is a turn off. What are we going to count? Sheep?

No. We will count strokes. "Strokes?" you say. Yes, those things that bring us to orgasm. Assume you are solo, masturbating. How many strokes does it take? 20? 50? 100? 500? You probably never counted. Who does? But now we will do some counting, at least until we can develop some discipline in front of orgasm. And the counting can help with that a lot, because it gets us used to stopping stimulation in front of orgasm. That is all it takes, you know. Just developing some familiarity with what it is like to stop stimulation in front of orgasm. It is not the end of the world. It is the beginning of a new world.

So, when you masturbate, do some stroking until it is starting to get exciting. You know, as that train is starting to speed up and run away. Then count ten strokes and stop for about fifteen seconds. Or stop for half a minute or longer if you want to. If ten strokes are too many, use five strokes and stop. If ten is not enough, use fifteen or twenty strokes and stop. But not close to orgasm. Not right on top of orgasm. Use the count method to give yourself some room. Allow yourself to become familiar with that space in front of orgasm. That is what the count method is for. In doing so you will be cultivating sexual essences higher in your nervous system, and after a while of doing this you will feel yourself entering a realm of peaceful ecstasy. Go there. Stay there for a time. The longer you do, the more your nervous system will be transformed into a pure vehicle of spiritual experience.

The count-based stopping is a regulated version of the holdback method, used in masturbation mode in this case. Just keep doing it. If the ten-count with fifteen second rests are moving you away from arousal, then up it to fifteen strokes. If you are moving closer to orgasm with each count, then make the count a little less. The idea is to find a balance-point of arousal in front of orgasm that is erotically pleasurable and then keep doing the strokes and holdbacks using the count method over and over again. See if you can keep it up for thirty minutes. That is good holdback practice, and you will notice much energy going up, and enter into that peaceful ecstatic state mentioned above. Most importantly, you will be developing the habit of knowing how to stop stimulation in front of orgasm and being okay with it because you will find the peace and ecstasy that come up in it. That is how to get that runaway train under control. It is a new and wonderful kind of stimulation and gratification we are developing. Both women and men can use the count method in masturbation with good results.

In practice with a partner, if the man is having difficulty with the holdback method, he can count strokes also to help develop the habit of staying in front of orgasm. And, of course, he has blocking available too. The count method is the same procedure in lovemaking with a partner as alone, except there are two people instead of one, so two sexual energies are being cultivated in front of orgasm instead of one. It is more stimulating and more complicated, and requires teamwork as discussed in previous lessons. That is where your boyfriend's reading of the lessons will come in handy for both of you. In the meantime, you can be practicing on your own, and it will help you tremendously in moving to tantric lovemaking. Whatever progress we make developing control in solo practice is directly transferable to lovemaking with a partner. When your boyfriend gets to be advanced in control of his ejaculation, then you can practice on top of him too. By then, you will probably be beyond needing to use counting in your tantric lovemaking, and you will both be making love in the higher realms of your nervous systems. By then you will know how to stay in front of orgasm by well-developed habit and be climbing the stairway to heaven with ease.

Counting is a good tool for developing the habit of staying preorgasmic. It is also a help for becoming very satisfied sitting aroused and preorgasmic in siddhasana throughout sitting practices. Of course, as you are finding, siddhasana is self-contained training for that in itself. It is okay that you go into masturbation sometimes in siddhasana. Don't worry about it. It is a normal transition everyone goes through in one way or another when developing siddhasana. Masturbation in siddhasana will gradually become less as experience advances. Over time you will find that slipping into siddhasana and doing your sitting practices preorgasmically all the way through is every bit as satisfying as having sex. Actually, it is much more satisfying because there is no let down – no cliff, just going higher and higher. It is orgasm reborn as unending whole body ecstatic bliss all through pranayama and meditation, and beyond. When experiences go so high like this, there is no need to give up sex. The principles of preservation and cultivation can be used to good advantage in either mode.

The count method can be used with your vibrator also, though you may not be able to count strokes if you are using it in a more or less stationary position. In that case, just count the seconds with your inner clock, and stop the vibrator stimulation at the appointed number. You may find that you need to use a lower count to stay in front of orgasm with the vibrator because it provides more stimulation. So maybe once you have the train going you will use a five count and stop, instead of ten or more using finger strokes only. It can be done like that, and there is no problem using a vibrator or other device for stimulation in this way if you are so inclined. The main thing is knowing how to stop to preserve and cultivate sexual energy, and the count method will do that for you if you are prudent in choosing your count numbers.

You are a tantric goddess in the making. In no time you will be taking your lover and yourself to new heights of ecstatic bliss inside. All of this will help make your sitting practices very enjoyable, and permeate your daily activities with increasing ecstasy.

The guru is in you.

Lesson T24 – Tantric Masturbation with Sitting Practices?

Q: After reading the material in the tantra lessons, it makes me wonder if I might help myself progress faster if I had more sexual arousal during sitting practice. Currently there isn't any. Siddhasana doesn't generate any sexual energy for me, possibly because I'm taking Prozac, which lowers the body's ability to get aroused, both flight-or-fight and sexually. I take it for both anxiety and depression, and it dawned on me today that maybe on the anxiety side, what needs to happen is not decreasing arousal/anxiety, but transformation of that arousal/anxiety into spiritual energy. It would be hard to provoke anxiety in myself before sitting practice, but not so hard to provoke sexual arousal. So I wonder if pre-orgasmic masturbation as part of sitting practice might be useful in increasing energy flow and getting to ecstasy?

I'm hoping that the practices you have been teaching will eventually enable me to stop taking the Prozac, but I'm not about to stop taking it precipitously.

A: I agree that you should not come off your medication just to become more sensitive in siddhasana. It is not essential, as much progress is being made bringing up inner silence in meditation with no sexual stimulation needed for that. As you know, inner silence is by far the most important ingredient for enlightenment.

Keep in mind that, in the tantra lessons, most of what is here is for those who have sex going on at a certain level already, and how to make the best use of it for yoga. It is not encouraged for everyone to become sexually active beyond their norm just to participate in more tantric sexual practices.

I can see how the idea of needing to promote sexual arousal for sitting practices could come up in your mind. It is in fact what siddhasana is for. However, it is not best to try and actively stimulate beyond siddhasana in sitting practices. Better to let it happen in siddhasana naturally. And don't forget mulabandha and the mudras, etc., higher up, which all tie in with raising ecstatic (sexual) conductivity in the nervous system.

You want to help your spiritual progress along, and that is fair enough. Better not to masturbate before or during sitting practices though. That is too much stimulation when you are wanting to let the nervous system come to stillness. You can use the tantric practices at other times though, and the results of that will accumulate in your nervous system and then naturally become more prevalent in siddhasana and sitting practices, as well as in daily life.

You can give siddhasana some help by cupping your genitals in your hand while doing sitting practices. This is not masturbation, just a little quiet help for your energy. Don't do it to the point of too much distraction from easy spinal breathing and meditation. A nice balance is what we want. That is where we end up with siddhasana too, with a nice balance between ecstatic energy gently washing up through us and deep inner silence coming up in meditation and other sitting practices. These two combine in us to create unending ecstatic bliss and overflowing divine love.

It is important to note that raising ecstatic kundalini isn't only about sexual stimulation, so all the preorgasmic stimulation in the world (including siddhasana) may not do it if inner silence is still formative and pranayama and other practices have not opened the nervous system enough yet.

If you are inclined to masturbate at times (other than during sitting practices), by all means take advantage of the tantra techniques. The count method just given can be used regularly with good effectiveness to coax sexual energy higher in long solo or partner sessions, and gradually cultivate the nervous system to be in that peaceful ecstatic mode naturally at all times. Then siddhasana will have increasing effects because the energy will be moving already.

So, if you work with sexual energy at times outside sitting practices on a regular basis, that will help siddhasana and all of your practices. It is a separate practice, which is how all tantric sex is discussed in the lessons, as separate rather than integrated with sitting practices. Let's not skew our regular sitting practices too far in the direction of tantric sex, or we will lose something there – balance...

Sitting practices are the bread and butter of yoga. We need them every day to progress. Tantric sexual practices are like the cake. We enjoy them when we can, but not as a twice-daily scheduled event. Tantric sex is not a substitute for daily spinal breathing and deep meditation.

The guru is in you.

Lesson T25* – Sri Vidya – The Fruition of Tantra

As was mentioned in the first lesson here, tantra has often been condemned as degenerate in the East and misunderstood (with great enthusiasm) as a sexual cult in the West. What we find as we travel our serious path of yoga is that tantra includes everything we are doing, and probably a lot we are not doing. Tantra is the most all-encompassing approach to yoga, leaving no stones unturned. But where does it all lead? What is the end of tantra? What is its fruition? In the main lessons, and here in the tantra lessons also, we have discussed the union of our inner polarities as being the end of all our yoga practice. There are many ways to describe this process – as many ways as there are spiritual traditions in the world. No matter how described, it is the same process of human spiritual transformation. On the level of our personal experience in the body it is the union of our blissful inner silence cultivated mainly in deep meditation, with our whole body ecstasy cultivated in spinal breathing and other pranayamas, mudras, bandhas and tantric sexual methods. On the level of tantric mythological metaphors it is the union of Shiva and Shakti, which correspond to the direct experiences of silence and ecstasy just mentioned.

The rise of Shiva, Shakti and their final union everywhere within us make up the three stages of enlightenment – First, 24/7 inner silence. Second, 24/7 whole body ecstasy. And third, 24/7 ecstatic bliss, the joining of the divine polarities of silence and ecstasy, yielding an endless outpouring of divine love, which is unity. (24/7 means 24 hours per day, 7 days per week) If you imagine the rise of a conscious ecstatic resonance vibrating in every atom of your body, occurring between every nucleus and its surrounding electrons, you will have an idea of the depth of the transformation. It is an unending cosmic orgasm within every cell and atom in us.

This fruition of divine transformation is recognized in a scriptural and experiential branch of tantra known as, "Sri Vidya," which means "glorious knowledge." It is the knowledge of ecstatic bliss, expressed with mathematical precision. If this seems like a paradox, then it is surely divine, for divine truth is a paradox. If truth is experienced as wildly ecstatic, it will be heading toward spiritual precision. If it is conceived to be mathematically exact, then it will soon to be undoing us in ecstatic reverie. Nowhere is this better expressed than in Sri Vidya's sacred diagram called *Sri Yantra*, sometimes called *Sri Chakra*. Here is one in black and white:

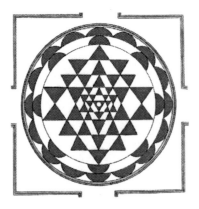

Sri Yantra

Links to several full color images can be found under "Sri Yantra" in the AYP links section on the web site. If you do a web search on "Sri Yantra" you can find many versions of *Sri Yantra*, and endless discussions about it. Perhaps you are familiar with it already.

Sri Yantra depicts the ongoing sexual union of Shiva (masculine white lingam bindu dot) and Shakti (feminine yoni triangles) in every atom of the cosmos. *Sri Yantra* in its entirety also represents the sushumna/spinal nerve tunnel, the nervous system, and the divine union occurring everywhere up and down inside us.

When you look at the *Sri Yantra* diagram, imagine you are looking up through the tunnel of the spinal nerve from the bottom, with each circle of half moons and triangles representing a layer of the seven chakras. The outside circle of half moons represents the root. The center triangle represents the crown where the union of Shiva and Shakti visibly occurs in the diagram (the bindu dot inside the yoni triangle). In fact, the union is occurring in every half moon and triangle of the *Sri Yantra*, representing union in every cell and atom of the body, and the cosmos which is contained within us and represented by the *Sri Yantra* also.

This union of polarities is behind everything that is manifest in us and the universe. We know this from modern physics – the unending electromagnetic and gravitational attractions between atomic particles and the physical objects of all sizes that make up our universe. Without the relationship of polarities, there would be nothing here but pure bliss consciousness. We human beings are both the universe and the pure bliss consciousness from which it is manifested, and we can realize our existence in both these aspects as ecstatic bliss and outpouring divine love.

We are like holograms – microcosms containing the whole of the macrocosm. This is why the effects of yoga practices are so profound. We open to and become the infinite that is within and around us. This is experiential – transcending the rigidity of intellectual theories. All we have to do is sit and meditate to get a taste of our infinite dimensions! *Sri Yantra* is a concise way of representing what already is.

Mathematically, *Sri Yantra* recreates the wave pattern formed by the vibration of *OM*, the sacred sound that is found humming naturally within the human nervous system as purification and opening occurs. *OM* emanates up through the medulla oblongata, the brain stem, forward through the center of the head, and out the third eye. *OM* is no small, quaint thing that happens inside us. It is "roaring devastating ecstasy" breaking loose inside us, and is synonymous with the highest stages of tantric sexual cultivation. *OM* is kundalini is full ecstatic swing. So here you have the link between Sri Vidya, *Sri Yantra* and tantric sexual practices.

How is one to use the *Sri Yantra*, if at all? Some traditions use it as an object of meditation. In these lessons we will not. When *OM* comes, *Sri Yantra* will be there in us. We become *Sri Yantra* when we naturally manifest the ecstatic vibration of *OM*, which is the sound of kundalini/Shakti ravishing her Shiva within us. As this occurs throughout our whole body, we become the *Sri Yantra* itself. The *Sri Yantra* is a representation of our nervous system in its highest mode of spiritual reverie.

When you look at the *Sri Yantra* from time to time, just be aware that this is a representation of your rising inner spiritual dynamic, as well as the ecstatic nature of the cosmos. It is both the microcosm and the macrocosm, and so are we. It is a confirmation and a reminder of what we are consciously becoming through our advanced yoga practices, including those we talk about here in the tantra lessons. Whole body union of ecstatic bliss is what we are cultivating ourselves toward, and this is what *Sri Yantra* is. Let there be no condemnation or misunderstanding about it.

No apology is necessary for cultivating human spiritual transformation to its highest level. So cultivate away!

The guru is in you.

Lesson T27 – The Quest for Infinite Intimacy

Q: Every so often I get this feeling that no matter what sexual or tantric practices I attempt I will never, in this body, be totally at union with my partner – never find infinite intimacy. It seems like if I were to stare into my partner's eyes I would never know exactly what they are thinking or feeling. I can't exactly express why but this is sometimes a very depressing thought for me. It sometimes makes me burn with passion as if I just keep trying to jump over the final hurdle that is to high to even see over, but it seems a useless/impossible passion. Is this a misguided feeling? Am I misinterpreting my subconscious will or God's will?

I haven't as of yet had the chance to try tantric practices with a partner but it seems as if no matter how divine the feeling is it will not surmount the personality gap that feels to me more significant as an obstacle. It doesn't even have to be a sexually related solution; though sex seems the most intimately possible attempt. Maybe I should try practicing clairvoyance of some sort? I'm not really sure. Any thoughts or words of advice on bridging this chasm in lovemaking or otherwise would be well spent.

A: True union is beyond thinking, feeling, clairvoyance, etc. It is beyond the idea of "the other."

It is a paradox. The best way to find true union with another person is by finding union in ourself. Then there is no personal agenda to get in the way. It is just Self in one serving Self in the other. Infinite intimacy is 100% service to the other, without expectation of receiving anything in return. Infinite intimacy isn't something that can be obtained or hurdled into. It is known by letting go, by surrendering, by giving everything. But more than that – it requires a transformation in the functioning of our nervous system at the most fundamental level. This can be accomplished through yoga.

Your desire for union is good. The frustration comes from pointing it outward to obtain something instead of letting go inward. Even looking into another's eyes is outward, unless we are looking from the perspective of inner silent pure bliss consciousness cultivated in meditation. If you use your desire as bhakti for motivation to do spiritual practices, then you will find what you are seeking, both in yourself and in your lover.

The only true infinite intimacy to be found is in our enlightenment. It is an internal affair in each of us – the divine union of our inner polarities. That is how we come to it. Then when we make love, we become the loving, and there is no question about someplace to get to, or hurdle to jump. It all melts away, as we become the caressing. Through practices we become it.

In yoga we don't surmount or overcome our obstacles. We dissolve them so the inherent inner light can shine through. This is the secret. Everything is changed by that one simple principle, and the practices that stimulate the reality of it in our nervous system.

It is suggested that you redirect your desire toward wanting to unfold your inner truth. Then things will happen. You must be willing to act – willing to engage in daily practices. With daily practices, your experience of life will expand in indescribable ways, and so will your lovemaking.

The guru is in you.

Lesson T28* – Advanced Siddhasana for Women and Men

In the main lessons (#33 and #75) we introduced a practice called "siddhasana," which is sitting with the heel under the perineum to provide gentle, steady preorgasmic sexual stimulation during sitting practices. The effect of this over time is to cultivate spiritually ecstatic energies throughout our nervous system, which is a prerequisite for the union of our divine inner polarities, leading to the final stage of enlightenment.

Activating sexual energies higher up in the nervous system has prerequisites also, the main one being the presence of resident inner silence (pure bliss consciousness), which is cultivated through deep meditation. This is why the main lessons begin with meditation and then move into spinal breathing and the other methods for systematically cultivating our inner life force (sexual energy), also known as "raising kundalini."

Yoga involving the use of various means for directly cultivating sexual energy for spiritual purposes has been around for a long time, and is controversial for obvious reasons. Sex gets much of the blame for the abuses and misdeeds of humankind, so has often been suppressed in spiritual practices, even though it has a crucial role to play in the neuro-biology of human spiritual transformation. The result of the denial of the role of sex in spiritual processes has been less enlightenment in the world.

The problem with sex is not sex. It is our tendency to become obsessed with the deeply intimate energies of sex, and with orgasm in particular. As we meditate and pure bliss consciousness rises within us, we are gradually able to become more objective about sexual energy, less obsessed, and begin to consciously stimulate it into the higher spiritual channels of our nervous system. Hence the usefulness of tantric sexual methods.

Siddhasana was described in an earlier lesson as being the best tantric sexual practice. This is because it can be done for extended periods during sitting practices with no effort, guaranteeing that tantric cultivation will be occurring every day at the most opportune time, while we are doing pranayama, meditation and other advanced yoga practices. This is ideal for producing the best results in yoga, yielding lots of permanently flowing ecstatic energy in our life. Our inner silence, cultivated in meditation, naturally comes to reside within our ongoing ecstasy, raising us to a state of permanent ecstatic bliss and outpouring divine love. The two, inner silence and euphoric ecstasy, become one. This leads to the highest stage of enlightenment.

Knowing there is such great benefit in using siddhasana to cultivate our ecstatic energy during sitting practices, the question arises, is there more we can do to help this process? Yes, there is. There are many things. In this lesson we will talk about enhancing siddhasana.

The version of siddhasana given in the main lessons and discussed here in the tantra lessons so far is the basic practice – simply sitting with the heel at the perineum. It can be optimized for more effect in sitting practices. It is done in slightly different ways for women and men, due to anatomical differences. In both cases, it involves positioning siddhasana for maximum effortless sexual stimulation, while remaining steadily preorgasmic. In doing advanced siddhasana, we do not enter into an active mode of masturbation. So besides being in preorgasmic mode, we are also in premasturbation mode. We are just sitting in a more sexually stimulating way, which is a boon to our sitting yoga practices.

For women, the shift to advanced siddhasana involves letting the heel come forward to rest snugly in the entrance of the yoni. It is a natural fit, and is easily accomplished by most enterprising yoginis. There is a second part to advanced siddhasana for women. This is to bring the toes of the outside foot up from under the shin of the inside leg and tuck the toes between the calf and thigh, bringing the heel of the outside foot to the yoni with the heel pressing against the clitoris. So, when accomplished, this form of siddhasana for women has the inside heel pressing comfortably up in the opening of the yoni, and the outside heel pressing comfortably against the clitoris. It is a very stimulating seat for doing advanced yoga practices. As with all advanced yoga practices, it takes some getting used to, and gradually settles in to be a steady and normal way of doing pranayama, meditation and the other advanced yoga practices. The result will be much more ecstatic energy moving up through the nervous system during and long after sitting practices. In time, all of life is illuminated by the ecstatic energies taking up permanent residence in the nervous system.

The second part of this siddhasana for women involving the outer leg and bringing the heel to rest effortlessly against the clitoris may not be easily performed by everyone. If it is too difficult, it is okay to leave the outer foot down with the toes tucked under the shin, while keeping the inner heel underneath at the opening of the yoni, as instructed. In this case, the yoni can be cupped with one hand during sitting practices, letting the appropriate fingers rest on the clitoris. This is not for active masturbation. It is just a gentle resting of the hand and fingers in such a way so as to provide some steady, mostly unmoving, stimulation. We want the attention to be free for pranayama and meditation, so if having the hand there is too distracting, then back off with it a bit. The stimulation is not for masturbation for its own sake. It is to support the cultivation of sexual energy for sitting practices. In time, the gentle preorgasmic stimulation will become normal in practices, whether the hand and the heel are used, or both heels.

Women who find it difficult to reach either the yoni opening or clitoris with their heels may choose to use prosthetic objects to achieve the same effects. It is perfectly okay and is valid yoga, as long as the principle of ongoing preorgasmic stimulation during sitting practices is achieved. So, if the legs do not fold well, or the heels do not reach, the effects of advanced siddhasana can still be achieved sitting in a chair, or anywhere, if the appropriate stimulating objects are used. The same goes for men, of course.

For men, the advanced siddhasana is similar. The inside heel is brought forward to rest comfortably in the soft place just behind the pubic bone where the urethra comes out. Anatomically, it is analogous to where the opening of the woman's yoni is. As the heel presses comfortably up into the soft area a direct stimulation of the inner energies is experienced. This is also where the heel can easily be used to block ejaculation by leaning forward on it. Once preorgasmic stimulation in siddhasana becomes stable, the blocking is not necessary. In some schools of yoga, siddhasana is taught as a tool to prevent erection. This requires a lot of pressure sustained in siddhasana, squeezing the root of the lingam against the back of the pubic bone, sometimes for extended periods. This is not recommended in these lessons. We always strive for comfortable, pleasurable practice. It is not necessary to try and strangle external expressions of sex that come up during practices. In these lessons, siddhasana is always used in a natural and healthy way to gently coax the ecstatic energies upward.

Erections will come and go during sitting practices, with or without siddhasana. As the nervous system becomes accustomed to cultivating sexual energy upward during yoga practices, external arousal and erections become less and less. This settling down of genital arousal and erection in yoga is not at the expense of our sexual relations at other times. It is just a different mode of sexual functioning that happens in sitting practices, where the energy is going up instead of down, so the genital energy turns in and up in that case. Then when it is time for sexual relations, the genitals will naturally turn outward. So we find our sexuality can go in one direction or the other. Of course, in full-blown tantric sexual relations, the sexual function is going both outward and inward at the same time, with the key process being the preorgasmic cultivation during sexual relations. That is what keeps sex in the realm of yoga. As soon as sex is primarily for the goal of genital orgasm, it is not tantric anymore. It is the conscious goal of preorgasmic cultivation (brahmacharya) that makes sex yogic.

There is also a second part to the advanced siddhasana for men. The toes of the outer foot are brought from under the shin of the inner leg up between the calf and thigh (or the foot can be put on top of the thigh by men who are used to doing padmasana). The heel of the outer foot is then brought to rest snuggly over the genitals in such a way that the genitals are held comfortably between the inner and outer foot. As with the outer foot maneuver for woman, this may not be easy for some men to accomplish in an effortless and comfortable way. If this is the case, then it is okay to leave the outer foot down with toes tucked under the shin, and use the hand to cup the genitals. This instruction was given a few lessons ago (#T24), and is being repeated now for those who have difficulty positioning the outer foot. Using the hand is just as effective (maybe more so) than using the foot, so there is no shortcoming here. The same goes for women using their hand instead of their foot. The idea is for steady preorgasmic stimulation with minimal movement in premasturbation mode. Siddhasana is a seat we want to be in without any attention required on it. This frees our attention to do pranayama and meditation, while effortlessly being sexually stimulated preorgasmically at the same time.

As was mentioned in the main lessons, either foot can be used for going under to the perineum, and the feet can be switched mid-routine if it helps to maintain comfort. Do not remain in siddhasana if it is uncomfortable to the point of distracting pranayama and meditation. If it is too sexually stimulating, then back off and give sexual stimulation a rest also. We can always come back later and resume. It is a process of developing familiarity. Along with familiarity comes an increasing ability to cultivate lasting ecstasy from head to toe. It will happen over a period of weeks, months and years.

Using advanced siddhasana in sitting practices will gradually change our relationship with our sexual energy to be much healthier. As our obsession with orgasm becomes less, we find ourselves more and more in a delightful relationship with our divine ecstatic energies. This change will not do away with our desire or ability to engage in normal sexual relations. Rather, siddhasana will expand our ability to have sexual relations that are more loving, much longer, and more spiritually regenerative. If we choose to engage in tantric sex, we will find that our ability to do it successfully will be enhanced because we have been using siddhasana for so many months and years in sitting practices. Our sex life will be naturally expanded into the spiritual dimension, and we will be walking around with divine ecstasy permanently caressing us inside.

This is the essential role of sex in yoga, and in our ongoing journey toward experiencing enlightenment in everyday life. And this is the reason for doing advanced siddhasana with our sitting practices.

The guru is in you.

Addition – This is a follow-up Q&A on advanced siddhasana:

Q: A quick question about Siddhasana: I had thought that the male spot you were speaking of to place the heel (in an earlier lesson) was against the perineum, but after reading Lesson T28, I am confused.

It sounds like you may be talking about the space between the base of the penis and the top of the scrotum instead of the perineum. If you could clarify this, I would appreciate it greatly, as I want to be certain about the placement before continuing.

Thanking you in advance

A: Yes, the perineum is the place where the heel (or substitute object) should go in siddhasana. In tantra lesson #T28, the instruction is to come a bit forward on the perineum, closer to the root of the lingam, but still behind where it goes up behind the pubic bone. So this is not on the lingam or scrotum. It is under and behind. Coming forward, closer to the lingam root, up into the soft area right behind it, increases the stimulation in siddhasana. This is analogous to the instruction for advanced siddhasana for women, where the heel goes into the opening of the yoni. It is the same location for both sexes, the soft area right behind the pubic bone.

The outside foot is brought up over the lingam with the outside heel resting lightly on top so the lingam and scrotum are between our two feet.

Please note the part in tantra lesson #T28 about not choking off the lingam excessively, allowing erections if they come up, and so on. We aren't moving forward with the heel to choke off the lingam (this is taught in some schools, but not in AYP). We are doing it to increase stimulation upward. Over time, this increased stimulation transforms from erotic to ecstatic energy going up and blending with our inner silence (pure bliss consciousness). You can review main lesson #235 for more on this blending process.

I wish you all success on your chosen spiritual path.

Lesson T29 – Sleeping Lingam

Q1: About Siddhasana, I was actually thinking I was doing well – the sitting didn't disturb my concentration at all. However, an unpleasant incident occurred this morning:

I was sitting in siddhasana during meditation and pranayama, as you instructed – heel at the soft spot of the perineum, not too much pressure applied, pressing mainly up into the perineum. As usual, It didn't feel too awkward, or stimulated. Then, when I ended the session, I had quite a bizarre feeling. I realized that my lingam was completely numb! Touching it, I didn't feel any sensation at all. Rather horrified, I immediately got up and started walking hectically around the room (looking back at it from a few hour's distance, it all seems quite comical, but it was definitely scary at the time). After about a minute I started to gradually feel it again. Now it still feels a bit weird, but I guess it should eventually be okay.

Obviously, I was doing something wrong, somehow cutting the blood supply to the area. Could you advise what had it possibly been, and how may it be avoided in the future?

A1: The numbness is from having the heel resting too firmly against the root of the lingam compressing it against the back of the pubic bone, putting it to sleep. It isn't harmful. Just back up the heel a little on the perineum and it won't happen. More austere versions of siddhasana go for this all the time, killing any chance of erection during yoga. It isn't necessary. This was discussed in the last lesson on advanced siddhasana.

Q2: About putting the lingam to sleep – are you certain it is not harmful? I do know that when an large pressure is applied on a certain nerve for a long period of time, it may eventually lead to its corruption. I realize that in your recommended form of siddhasana, the pressure isn't very severe. Still, I don't know how I may monitor it during practice. I considered trying to get used to the traditional, "complete" siddhasana pose – in which the body appears to be more static and stable (not dependent on varying levels of back support and leaning back). Do you recommend it?

A2: The lingam falling asleep is not more harmful than any other limb falling asleep. Anyway, I don't recommend you sit in such a way that it happens, and more formal versions of siddhasana without back support, etc., may do that. If you are asking me if it is okay to undergo physical effects from a way of sitting that I do not recommend, there is not much I can say. Neither the numbing effect, nor the formal way of sitting, have much to do with our approach in the lessons.

The advantage of using back support is that we can more easily regulate both the angle and pressure of the heel at the perineum by sharing our weight with the pillow behind us. It is easy to get the right effect of siddhasana this way while maintaining comfort, so our attention can go to spinal breathing and meditation. This goes for both men and women.

If you want to go with formal siddhasana, that's fine, but I am not necessarily the right one to ask about it. For whatever it is worth, I think formal siddhasana is not harmful. I did it for many years myself with no ill effects. But, along the way, I found that the same results could be achieved without the extra effort, so I am for informal practice of siddhasana, especially with so many people needing to learn it for their rapidly advancing yoga these days. Siddhasana is excellent tantra, so let's keep it as easy as possible for everyone.

The more preoccupied we are about things like that, the less attention we have for the very important core practices of meditation and spinal breathing. These require our attention. Siddhasana should not require any attention at all, once comfortably established. It is good to keep the priorities straight. I know you are in the formative stages, and are detail oriented. Still, try and be as easy about all this as possible. There are many more practices to come after siddhasana, and none of them has to be done perfectly. It is the basic principles we wish to take advantage of, without knocking ourselves out. This is supposed to be fun!

You are doing very well, and your feedback is appreciated. Keep going. Your persistence assures your success in yoga.

The guru is in you.

Lesson T30* – Vajroli Mudra

Q1: I have a question on a mudra – vajroli mudra with mastery of retrograde ejaculation. Could you provide some light on how this mudra can be practiced?

A1: Vajroli mudra, the drawing in of the sexual fluids, is one of those practices that occurs naturally through the connectedness of yoga as one progresses in siddhasana and tantric sexual practices. This is not to say that you could not work on developing it at any time. However, it is only useful once inner silence and ecstatic conductivity have come up to be resident in our nervous system. That is when sexual energy has its greatest spiritual effect in the body. The blocking method given here in the tantra lessons is a "poor man's" version of vajroli, and is a lot easier to do from day one. As the nervous system purifies and opens, blocking leads naturally to full vajroli.

Q2: You mention that with the continued practice of siddhasana, vajroli naturally happens. Has this happened in your experience?

Also, in vajroli, the effort is in drawing back the sexual fluids into the bladder, which is promptly thrown out when urinating. So what really is the point in vajroli if there is no sublimation of the sexual fluids to the brain (this question applies to the poor man's vajroli that you have described).

I have attained some success in vajroli – I do not need to press the perineum for blocking when asvini, mulabandha and uddiyana are simultaneously done with slow breathing. It has the same effect as pressing the perineum. But in both these cases, the seminal fluid promptly goes into the urinary bladder. I can feed the drain of ojas as soon as this happens. How can we truly sublimate the sex energy rather than let it drain out eventually.

A2: Real vajroli is not only about retaining semen during ejaculation, though this is what gets all the press coverage. With inner silence and ecstatic conductivity (kundalini) coming up in the nervous system, there is a constant release of semen at the root, and constant absorption up into the bladder, and beyond. Then inner lovemaking never stops. The bladder has a higher function, which is processing the energy upward into the higher neuro-biology. This was covered in lesson #T11 also. Spiritual biology happens in the GI (gastrointestinal) tract also, and is very noticeable once kundalini is moving significantly – a mixing of air, food and sexual essences. It can be traced from the GI tract up into the head, and back down into the GI tract again in the form of nectar.

Yes, I have vajroli of that natural ongoing variety, and also to a large degree during ejaculation, though I still use some blocking to aid it when necessary. The main thing is that the flow of sexual energy is being drawn up constantly, 24/7, and this is best stimulated by long term daily practice of the full range of advanced yoga practices. (24/7 means 24 hours per day, 7 days per week)

Just as we continue to evacuate the bowels even as the spiritual biology is actively going on in the GI tract, so too do we continue to urinate even as the spiritual biology is going on in the bladder. Once the higher spiritual biology is established and stable, these functions become very strong and unshakable. Then there is not so much worry about performances like vajroli. Like with siddhasana, the mechanics of vajroli practice fade into the ongoing functioning of our spiritual biology, and we don't give it much thought once that stage is reached. We are off into ecstatic bliss and divine love bubbling out by then. That is how we are illuminated by sexual energy coming up inside.

Undoubtedly it is better to be having a constant, steady feed of sexual essence going up into the higher biology that is little affected by urination, than to have a large infusion from a recovered ejaculation, by either blocking or vajroli, which is then mostly lost in the next urination. Hence the rationale for developing preorgasmic and holdback-style tantric practices which stimulate the long term upward cultivation of sexual energy as a natural ongoing neuro-biological function.

All of this applies to women also, with the mechanics being nearly the same.

The guru is in you.

Addition – And another question on vajroli:

Q: I will be going to India this January, as I do each year. Can you recommend any places where I could get reputable training in vajroli mudra? It is to be done under guidance, as I am sure you would agree.

A: I don't know any place you can go specifically for vajroli training. Most of the traditions are such that coming in for training on a specific item like that is not in the cards. The expectation is that one should be a dedicated disciple for some time before receiving techniques – and then in the prescribed order over a long period of time.

As you know, AYP is a departure from that. I don't agree that such things must be learned according to external discipleship or a schedule, or even necessarily be learned under close supervision, though it certainly wouldn't hurt if it were available. It is the spiritual evolution of the human nervous system we are talking about here. What human being should be in charge of that? The aspirant! With strong bhakti, some clear instructions, and good common sense, just about any spiritual technique can be mastered by the practitioner well enough to achieve good results. With regular practice, nature will take care of the rest.

In the case of vajroli, it is not a discrete training event. It is part of a natural evolution toward brahmacharya (not necessarily of the celibate variety – see lesson #T9 on that). The occurrence of vajroli has more to do with bhakti and the rise of ecstatic conductivity than a lesson we might get on it. You obviously have bhakti for this. If you are regular in your practices, including mulabandha/asvini, uddiyana/nauli and siddhasana, you will be well on your way to natural vajroli. If you have been moved to engage in blocking of ejaculation by the method in the lessons (#T5), you will be even closer. Of course, meditation and spinal breathing come before these physical methods. All of these things are prerequisites to vajroli. It is a natural progression.

Just a reminder – vajroli is not mainly about recovering semen during or after orgasm. If our motivation for learning vajroli is to prevent the loss of semen during lovemaking, then our purpose will be far better served by learning the holdback method, which not only preserves semen, but cultivates lasting ecstatic bliss in both partners as well.

Vajroli is about constant, automatic absorption of sexual essences up into the bladder and the surrounding neuro-biology. For those with ecstatic conductivity (kundalini) in full swing, vajroli is a 24-hour process that is hardly noticed. In that situation, the practitioner is experiencing "constant coming" (next lesson). Wishing you success on your path. Follow your bhakti, and enjoy!

Lesson T31 – Constant Coming

Q: What you say makes sense and in true essence, it is the ojas that we take up derived from the muladhara fire.

But it does happen especially when we are fully perched above at the third eye, and as our body is played as a divine instrument. The "orgasmic" waves are brought upward and centered into the third eye ... the muladhara climbs up ... and then when we come ... the whole body resonates and, surprisingly, sperm does not come out. The process also requires us to roll our tongue as a straw and suck up the pleasure with every inhale and closing our eyes, guide it to the third eye.

A: Thank you for your clear perspective on vajroli, and root to third eye orgasm. I agree, true vajroli (upward absorption of sexual fluids), beyond the managed mechanical technique of it, is an automatic part of a much bigger process that involves the third eye to root connection. I call it ecstatic conductivity. You call it the muladhara (root) climbing up to the third eye. That is an interesting description you give, because one of the observations we have in spinal bastrika, where attention and breath are rapidly oscillating between the third eye and root, is that the third eye and root "merge" into one. This merging of root and third eye is what is occurring in slow spinal breathing as well, though it may be less noticed in the early stages. This is the ecstatic connection being cultivated between the root and third eye, just as you have described.

There is another element we can observe, and that is the phenomenon of the change that occurs in "coming." In sex, "coming" is orgasm, both before and after the vajroli effect naturally joins into the spiritual-sexual equation. With rising ecstatic conductivity between the root and third eye, the event of "coming" into the third eye you describe creeps into our life as an ongoing experience. In other words, "coming" or "orgasm" becomes an ongoing whole-body event that never stops, and requires no external stimulation. A mere raising of the eyes, an entering into kechari, or a small flex at the root will keep waves of ecstasy coursing through the nervous system like a rolling sea. And that isn't all. Over time, the whole process migrates upward from the third eye to the crown as well. That process of opening the crown with stability is covered in the main lessons (see "crown opening" in topic index, and lesson #199 especially).

Can "coming" be sustained like this? Can we continue to function under the influence of constant whole-body orgasm? Is it exhausting?

In fact, this ongoing experience of "coming" is the fruition of yoga, the rise of an unending state of ecstatic bliss and divine love in the nervous system. We can continue to function in this situation, because our nervous system acclimates to it, just as it does to all other enhancements in our spiritual neuro-biology that occur with long term practice of yoga.

It is not exhausting. Just the opposite. As divine energy surges through us, it continuously regenerates every cell in our body. In this situation sex has become the source of unbounded energy, creativity and happiness in the body. There is so much divine love surging up inside that it flows out to everyone around us in the form of uplifting energy and loving service.

This is why we pay close attention to the management of sexual energy as we move along our chosen path in yoga.

Does this eliminate the need for sexual relations? It certainly makes us less obsessive about reproductive sex. That is a good thing. At the same time, this transformation turns all sex into spiritual practice. Preorgasmic tantric sex can offer support to the process of spiritual transformation. So, the advances that occur in our nervous system as a result of yoga make sexual activity all the more precious whenever we are inclined to engage in physical lovemaking. Sexual activity then becomes a stepping-stone to permanent ecstatic bliss.

Reproductive sex is not mandatory for enlightenment, but under the right circumstances it can be a significant help.

The guru is in you.

Lesson T32* – Menstruation, Yoga and Amaroli

Q: I have really enjoyed and learned from the wisdom you have passed on in these lessons and the main ones. How blessed we are that you are willing and able to answer so many questions whose answers have evaded us for so long.

I am wondering if you know about a tantric or yoga practice that a woman can use to minimize or temporarily eliminate menstruation. I have read in several sources that women have practiced the Taoist microcosmic orbit to do so and have thereby prevented the energy loss that comes with menstruation. If you know of such a practice, is there one for celibates?

A: The effectiveness of using the Taoist microcosmic orbit (breathing) for relieving the menstrual cycle may be so, but I can't say for sure. I have not done much with the microcosmic orbit for many years because I moved to yogic spinal breathing methods, which are simple and effective for spiritual transformation. These are the methods in the lessons – spinal breathing and spinal bastrika in particular. These, along with deep meditation and the other practices in the lessons, will gradually expand the sexual function upward in the nervous system, including an upward shift in energy flows in the menstrual cycle.

Another thing to look at that is not in the lessons so far is "amaroli," which is urine therapy. Some good health benefits can be achieved with it, including normalizing difficulties with menstruation. You can do some web searches on amaroli and find a lot of good information. You can also find some links on amaroli in the AYP links section on the web site. I wish you all success on your chosen spiritual path.

The guru is in you.

Addition – Here is a Q&A which expands on the subject of amaroli:

Q: Being a long time yogi, I have found your writings to be first class. Yet, if the lessons are truly "advanced," why haven't you gone into more detail on amaroli? I not only owe much of my spiritual progress to amaroli, but my good health as well. If there ever was a place to be sharing about the spiritual benefits of this little-appreciated practice, it is in the AYP lessons. What do you say?

A: Admittedly, the lessons have held back, so far, on going deeper into amaroli. Why? Stigma. You are right. It should be covered in more depth. It is only fair, because I too have been benefiting from this practice for quite some time. We have taken on some controversial practices in these lessons – siddhasana, kechari, kumbhaka, tantric sexual practices and so on – and hopefully unveiled the essential principles and practices sufficiently so that anyone can put them to good use in their yoga routine. Amaroli is in a class by itself, because it straddles a great paradox.

On one hand, amaroli walks headlong into one of the great negative stigmas of Western society – the revulsion so many have at the thought of drinking their own urine. It is not such a stigma in the Far East, as practice and knowledge of the benefits of amaroli have been around for thousands of years. Even so, it is easy nowadays to find Western-educated Far Easterners who have developed the same aversion.

On the other hand, amaroli has been proven clinically to have tremendous health benefits, and is perhaps one of the greatest healing tonics of all time. So much so that the pharmaceutical companies are, in some cases, selling back to us in pill form what we could have gotten at a higher quality for free in the privacy of our own bathroom. Shhhh … that is an industry trade secret.

The truth is that daily urine therapy is one of the best things any of us can do as a preventive measure to ward off disease, and heal faster if we are suffering from just about any malady. Why is this? While it is still not fully understood, it is generally agreed by researchers that urine therapy enhances the presence of hundreds (or possibly thousands) of vital elements and compounds in our body, and builds our immune system to a strength beyond what it would be otherwise. Though less understood, amaroli also has been shown to have a purifying effect in the body. All of that is pretty impressive, and we have not even begun to assess the spiritual benefits yet. So what about the spiritual benefits? Let's work into it a step at a time.

It is notable that amaroli comes to us from ancient sources, not primarily because of its medicinal value, but for its value as a spiritual practice. The 500 year-old *Hatha Yoga Pradipika*, a comprehensive scripture on yoga, covers amaroli. A 5,000 year-old scripture called the *Damar Tantra* contains much detail on amaroli. In both of these, the goal of amaroli practice includes cultivating physical wellbeing, but reaches far beyond it, out into the realm of enlightenment. How can our daily experience of life be changed by practicing amaroli? Is it worth trying to overcome our long-held revulsion for such things? You bet.

If we get up the courage to try, we will be wise to start small and build up. Isn't that how it is with most things in life, including our yoga practices? A full daily dose of urine is considered to be a glass full, or about 6-8 ounces. But we can start with a few drops, mixed with some water in a glass, if we need to do that. When we engage in amaroli practice, the guideline is to do it first thing in the morning, whenever that is for you. When collecting urine, catch it "midstream," which means after it starts and before it ends. As with many things, the first time will be the most daunting, even mixed with water. Take my word for it, it won't kill you. Down the hatch!

Still there? Good. Not so bad, was it? If you do this in the shower and/or right before doing your oral hygiene in the morning, there will not be a trace of any odor or anything by the time you leave the bathroom. Not that you will mind much after a few weeks. It is an acquired taste, and is soon not offensive to the practitioner. But your mother-in-law might notice something if you give her a big kiss right after doing amaroli, if you have not brushed your teeth or had a glass of juice or something first. After a few days, you may be surprised to find that this is much easier than you thought it would be. It is really a breeze to do once the psychological barrier is broken. It's much easier than siddhasana or kechari, and definitely easier than learning tantric sex. It is a relatively quick journey from a few drops to a couple of swallows. Before you know it, the glass will be practically full, and disappearing back into you again. That's daily amaroli practice. There isn't much more to it than that – except time. The longer we are doing it as a daily practice, the more the benefits accumulate.

It is not necessary to be drinking a full glass of urine every morning. In fact, it could be undesirable at certain times, or for certain people. There are several factors that could vary the dose. One is the quantity available. Another is the quality. If we have been eating heavily seasoned, salted, or fatty foods, the urine will not be so good, both to the taste and in its effect. Our old friend, "self-pacing" will get into the act also. If we are doing too much amaroli, we can have symptoms similar to those experienced when we do too much of any advanced yoga practice – too many impurities coming out of the nervous system at once due to excessive purification going on inside. If we are any feeling discomfort related to amaroli, then we know we should back off until things smooth out. We all know how to do that by now, right? We don't do practices at a level that makes us feel uncomfortable. Amaroli is no different than other yoga practices in this respect. So, if a full glass is proving to be too much, then try half a glass. If that is too much, start measuring swallows, and zero in on the right dose for yourself. It may be very little for some people, and more for others. Everyone is different. You won't find out what it is for you until you get into it. In all of yoga, finding a balance between practices and our daily activities is an important part of the process. Fortunately, once we have been on the path of yoga for a while, the right guidance always seems to come. Be flexible in that regard.

Once we have been doing amaroli for a couple of weeks, we may notice something happening. Somehow we feel stronger inside – like some weak spaces inside us have been filled in. "Inwardly robust" is a phrase that comes to mind. We may not have noticed the weak spaces inside before, but we can feel that something has been filled in. That we will feel healthier goes without saying. Yes, definitely healthier. But there is something more, something beyond the feeling of a stronger, more stable physical presence. We can feel our awareness becoming more stable also. One way to understand it is to think of our body and nervous system as the vehicle of our consciousness. When we strengthen the quality of our body and nervous system on the most subtle level of physicality, on the cellular level, we come to find ourselves living in a stronger and more reliable vehicle for our conscious self.

When we sit to do practices, this gradual change in us that is being brought about by amaroli is noticeable also. The quality of our inner silence in meditation deepens and expands. The ecstatic energies we cultivate in spinal breathing, kumbhaka and related practices, become more lively and luminous. The whole thing goes up a few notches with amaroli added into the daily schedule. And it keeps getting better, you know. As with the rest of our yoga, the effects of amaroli are cumulative, going ever deeper experientially over the months and years of our daily practice.

What is it that sets the condition for enlightenment in the human being? We have often said that it is a neuro-biological change involving our nervous system and the overall biological functioning inside us. In other words, a primary prerequisite for enlightenment is raising the inner functioning of the human body to a much higher level. Then our vehicle of consciousness becomes capable of extraordinary expressions of the divine possibilities that lie within us all. Bringing this change about is the purpose of yoga. We work systematically with our mind, our body, our emotions, our breath, and our sexuality to accomplish this transformation. With amaroli, we are enhancing the chemical composition of our body on the most refined level, right down to the atoms and molecules. This creates a physiological foundation that adds an advantage as we engage in all of the other advanced yoga practices that propel us along our road to enlightenment.

And, of course, we enjoy the benefits of our yoga practices in daily living every step along the way. That is the role of amaroli.

Lesson T33 – Spinal Breathing during Tantric Sex?

Q: There is a vama (left-handed) form of kriya that is practiced during copulation, called cobra breath, which has 4 stages of practice. This appears to be a fast-track method of the regular kriya, with rapid benefits. Yet in these lessons you have told us to practice the spinal breath outside of tantra practice. But if spinal breath can be done during tantra practices with immense benefits, then why have you not recommended spinal breath with sexual practices?

A: Obviously, it is possible to do spinal breathing during tantric sex. There are several reasons why we have not jumped into it before now. The reasons have been touched on in the lessons.

First, sexual relations do not lend themselves to being done by the clock – not at a certain time twice each day, and not every day without fail.

Second, sexual relations do not lend themselves to being regulated in duration – so many minutes of this practice and so many minutes of that practice.

Third, combining sitting practices with tantric sex can lead to additional releases of obstructions that must be regulated in some way so as not to become excessive.

Fourth, the occurrence of sexual relations is most easily left to serendipity, which is how it naturally happens. This is not in sync with any of the above, but can be overridden by the discipline of mutually dedicated practitioners.

The time-related matters are of great importance in yoga. Without regularity and correct measurement of practices, yoga can quickly fly out of control, and quite a few people in the main lessons have commented in the Q&As on aspects of experience from sitting practices related to this. In fact, most of the Q&As are about pacing practices to accommodate experiences. It can be a tricky business to keep balance in advanced yoga practices. For this reason, using sexual relations as a primary means for yoga is like trying to row a small boat across the ocean in a hurricane.

Does this mean spinal breathing should not be done in sexual relations? No, it doesn't mean that. It means that it should not be considered to be primary practice, which, in the main lessons, is measured by the clock, twice-daily before breakfast and dinner.

If we engage in sexual relations, whenever that happens to be, then we can consider using spinal breathing, or, for that matter, any other practice we have discussed in the main lessons. I'm sure many have thought about this already, as you have. There are a lot of practices to choose from. But there is a challenge, you know, and that is the matter of the possibility of stimulating excessive release of obstructions in the nervous system.

We will know it has happened by how we feel later on after sexual relations that have been blended with spinal breathing or other practices.

Being in sexual union during spinal breathing is powerful indeed. But power does not translate immediately into progress. After all, we have huge power available already in our sitting practices, if we could only absorb and use it all. But we can only go as fast as our nervous system can accommodate the release of obstructions, and therein lies the limiting factor. There is no limit on power in these practices, with or without sexual union. So, again, it gets back to regulation of practices through self-pacing.

The same thing applies in tantric sex, though not so much in using the holdback method to facilitate long preorgasmic unions. This does not usually lead to excessive releases – just more and more ecstatic bliss, which stays with us even as we enter our sitting practices later on. This is why the focus in the tantra lessons has been on holdback and long preorgasmic unions. It does not usually cause imbalances in our internal energies, and sets up our nervous system for wonderful sitting practices later on, the next day, or whenever our sitting practice time arrives. This is the real payoff that comes from tantric sexual union, and only long preorgasmic unions are necessary to produce it. There is a lot to be said for doing tantric sex and sitting practices separately, rather than at the same time.

With spinal breathing added to sexual relations, there will be additional release of inner obstructions in the nervous system, and you will find a need to regulate the practice to avoid the excesses that can happen. This is a bit tricky when in the throes of lovemaking, unless two people are so in tune that they can sit in union face to face, propped up with pillows in a "V" formation (or other semi-vertical position), doing spinal breathing for 5, 10 or 15 minutes. It doesn't sound very romantic, does it? Well, to let it go on and on could lead to too much release for one or both partners, and much crabbiness later on after the lovemaking is over. Try it and see. Powerful spiritual practices are powerful spiritual practices no matter when they are done.

So, do you see why we have not gotten into this before? It leaves the door open for complications and potential difficulties. In the lessons we want to stick with approaches that are simple with minimal difficulties, while at the same time very effective for purifying and opening the nervous system to divine experience.

So, instead, what we do is bring sexual stimulation gradually into our sitting practices in a measured way using siddhasana, mulabandha and sambhavi (very sexy with ecstatic conductivity). Practices such as nauli/uddiyana, chin pump and spinal bastrika become quite sexual in the middle to later stages also. All of this we can regulate within our sitting practices. There can also be good regulation when combining practices with masturbation. But even that can get out of hand, leaving us crabby and with a headache. It is all in the measuring. If we do too much we can be stymied and uncomfortable for a while as the energy excess and imbalance corrects itself. Yoga practice is about releasing obstructions in a way that we can continue day by day over the long run, with ecstatic bliss gradually building up and overflowing into our daily activity.

If you have a partner you can work with in a measured way during sexual intercourse, you may be able to self-pace additional practices during lovemaking with smooth results. If so, then by all means go for it. But be mindful that lovemaking is a serendipity event, a nice extra boost on the path of yoga at best, and it is wise to always regard daily sitting practices as the primary yoga.

If we can handle the huge extra energy generated by combining spinal breathing, kechari, chin pump, spinal bastrika or yoni mudra kumbhaka with preorgasmic sexual relations, it can be a good boost. On the other hand, it can end up fizzling for the reasons mentioned above. Experiment and see what happens. And then – apply self-pacing.

Or, just enjoy long preorgasmic sex with your lover whenever it happens, and be assured that the ocean of ecstatic bliss you both have gained will still be available when you sit on your respective meditation cushions for twice-daily practices.

The guru is in you.

Lesson T34* – Kechari and the "Secret Spot"

Q: I have finally made it above the soft palate ... thanks as always for your support.

It's funny how kechari is so couched in sexuality. I was going to say "sexual metaphor," but really, it is quite literally sexuality. The tongue and pharynx resemble lingam and yoni, only here we're all complete with both genders. Then there are the erectile tissues in the nasal passages...

I feel as though I've lost my virginity again. It wasn't really as much fun as the first time, but I'm willing to give it a chance.

A: Congratulations on your entry into stage 2 kechari! You've just crossed a major milestone on your journey in yoga.

The sexual metaphor is appropriate. Kechari is directly tied in with higher sexuality, just as sambhavi and all the other mudras and bandhas are. All of these link directly into our sexual neurobiology in the pelvic region, expanding its function upward throughout the body, and beyond.

While "losing virginity" with kechari may not be as much fun as losing it the other way, kechari makes up for it in the long run. As ecstatic conductivity rises, we eventually end up in a kind of constant simmering whole body orgasm. Then all of these yoga mudras are functioning naturally in reflexive coordination. See lesson #212, "Whole Body Mudra."

Kechari is both mysterious and conspicuous in its role in cultivating higher ecstatic experiences. Part of this is because it is a "new place" where the vast majority of human beings have not been yet, even though getting into it is just a centimeter or two away from the everyday travels of our tongue. The means for entering it are controversial, at least in these times of little (but increasing) understanding of kechari. It is likely that many will be going there in the coming years.

Why?

Up in the cavity of the nasal pharynx, within easy reach of an inquiring and liberated tongue, is an organ that is erogenous on a level similar to the genitals. "Spiritually erogenous" is a good qualifier for that, as kechari stimulates ecstatic/sexual energy upward in the body, while the genitals, if not brought into tantric preorgasmic practice mode, will lead our energy out to serve the reproductive function.

Let's call the spiritually erogenous focal point up there in the nasal pharynx, the "secret spot," since we have known so little about it before now.

Once the word gets out, the erogenous aspects of kechari alone will draw the pleasure-seeking masses to it. And why not? Who would have babies if it were not so enjoyable to make them? Should becoming enlightened be less enjoyable? When the spiritual path becomes widely known for what it really is, a constant internal orgy of radiating ecstatic bliss, then the roads to enlightenment will be crammed full with practitioners, just as the roads to reproductive sexual experience are crammed full now. Interestingly, the two roads intersect, right here in the world of tantra, which is why this lesson is being posted here instead of in the main lessons. It is time to let our hair down a little on the subject of kechari.

So what is this secret spot?

In main lesson #108 on kechari, the edge of the nasal septum was described as being "ecstatically sensitive." It was also called an "altar of bliss." Here in the tantra lessons we call it "spiritually erogenous." With all of these descriptions, it should be clear that there is something special going on with the septum in kechari practice.

The septum is the flat, thick membrane that divides our left and right nostrils. The back edge of it runs up the middle of the front of the cavity above our soft palate called the nasal pharynx. When the tongue finds its way up into the nasal pharynx, it also finds the edge of the nasal septum. About half way up the edge of the septum is a small protrusion, a small bulge. It is extremely sensitive. That is the "secret spot."

As with our regular sexual anatomy, there is a lot more going on in the nasal pharynx, inner nostrils, etc., than at that one spot on the edge of the septum. But the secret spot is a neurological focal point, much as the clitoris is for a woman, or the head of the lingam for a man. The secret spot is like that. But there are some fundamental differences between the secret spot and our genitals.

First, unlike with the unconditioned genitals (though they too can be made spiritually ecstatic through tantric practices), it takes stimulation over time to fully awaken the secret spot. The length of time will depend on our overall progress in purifying and opening our nervous system using the full range of yoga practices we have available. The rise in ecstatic conductivity in the nervous system greatly increases the sensitivity of the secret spot. Kechari practice itself is a stimulator of ecstatic conductivity throughout the body, and the rise in sensitivity of the secret spot is an effect of this. Cause leading to effect, and effect leading to cause. The more the secret spot is stimulated, the more sensitive it becomes, along with the increasing ecstatic response throughout the entire nervous system. On it goes, without limit! This rise in ecstatic response is an important part of the road to unending ecstatic bliss in the body, which radiates outward to saturate the surrounding environment with divine love. So, there are good incentives to develop the capability to practice kechari throughout our sitting practices, and longer. It is a primary way to cultivate endless inner pleasure, and at the same time a way to cultivate worldwide illumination. This is why kechari has been called "a giant leap for humankind."

Second, unlike with reproductive sex, kechari and stimulation of the secret spot does not lead inevitably to reproductive genital orgasm. While the secret spot becomes highly erogenous over time, it is a different kind of sensitivity. That is why the term "spiritually erogenous" is used. The stimulation in kechari of the secret spot touches all of our erogenous areas from the inside, luring our passion inward and upward to the main pleasure centers in the brain. Imagine being sexually stimulated from the inside. Being highly aroused with no external stimulation to speak of at all, and having all that pleasure rising up through the body in waves, culminating in the pleasure centers of the brain, and then undulating back down to the end of every nerve. What are these pleasure centers in the brain? They are components of the third eye, the ajna, which occupy a region including the medulla oblongata (brain stem), pituitary and pineal glands, and the surrounding nerves. The influence spreads naturally to the crown (corona radiata) also. All of these participate in the ecstatic processes rising in the nervous system.

So, with kechari, combined with sambhavi (the powerful third eye technique), the other mudras and bandhas, and siddhasana, we are engaging in a powerful inner lovemaking. Combine all of that with the underlying influences produced in daily deep meditation and spinal breathing techniques, and we have a formula for cultivating endless ecstatic bliss and outpouring divine love – enlightenment!

When we are meditating, kechari can be done quietly with the tongue resting gently on the secret spot. At other times, we may be inspired to actively stimulate the secret spot with various movements of the tongue. Here the sexual analogy becomes very close, and probably not much advice is needed. We each have our own ways of achieving maximum stimulation. Kechari offers this opportunity as well. But, as with using external sexual stimulation in sitting practices, we want to be careful not to totally disrupt our routine. So "dynamic kechari" should be reserved for times when it will not distract our deep meditation. There is no reason why kechari cannot be dynamic during spinal breathing, as long as we continue to travel the spinal nerve with our attention. It can also work well with spinal bastrika, targeted bastrika, yoni mudra, and even in tantric sex, or at any other time we are not engaged in deep meditation, samyama, or other activity where our attention is being delicately applied. It is at the practitioner's discretion.

As with any advanced yoga practice, self-pacing should be applied when the energy flows associated with kechari become excessive.

In the early stages of kechari, beginning active stimulation of the secret spot, we will likely become sexually aroused. Later, it will not happen much externally, and we will be lit up with ecstasy inside. That is how it goes. As we carry on with our internal lovemaking, joyful pleasure will be pulled up from within our genitals, and from every erogenous zone in our nervous system. Then we will shiver with joy as the waves undulate up and at the same time back down through every cell in our body. We may be covered with goose bums, cry out with ecstasy, dance around like a whirling dervish, or whatever the energy moves us to do. It is an unending inner orgasm! Meanwhile, palpable waves of love will be shooting out of us, uplifting everyone in the neighborhood. That is a pretty good use for our sexual energy. Just as good as making babies. We can do both if we want. It is making the most of all that we have in us.

Lovemaking is the joining of the two polarities of life to fulfill the purpose of creation. It happens automatically externally, and that leads to reproduction. With conscious participation, it can be cultivated to happen automatically internally, and that leads to enlightenment.

The guru is in you.

Addition – There are two follow-up Q&As here – one from a woman, and one from a man.

First, the woman:

Q: A few days ago, after doing my pranayama and then yoni mudra kumbhaka with the head falling forward to the chest, three times, I then added three rounds of the nadi shodana. Then I did my meditation sitting on my rolled up sock with another ball closer to the front.

While I was doing the nadi shodana, my tongue once again started trying to climb up my nasal cavity. This time, it curled vertically, like a tube as it went up. I think it went further up than it has been before but was only as far as the farthest part of my upper throat where it starts to curve up. (I don't know the anatomical term for the area).

Then, almost immediately after completing the nadi shodana, I went into my meditation. My tongue continued to stretch as far as it could up into my nasal cavity in its tubal shape and then it started to massage a spot somewhere up there in my upper throat or where the roof curves up. I'm sure I was not at the spot that is reached in the advanced stages, but whatever spot I had was unbelievable. As my tongue massaged this spot, I felt it in my clitoris. It was like that spot was directly connected to the clitoris! Normally I'd be embarrassed to write about this but after reading more of your lessons I see that this in nothing to be embarrassed about. The sensation was so ecstatic! After it was all over, I wasn't sure later if I'd had an orgasm but it didn't feel really like an orgasm. In orgasm, you reach a finish line and then it's over and you want to end it. Whereas this didn't have that need to finish, it just went on and on and on and did not seem to have any end that needed to be reached. It was more ecstatic than orgasm. Is this spot always able to produce this if people could get there tongue there, or is it only after practicing yoga that such a result can occur?

I wanted to share that experience, but also to ask if I want to continue the nadi shodana, when should it be done? Though I did it after pranayama and yoni mudra kumbhaka on that one day, I haven't done it that way since. Now I do it at other times rather than my meditation time since the *Hatha Yoga Pradipika* book stated it should be done morning midday and midnight. (I'm only doing three rounds about twice a day.) I wanted to check with you before I did it in that order again with my meditation in case this is wrong. I think I read somewhere in the *Pradipika* book that it should be done to properly do pranayama, which leads me to think it should be done before the spinal breathing. In any case, it did produce some very powerful automatic yoga responses by doing it after the yoni mudra kumbhaka.

Also since starting it outside of my yoga practice, (I'm now at lesson #91), I'm also having some really strong automatic yoga. It almost feels like my body is possessed. Like someone else is moving my body. Sometimes my head makes a full circle of neck rolls from right to left for a while and then the other way. It feels like invisible hands are moving me into various exercises and stretches.

Lastly, each time my tongue tries going up my nasal cavity, it seems it reaches a little further. Is it possible that it will eventually stretch enough by continually trying to move to that spot you wrote about? And how will I know when its there if it does?

Thank you!

A: That's really terrific. You are finding your ecstatic conductivity early on here – further evidence of your previous unremembered work in yoga. Your nervous system remembers.

If you mean by nadi shodana, easy alternate nostril breathing, it is not generally regarded as a high-octane practice, unless combined with kumbhaka, which is not recommended in the lessons because we are applying kumbhaka in other practices, and don't want to complicate things too much. (See the addition to lesson #41 for more on nadi shodana.)

If you just started kumbhaka with yoni mudra (lesson #91), that is the more likely the cause of the big leap you are experiencing. It doesn't take much kumbhaka to move mountains of impurities in the nervous system. Yoni mudra kumbhaka is a very powerful practice, even in small doses. Starting two or more practices in the same time period can cloud the issue of what is doing what, so be careful about that. Make sure you settle in with one practice before taking on another, or you could find yourself exposed to burgeoning energy flows (a la your automatic yogas) and not know what is causing it. Remember self-pacing – it is the most important practice of them all.

On kechari, if your tongue is behind and on top of the soft palate (the soft part of the roof of your mouth in the back), then you may be finding the "secret spot" already. You will know it as being an "edge" – the vertical edge of the back of the nasal septum, which is the divider between the left and right nostrils. The front of the septum is the divider between the left and right nostrils on our outer visible nose.

Another possibility is that you are pressing the soft palate up and forward (like a flap) with your tongue from underneath so it is touching secret spot. Either way the stimulation is there. The sensation of erotic connection to the genitals is the beginning of ecstatic conductivity. At some point it will start to happen with sambhavi also. Then the ecstatic response can be elicited at will, anytime, anywhere.

The degree to which the ecstatic response occurs in kechari is a function of purification in the nervous system, and past work in yoga in particular. It is entirely possible to enter stage 2 kechari, be touching the secret spot, and not have much of a connection to the pelvic region for a long time. It that case, it would gradually evolve over time after entering stage 2 kechari. Each person has a different structure of obstructions in the nervous system, but we are all going in the same direction. It is only a matter of time, because everyone is wired for divine ecstasy.

With regard to the sexual aspect of kechari, it will move on from being a sexual experience as it gradually encompasses the whole nervous system. I call it going from erotic to spiritually ecstatic. From your description, it's clear you are seeing this already. The progress of this is not toward genital orgasm (though it can happen in the beginning). It is toward unending ecstasy in the whole body. This ecstatic condition blends with inner silence cultivated in meditation and samyama, and that combination is unending ecstatic bliss. The later lessons get into the implications of this – not so flashy, really. Life gradually becomes about serving others from within our endless overflowing river of ecstatic bliss. There is nothing more to do but be a channel of divine love. It is total freedom in this life, and beyond.

And now, the man:

Q: In my new experience with stage 3 kechari I have found a sensitive spot just about the nasal septum that feels a bit pulpy and soft and has a higher level of sensitivity and effect on the breath than the other areas. I did get the feeling that it feels somewhat similar to sexual tissue but am not sure what the result of stimulation is. At first I thought it might be possible to have an orgasm of the crown chakra but it feels different than that. I don't really know though. It reminds me of the fact that many women do not realize that a woman can ejaculate when they orgasm until they actually have the experience. Kechari is an exploration that seems to have very few to share and guide in the experience. My suspicion is that even among those who share that many mention it in passing, but very few have tried it, and fewer still have achieved its deeper levels.

Kechari, and particularly keeping the tongue tip on the "secret spot" really makes a change, and that is a wonderful one and will take some time to integrate. It seems to create an automatic lift of the bandhas and I can feel that kechari combined with sambhavi creates a streaming energy sensation that moves from the pelvis to the head without my doing anything but feeling my breathing.

The sensation is that the energy streams up my spine on the inhale but doesn't drop so much on the exhale, or maybe drops towards the belly a bit on the exhale. The streaming energy doesn't actually fall back to the pelvis until I release kechari. So far I am a beginner at this, but since I am experienced at pranayama I suspect that kechari and sambhavi will rapidly transform pranayama as I know it and make the stages of inhale/retention/exhale less physical and distinct, but along with the bandhas, integrate it all much more into an energy flow.

Your help is much appreciated.

A: That sensitive spot on the septum is what I call the "secret spot," and is really at the heart of kechari stimulation. Entering the nasal passages from the inside (kechari stage 4) adds to it significantly, but the secret spot is the focal point, similar to the way the clitoris is for a woman.

Speaking of which, female practitioners have reported that the secret spot is directly connected neurologically with the clitoris. Both women and men who have reached the secret spot have quickly realized that it is not for genital orgasm, though it can happen in the early stages. Neither is it for "sahasrar orgasm," not in the way we think of orgasm being climactic. It is for cultivating the gradual rise of what I call "constant coming," which is the title of one of the other tantra lessons. Constant coming is a permanent state of ecstatic bliss and outpouring divine love – enlightenment.

Your symptoms of the physical experience shifting to an energetic connection between head and pelvic region is a classic birth of the rise of ecstatic conductivity. That is how it happens. From there it just keeps going, and going, and going. And, yes, the kechari secret spot and sambhavi are instrumental in this, and do change the whole nature of pranayama and kumbhaka for the better. Meditation too ... and then it comes back around from all of those practices, re-amplified ecstatically again.

If you let the energy cycle the full range of the spinal nerve from the point between the eyebrows to the perineum with breathing, you will find a much more balanced purification and opening effect over time. That is the essence of spinal breathing. If you are making partial journeys with the energy, or going to the crown instead of brow at this stage, there is the possibility of some kundalini imbalances building up. Clearing the sushumna between the third eye (brow) and root (perineum) is the key to advancing smoothly with ever-expanding ecstatic conductivity. Without the spinal breathing component, it can get kind of messy with too much kundalini energy running around. Spinal breathing takes care of that.

Yes, there are few who have made this transition, but I think many are coming to it in the years ahead. It is too important (and fulfilling!) for serious yogis and yoginis to ignore. I hope that the free and open integration of practices in AYP will help it along. It is about time for all this to come out of the closet, don't you think? It is the destiny of humanity we are talking about here, and there is no time to waste.

Lesson T35 – Ecstatic Reflex during Sex

Q: Thank you very much for your remarkably lucid writings on kechari. It is of tremendous value to me. I have been in stage 1 kechari for many years. The truth is, I never actually knew how to get to stage 2, since I did not know about the "side approach." My tongue seems nearly long enough to get to stage 2 soon and I feel ready. If I had not read your message (main lesson #108), it would have been delayed for some years, since I was going through the middle.

I have a question for you if I may. As I approach sexual orgasm, (during ordinary sexual activity not in any way approached as yogic) I find the instinct to roll my eyes upwards and push the tongue back and up as in kechari. I have followed this instinct on many occasions. I do not know how to describe the affect well, but it seems to integrate the ajna and the sexual impulse. It seems as if the sexual urges become more powerful under ajna control as the result of the practice. It is fulfilling, intense and pleasurable.

Have you any comments on the practice?

A: I am very happy to hear that the kechari discussions have been helpful to you. This practice has been shrouded in mystery for so long, and barely heard of by so many yogis and yoginis, even though it is a key factor in the development of ecstatic conductivity in the body. It is time to bring kechari out of the closet, so we can intelligently follow the natural impulses that are coming up in so many of us these days.

Even stage 1 kechari carries great power, because the sensitive nerves in the septum come down to the roof of the mouth right where the hard and soft palates meet. That is where the bottom of the edge of the nasal septum is. Putting the tip of the tongue there is like closing an energy switch. As soon as some ecstatic conductivity is rising in our nervous system, the pleasure of putting the tongue there is quite obvious. Of course, when kechari evolves to stage 2, going behind the soft palate and up, our tongue is directly touching the "secret spot" on the septum (see tantra lesson #T34), and the long term results of that are beyond description, though we try our best to explain it. Yoga will make ecstatic poets out of all of us yet!

The tendency to raise the eyes and roll the tongue back during sexual activity and orgasm is a natural reflex that occurs when ecstatic energy is coursing through the body. It is an automatic yoga. The energy moving in sex is the same energy we are cultivating in advanced yoga practices. The fact that many (even those not doing yoga) experience this reflex during sex is a testament to the latent ecstatic conductivity that exists in everyone. Promoting it systematically through yoga practices is not only an important part of how we move toward enlightenment, it also unravels the mystery of how sexual energy functions in us on every level.

Yes, the most effective control and inner stimulation of sexual energy in the nervous system is exercised through the ajna (third eye), as you are finding. Kechari (rolled back tongue) is part of this, and a close bedfellow of sambhavi (eyes rolled up toward a slightly furrowed center brow). Spinal breathing and many of the other techniques are for developing the third eye to root connection. You are experiencing indications of this important connection in the ecstatic reflex during your sexual activity.

I suggest you take this reflex of the eyes and tongue as an indicator of the possibility for cultivating the experience of ongoing ecstatic conductivity in your nervous system. Such an experience does not end with orgasm. It just keeps going around the clock. The methods of yoga aim to promote this, as discussed throughout the main and tantra lessons.

The overall process is pretty simple, really. Cultivate inner silence in daily deep meditation. Then overlay the stimulation of ecstatic conductivity with spinal breathing, mudras (including sambhavi and kechari), bandhas, siddhasana, samyama, chin pump, spinal bastrika, tantric sexual methods, and so on. When blissful inner silence and ecstatic conductivity rise and meet in us, the result is an endless lovemaking on the cellular level. Then we bubble over in the ecstatic bliss and outpouring divine love that is the natural fruition of human evolution. No more struggle. Just pure joy through all circumstances in life. That is what we are, and it unfolds as we go through the process of purification and opening of our nervous system.

Once we get to that stage, a simple lifting of the eyes at any time will send us into a reverie of ecstatic bliss. All of life is divine to one who is constantly in love and in lovemaking.

Regarding your question on practice during sex, it is suggested you see how long you can stay in front of orgasm in a lovemaking or masturbation mode. In other words, let that state of ecstatic conductivity that draws your eyes up and tongue back continue for some time without taking it to orgasm. There are techniques to help with this. Consider reviewing the tantra lessons on holdback (#T4), blocking (#T5), and the count method (#T23). As we develop familiarity and skill at staying in front of orgasm, we find that the ecstatic conductivity in our nervous system will stay with us much longer during the day. If we are doing daily meditation, spinal breathing and other practices, then we will be setting the stage for ecstatic bliss to take up permanent residence. It's well worth the effort.

No doubt you are doing many of these things already, so please regard all of this as a reminder. I wish you all success on your chosen spiritual path. Enjoy!

The guru is in you.

Additional Resources

Topic Index

This index provides multiple references, by lesson number, for topics covered in the Advanced Yoga Practices lessons. The main techniques are listed first, in the order given, followed by many related topics listed in alphabetical order for easy reference.

Advanced Yoga Practices – Main Techniques (in the order given):

Related Topics (listed alphabetically):

Breath Suspension – 45, 46, 51, 52, 62, 91, 106, 144, 167, 175
Buddha – 20, 134

Caduceus – 89, 90
Carl Jung – 134
Celibacy – 101, T9
Chakras – 21, 47, 73, 77, 206, 220
Chanting – 37, 59, 186
Chiropractic – 104
Connectedness of Yoga – 104, 149, 150, 169, 178, 180, 183, 185, 191, 204, 212
Crown Opening (avoiding premature) – 69, 77, 125, 181, 188, 199, 201, 208, 230

Daily Practices
    Establishing – 58, 86, 147, 148, 187
    Maintaining – 102, 148, 187
    Expanding – 148, 193
    Compressing – 18, 50, 209
Deepak Chopra – 69
Destiny – 103
Devotion – 12, 67, 68, 88, 109, 112
Dharma – 178
Diet – 30, 69, 167, 200, 216, 220
Digestion – 51, 133
Divine Love – 110, 113, 138, 143, 182
Divine Union – 69, 113, 169
Doshas (Ayurveda: vata, pitta and kapha) – 69, 200

Ecstasy – 64, 66, 78, 95, 113, 138, 143, 203
Ecstatic Bliss – 78, 113, 120, 139, 143, 169
Ecstatic Confessions (by Martin Buber) – T22
Ecstatic Conductivity – 64, 65, 143, 169, 170, 191, 198, 212, T35
Ecstatic Radiance – 42, 44, 90, 139, 152
Eight Limbs of Yoga – 149, 151, 153, 156, 176
Energy Blockages – 104, 134, 171, 194, 198
Energy/Chakra Healing – 73, 77, 104, 124
Enlightenment Milestones – 35, 85, 100, 120, 138
Esoteric/Secret Yoga – 93, 105, 108, 189, 201, 214

Fifth Dimension – 36
Free Will – 103

Gopi Krishna (kundalini excesses) – 73, 99, 181, 188, 208
Grieving Process – 68
Group Practice – 37

Glossary of Sanskrit Terms

This glossary of Sanskrit terms is designed primarily to support the Advanced Yoga Practices lessons. Since the lessons were written with a mind to simplify things, including minimizing the use of Sanskrit terms, this glossary should not be considered to be a complete general purpose one for use in academic studies. Nevertheless, there are over 100 Sanskrit terms here, which is not too skimpy. Nearly all of them are related in some way to the conduct of yoga practices.

Advaita – The same as vedanta, the monistic (non-dual) branch of Indian philosophy discussed mainly in the *Upanishads*, the *Bhagavad Gita* and the *Brahma Sutra*. Advaita upholds the oneness of God, soul and universe.

Ajna – Means, "command." The sixth chakra, also known as the third eye, encompasses the neuro-biology from the center of the brow to the center of the head, and the medulla oblongata (brain stem). The third eye is the command center controlling the ecstatic aspects of the enlightenment process, which is the orderly awakening of kundalini.

Akasha – Means, "space." Inner, omnipresent space in particular. When used in samyama, akasha reveals the body to be one and the same as inner space, allowing it to be effortlessly transported anywhere.

Amaroli – Urine therapy, an ancient spiritual practice described in the *Hatha Yoga Pradipika* and the *Damar Tantra*.

Amrita – Means, "nectar." In yoga, most often associated with fragrant secretions coming from the brain, down through the nasal pharynx and into the GI (gastrointestinal) tract.

Anahata – Means, "unstruck sound." The fourth chakra located in the heart area. This is where the yoga practitioner first experiences the vastness of inner space, which is often filled with celestial sounds and other inner sensory experiences.

Ananda – Means, "bliss." One of the three characteristics of sat-chit-ananda, our blissful inner silence.

Asana – Means, "posture." The third limb of the eight limbs of yoga from the *Yoga Sutras* of Patanjali. Asanas are used to physically loosen and open the subtle nerves of the body, particularly the sushumna/spinal nerve. Asanas are generally practiced immediately before pranayama and meditation.

Ashtanga Yoga – Means, "eight limbed yoga." A system of yoga practices based on the eight limbs of yoga from the *Yoga Sutras* of Patanjali.

Asvini Mudra – A dynamic version of mulabandha (root lock), where the anal sphincter muscle is gently flexed and released periodically. This happens automatically as ecstatic conductivity rises in the nervous system.

Atman – The immortal soul of a human being. The divine Self that exists in every person. Upon beginning meditation, it is first experienced as stillness, peaceful inner silence, and, later, as ecstatic bliss and outpouring divine love.

Avatar – Means, "incarnation of God in human form." Also is regarded to mean a spiritual savior of humankind. The birth of an avatar is sometimes foretold beforehand, and he or she typically undergoes the trials of achieving final enlightenment, and then takes on a mission to help many others advance spiritually. Well known avatars in the East include Krishna and Buddha, and in the West, Jesus. Many avatars have come to earth, and most are little known. Everyone has the inherent ability to become an avatar because everyone contains the same divine potential. The primary mission of an avatar is to show us that this is so.

Ayurveda – The ancient yoga-based system of medicine that focuses on balancing the doshas (constitutional elements) and pranas (energies) in the body. The great strength in this system is in the application of natural modalities and preventive measures that pre-empt illnesses, or resolve them before they can become chronic. Ayurveda can aid in resolving imbalances and internal energy excesses that can crop up on the path of yoga.

Bandha – Means, "lock." A fixed muscular position that is applied in the course of yoga practices. Examples: mulabandha (root lock) and uddiyana bandha (abdominal lock).

Bastrika Pranayama (also spelled **Bhastrika**) – Means, "bellows breathing." A rapid (panting) breathing technique used in advanced stages of yoga practice. In the AYP lessons it is used while tracing up and down the spine with the attention, and is called spinal bastrika pranayama.

Bhagavad Gita – Means, "song of God." The most widely read scripture in India, sometimes referred to as "the Hindu Bible." It is part of the much longer epic, the *Mahabharata*, and details a dialog between Krishna and the great warrior, Arjuna. In the *Bhagavad Gita* the path to enlightenment is described, including many of the methods found in the AYP lessons.

Bhakti Yoga – Bhakti means, "love of God" or "love of Truth." The first manifestation of this is desire for something more in life, for an ideal (ishta). Bhakti yoga practice systematically channels desire and emotion toward the practitioner's highest ideal, beginning with the question, "Why am I here?" and ending with ecstatic union with the divine within.

Brahma Sutra – A primary scripture of vedanta's non-dual philosophy. The others are the *Bhagavad Gita* and the 108 *Upanishads*.

Brahmacharya – Means, "walking in Brahma" or "walking in the creative force of God." Commonly interpreted to mean celibacy, but it means more that that. It means preservation and cultivation of the vital force (sexual energy) in the yoga practitioner, which can be accomplished by both celibates and non-celibates through yogic methods.

Brahmari Pranayama – Means, "bee sound." A supplemental pranayama that involves using the larynx (voice box, located below the epiglottis) to restrict the exit of air on exhalation while making a sound deep in the throat like the high pitched hum of a bee. This is a powerful stimulator of the *OM* vibration emanating from the medulla oblongata (brain stem), and is most effective once ecstatic conductivity has arisen in the nervous system. In AYP, Brahmari optionally can be used instead of ujjayi during spinal breathing pranayama.

Chakra – Means, "wheel." Chakras are neuro-biological/spiritual energy centers in the human body, connected together by thousands of subtle nerves/nadis. There are seven major chakras and numerous minor ones. The seven major chakras are muladhara (perineum), svadhisthana (inner reproductive organs), manipura (naval/solar plexus), anahata (heart), vishuddhi (throat), ajna (brow to medulla) and sahasrar (crown).

Chit – Means "consciousness." One of the three characteristics of sat-chit-ananda, our blissful inner silence.

Darshan – Means, "to see or experience." To see or experience the presence of one's chosen ideal. It also means, generally, to be in the presence of and receive spiritual energy from an enlightened person.

Dharana – Means, "focused attention." The sixth limb of the eight limbs of yoga from the *Yoga Sutras* of Patanjali. Dharana is the first stage of meditation, and also of samyama, when the attention is focused in a particular way on either a mantra or a sutra.

Dharma – Means, "that which sustains." In yoga, this refers to activity one does in the world that is naturally supportive their spiritual evolution – one's dharma. In Buddhism, this refers to the entire teaching of the Buddha – the dharma.

Dhyana – Means, "meditation." The seventh limb of the eight limbs of yoga from the *Yoga Sutras* of Patanjali. Meditation is the process of attention expanding from focus on an object (like a mantra) to an unbounded undifferentiated state of blissful awareness called samadhi. The process of meditation, correctly practiced, leads to profound stillness and purification in the human nervous system.

Doshas – The three basic types of biological humors in Ayurvedic medicine, which determine an individual's constitution: vata (movement), pitta (heat) and kapha (structure). The therapies of Ayurveda promote balance of the doshas, which provides the foundation for good physical and spiritual health.

Guru – Means, "dispeller of darkness." The guru is that within us, and also reflected outside us, that leads us gradually toward the experience of enlightenment. Our innate desire for Truth and God (bhakti) is the most fundamental manifestation of the guru. There is a common belief that the guru can only be found in the form of another person. In fact, it is the inner guru that leads us to all other forms of the guru. We are never more than a heartbeat away from the illuminating power of the guru.

Hatha Yoga – Means, "joining of the sun and moon." A system of yoga practice focusing on purifying the nervous system through physical postures (asanas), breath control (pranayama) and related means.

Hatha Yoga Pradipika – A five hundred year old scripture detailing many of the practices of Hatha Yoga.

Ida and Pingala – Two of the primary spiritual nerves (nadis) in the body. Second in importance only to the spinal nerve (sushumna).

Ishta – Means, "chosen ideal." Ishta is at the heart of bhakti yoga, and is that which each person chooses as the ideal to inspire active engagement on the spiritual path. The ishta can be as simple as the constant question, "Who am I?" and its gradually unfolding answer. Or as complex as a guru in human form. Any object or idea can serve as the touchstone for a person's ishta – statues, philosophical concepts, the beauty of nature, etc. What all ishtas have in common is their ability to inspire the aspirant to diligently pursue spiritual practices.

Jalandhara Bandha – Means, "chin lock." Practiced during certain stages of kumbhaka (breath retention). A more advanced version in the AYP lessons is called dynamic jalandhara, or chin pump.

Jiva – The individual soul. Body and ego-bound consciousness. An unenlightened human being.

Jivan Mukti – A liberated soul, merged with the infinite. An enlightened, living human being. One who has attained Christ consciousness.

Jnana (or Chin) Mudra – The well-known hand mudra where the thumbs and index fingers of both hands are joined to form circles with hands resting, palms upward or downward, on the knees during sitting practices. This mudra is more effect than cause, since it arises automatically with the awakening of kundalini energy in the nervous system.

Jnana Yoga – Path of the intellect. A system of yoga practice based on inquiry and intuitive reasoning. Jnana yoga is commonly misunderstood to be the collection of intellectual knowledge about spiritual matters. In reality, it is a close cousin of bhakti yoga, where the mind and heart both melt in the tapas (heat) of the ever-penetrating inquiry, "Who am I?"

Jyotish – The Indian system of astrology.

Kama Sutra – An ancient guidebook on social and sexual relations between men and women. While it is commonly believed in the West to be a tantric scripture, the *Kama Sutra* does not contain the core principles or sexual techniques of tantra yoga, which are embodied in brahmacharya – the preservation and cultivation of sexual energy by celibate or non-celibate tantric methods.

Karma – Means, "action and its effects." This is the idea that our past actions have created current tendencies, limitations and opportunities in the present. This is sometimes referred to as "the law of karma." In Christian theology, it is contained in the phrase, "As you sow, so shall you reap." Karma is the basis for the doctrine of reincarnation, and the idea that dissolving stored karma (samskaras) in the nervous system through yoga practices will unfold more happiness in this life, the next life, and eventually lead the soul to eternal life in the higher realms, freed from the necessity of taking human birth.

Karma Yoga – The path of action. This is the spiritual method of acting in the world in a spirit of service (seva), while systematically letting go of the expectation to receive anything in return, thereby promoting a positive cycle of causes and effects. Living a lifestyle of karma yoga emerges naturally as yoga practices have been engaged in over a period of time. Some are born with the gift of karma yoga, and spend their lives lifting up all of humanity (and themselves) through their good works.

Kechari Mudra – Means, "to fly through (inner) space." Kechari is the practice of raising the tongue to the soft palate, and eventually above it into the spiritually erogenous nasal pharynx. This closes a neurological circuit in the body, enabling ecstatic energy to flow between the pelvic region and the head. Kechari, practiced in coordination with sambhavi and other yoga methods, leads to opening of the ecstatic celestial realms within the heart, and throughout the subtle levels of the nervous system.

Kriya Yoga – Means, "the yoga of techniques." It comes in many forms through the various traditional lines of teaching. The main teachings of kriya yoga focus on pranayama, with spinal breathing being the core practice. Kriya yoga also utilizes many of the methods of hatha yoga.

Kumbhaka – Means, "suspension of breath." The breath is held in (internal kumbhaka) and out (external kumbhaka) at different times during yoga practices. When practiced in conjunction with other yogic methods, such as mudras and bandhas, kumbhaka plays an important role in awakening the kundalini energy located in the pelvic region. Kumbhaka also occurs spontaneously at times during yoga practices, especially during deep meditation when the metabolism comes to a near standstill.

Kundalini – Means, "coiled serpent." A metaphorical word and concept used to describe the latent and active states of sexual energy in the overall process of human spiritual transformation. When kundalini is "awakened," it is the activation of sexual energy in the pelvic region in an upward flowing direction, permeating the entire nervous system with great transforming power. The feminine name, Shakti, is often used interchangeably with kundalini once the energy becomes dynamic. In the Christian tradition, it is called the Holy Spirit.

Kundalini Yoga – A system of practices designed primarily to awaken kundalini energy throughout the body. Techniques used are taken mainly from hatha yoga, focusing more on the use of pranayama, kumbhaka, and mudras and bandhas, and less on asanas.

Lingam – The male sexual organ, both literally and energetically as the Shiva power in the yogic merging of Shiva and Shakti energies throughout the nervous system.

Maha Mudra – Means, "great seal." An advanced yoga asana designed to purify and open the sushumna (spinal nerve).

Mahabharata – The great epic poem of India covering the life of Krishna and a war between two rival families, the Pandavas and the Kauravas. The *Bhagavad Gita* is part of the *Mahabharata*.

Mala – A string of beads (like a rosary) containing 108 beads, used for counting repetitions of spiritual practice. Also sometimes worn for ceremonial and devotional purposes.

Manipura – Meaning, "city of gems." The third chakra, located in the naval/solar plexus area, associated with digestion, including the higher metabolism associated with the production of enlightenment-promoting organic compounds in the GI (gastrointestinal) tract that radiate sparkling energy. Hence the reference to gems.

Mantra – A specially chosen syllable or series of syllables that is used in the practice of deep meditation.

Mantra Yoga – A system of yoga practice based on mental techniques that utilize mantras and sutras.

Maya – Means, "illusion." Refers to the illusory nature of the world experienced by an unenlightened person. Acts of ignorance and death are regarded as part of maya. An enlightened person has a different experience, seeing maya as a play (lila) on the infinite, immortal field of pure bliss consciousness, which is known to be one's Self. Though an enlightened person is affected by acts of ignorance and death on the earth plane, he or she lives a radiant reality that is forever untouched by maya. That is the outcome of yoga – a purified nervous system that has been opened to the infinite within – pure bliss consciousness and outpouring divine love.

Moksha – Enlightenment. Liberation in this life in the form of ongoing ecstatic bliss and outpouring divine love. Freedom from the wheel of birth and death.

Mudra – Means, "seal." Various physical postures and maneuvers that direct ecstatic energy toward higher levels of manifestation in the nervous system.

Mulabandha – Means, "root lock." Systematic stimulation of sexual energy upward in the nervous system during yoga practices through gentle compression of the anal sphincter muscle.

Muladhara – Means, "root or foundation." The first chakra, located at the perineum, where kundalini energy is first awakened.

Nadi – Means, "channel." Nadis are the subtle (spiritual) nerves corresponding with the physical nerves. There are thousands of nadis in the body, but only a few are deliberately purified and opened to achieve the broad effects of yoga throughout the entire nervous system.

Nadi Shodana – A simple and relaxing form of pranayama involving use of the fingers to achieve alternate nostril breathing.

Nauli – Means, "to churn." A yoga practice involving the twirling of the abdominal muscles first in one direction, and then the other. This practice stimulates the higher functioning of the digestive system and raises kundalini.

Niyama – Means, "observance." The second limb of the eight limbs of yoga from the *Yoga Sutras* of Patanjali. The niyamas are aspects of conduct that support the process of human spiritual transformation. They are saucha (purity and cleanliness), samtosa (contentment), tapas (heat/focus/austerity), svadhyaya (study of spiritual writings and self) and isvara pranidhana (surrender to the divine).

Ojas – A luminous substance/energy that ecstatically permeates the human body as sexual energy is cultivated and refined to a higher spiritual purpose.

OM (also spelled **AUM**) – The most sacred mantra syllable in India, and found in other cultures as well. The primordial vibration of God in human beings. *OM* is used alone and with other syllables for meditation. As yoga practices advance, *OM* can be heard as a natural spiritual vibration emanating ecstatically from the medulla oblongata (brain stem). The medulla, which is part of the ajna/third eye, is also called, "the mouth of God."

Padmasana – Means "lotus posture." A way of sitting for pranayama and meditation that involves crossing the legs and resting both feet on top of the opposite thighs.

Prana – Means, "first unit." Prana is the first manifestation of consciousness in the nervous system. It is experienced as moving energy, and it is moved in yoga practices to advance the process of human spiritual transformation.

Pranayama – Means, "restraint of prana." Prana is the first manifestation of consciousness in the body, and can be encouraged toward higher spiritual expression. This is accomplished with the breath through a variety of pranayama (breathing) practices to stimulate the flow of prana in the body. Pranayama cultivates the subtle nerves (nadis), making the nervous system a much more receptive vehicle for meditation.

Prasad – A spiritual offering or gift offered to one's ishta, guru, or teacher, which is returned bearing a spiritual blessing.

Pratyahara – Means, "withdrawal." Withdrawal of the primary focus of attention on the external senses. This is caused by the expansion of inner sensuality due to yoga practices and the awakening of ecstatic conductivity. The attention is naturally drawn inward to more enjoyable levels of inner experience. Over time, inner sensuality expands back out into sensory perception of the everyday world. Pratyahara (the withdrawal) is the first step on the journey of attention going inward toward divine perception, and then back outward again to divine perception everywhere.

Raja Yoga – Means, "royal yoga." A name given to the systematic application of the practices contained in the eight limbs of yoga described in the *Yoga Sutras* of Patanjali.

Rishi – Means, "seer." One who has raised ecstatic conductivity (kundalini) in the nervous system and experiences refined sensory perception inside and outside the body. Then the relationship of consciousness and prana (refined energy) can be observed directly. Hence the term "seer." Rishi is also a general term that is used describe a sage, sadhu, hermit, or mendicant.

Ramayama – A great epic poem of India, telling the story of Rama and the path of right action – the Dharma.

Sadhana – The regular practice of spiritual disciplines.

Sadhu – An ascetic practitioner of yoga. A mendicant. A holy person.

Sahasrar – Means, "thousand-petaled lotus." The seventh chakra, located at the crown of the head (corona radiata). Awakening and entering it leads to the merging of individual consciousness with infinite divine consciousness. Awakening the sahasrar prematurely leads to many troubles in a nervous system that has not been sufficiently purified beforehand. Awakening the ajna (third eye) first prepares the nervous system, while at the same time slowly and indirectly opening the sahasrar with much greater safety.

Samadhi – Absorption in the inner silence of pure bliss consciousness. The repeated destination of meditation, and, ultimately, a state which is sustained throughout daily living. This is the eighth limb of the eight limbs of yoga described in the *Yoga Sutras* of Patanjali.

Sambhavi Mudra – The practice of lifting the eyes to the point between the eyebrows while slightly furrowing the brow, producing physical stimulation back through the brain to the medulla oblongata (brain stem). When used in coordination with other yoga practices, sambhavi is a primary means for purifying and opening the ajna (third eye). This is first experienced as an ecstatic connection between the head and the pelvic region.

Samkhya – The dualistic branch of Indian philosophy which is closely integrated with yoga. In it, unmanifest pure bliss consciousness and the manifest universe are seen as two sides of the whole of life, and can be experienced as one by the yogi and yogini. This "two becoming one" is the intersection of the dual (samkhya/yoga) and non-dual (vedanta/advaita) philosophies if India. It is through yoga practice and direct experience that the apparent inconsistency is resolved.

Samyama – A practice which utilizes the characteristics of the last three limbs of the eight limbs of yoga in the *Yoga Sutras* of Patanjali – dharana (focus), dhyana (meditation) and samadhi (absorption in inner silence). Through the initiation of sutras (particular words and phrases with meaning), in the quietest levels of awareness, consciousness is moved through the nervous system with great purifying effects. Samyama is the source of miraculous powers exhibited by human beings. These are called siddhis, and are effects rather than causes of rising enlightenment, and are best regarded as such.

Sanskrit – The ancient language of Indian spiritual culture (the vedas) and of the great scriptures that have emanated from it.

Sat – Means "eternal existence." One of the three characteristics of Sat-chit-ananda, our blissful inner silence. It is that in us which never dies.

Sat-Chit-Ananda – Means, "eternal bliss consciousness." Inner silence. Immortal Self. Pure bliss consciousness. The witness. the Tao. God the Father. It is that in us which is our self-awareness in every moment. Through yoga practices, our nervous system is cultivated toward its natural evolutionary transformation to provide the direct, permanent experience of this, our essential nature.

Satsang – Means, "association with truth." Keeping company with those of high spiritual aspiration. Also, association with enlightened persons. *Bible*: "If two or more are gathered in my name I will be there in their midst." Any contact or communication with others on matters pertaining to human spiritual evolution will stimulate the inner energies of bhakti. Reading spiritual writings can be a form of satsang also.

Shakti – The dynamic, feminine creative force in the human body and in nature. Shakti is awakened kundalini. In order to create, Shakti must merge with her counterpart, Shiva, who is the silent seed behind all manifestation. The movement of kundalini/Shakti in the human nervous system is toward that end, and yoga practices are designed to facilitate the union of Shiva and Shakti everywhere in the body, leading ultimately to an ecstatic overflowing from the head down to the melting heart. The Christian name for Shakti energy is the Holy Spirit.

Shaktipat – The awakening of the kundalini/Shakti power in an aspirant by a guru or spiritual teacher. While this may have benefit, the ultimate responsibility for spiritual progress remains with the aspirant, who can carry the process forward through the conduct of daily yoga practices.

Shiva – In yoga, Shiva is analogous with inner silence, the silent, blissful aspect of experience gained through meditation and other yoga practices. Shiva is the silent seed from which all is manifested, and to which all must return. It is the blending of inner silence (Shiva) and the dynamic ecstatic energy (kundalini/Shakti) in the body that produces enlightenment in the human nervous system. In Hinduism, Shiva is personified in the trinity of Brahma (creator), Vishnu (sustainer) and Shiva (dissolver/destroyer), and plays a major role in the religious heritage and customs of the culture. The Christian equivalent of Shiva is God the Father.

Siddhasana – Means "posture of the perfected ones" or "perfect posture." A way of sitting for pranayama and meditation that involves crossing the legs and sitting with the perineum firmly on the heel of one foot. This seat provides stimulation of sexual energy upward through the nervous system, ultimately creating a constant fountain of ecstasy throughout practices. Over time, siddhasana, practiced in coordination with other yoga methods, will lead to ecstasy naturally being experienced throughout daily life. This is so because the nervous system can be cultivated to naturally sustain a condition of ecstatic conductivity. This is one of the primary prerequisites for enlightenment.

Siddhi – Means, "perfection." Siddhis refer to powers, which result as a by-product of yogic purification occurring in the nervous system on the path to enlightenment. This is especially so in Samyama practice, which cultivates the movement of consciousness in the nervous system in particular ways for the purpose of enhanced purification and opening to the divine within.

Soma – A substance produced in the GI (gastrointestinal) tract that greatly enhances the processes of yoga. Soma arises from the alchemy of food, air and sexual essences blending naturally in the digestive tract, giving rise to a luminosity that begins in the belly and travels throughout the body. The production of soma is stimulated by kumbhaka (suspended breath) and mudras and bandhas, and is closely related to the raising of kundalini energy. Soma is also a hallucinogenic plant in India, which is referred to in the ancient Vedas.

Sri Vidya – Means, "glorious knowledge." In tantra it is the scriptural and experiential fruition of human evolution. Sri vidya is ecstatic bliss and outpouring divine love, expressed through the enlightened nervous system, and in the mathematical precision of the ancient *Sri Yantra* diagram.

Sri Yantra (or **Sri Chakra**)– Means, "glorious diagram" or "glorious wheel." Represents the spiritual structure of the human nervous system and the universe. Mathematically, the *Sri Yantra* recreates the wave pattern formed by the vibration of *OM*, the sacred sound that resonates naturally within the human nervous system as purification and opening occur.

Sushumna – The spinal nerve that extends from the perineum to the head. It is the most important spiritual nerve (nadi) in the body. By purifying and opening the sushumna, the entire nervous system is transformed to higher spiritual functioning. All of the practices in yoga are designed to cultivate, in one way or another, the purification and opening of the sushumna.

Sutra – Means, "stitch." A short verse containing potent spiritual knowledge. When a group of such short verses are brought together, they "stitch" together the whole of knowledge. Particular sutras can be used for the purpose of structured samyama practice, as described in the *Yoga Sutras* of Patanjali. The use of sutras in samyama can have dramatic effects on the course of the enlightenment process in the nervous system, and can also lead to the manifestation of siddhis (powers).

Svadisthana – Means, "dwelling place." This is the second chakra, located in the area of the internal reproductive organs. It is the dwelling place of the great storehouse of pranic energy, the sexual vitality. Once activated, vast energy flows up from there and spiritually illuminates the entire nervous system.

Swami – Means, "master or owner." A title given to indicate a teacher who is enlightened. More commonly, it is a title given to indicate rank in the religious hierarchy, like the title of priest, rabbi, or mullah.

Tantra Yoga – Tantra means, "two woven together." The meaning is similar to that of yoga, "to join." Tantra is the broadest known system of yoga, encompassing the methods of all other systems. While tantra includes the eight limbs of yoga from the *Yoga Sutras* of Patanjali, it goes beyond them by addressing sexual practices that have been controversial for hundreds of years. Hence, tantra has been known as the yoga of sex. But sex is only an aspect of the whole of tantra, so the label is misleading. Tantra is concerned with meditation, pranayama, mudras, bandhas, asanas and every other useful practice in yoga, including methods that promote the expansion of sexual energy upward to facilitate the enlightenment process.

Tapas – Means, "heat or intensity." This is an aspect of bhakti (devotional desire), which determines the spiritual force behind the desire for union with the divine, and enlightenment. Tapas is commonly associated with austerity and self-sacrifice (sometimes extreme) in spiritual practices. There is no standard to meet for tapas. Each aspirant will experience and apply tapas in their own way.

Turiya – means, "the fourth state." This is the experience of inner silence cultivated in meditation. It is called turiya because it is distinct from the first three states of consciousness – waking, dreaming and deep dreamless sleep. As yoga practices advance, turiya gradually comes to coexist as a constant condition during the other three states of consciousness. It is the beginning stage of enlightenment. In that situation, one is never unconscious, whether awake, dreaming, or in deep sleep. That is called witnessing.

Uddiyana – Means, "to fly up." A yoga practice involving the lifting of the abdomen with the diaphragm while the lungs are empty. This practice stimulates the higher functioning of the digestive system and raises kundalini. It is also a preparation for Nauli practice.

Ujjayi Pranayama – This is an additional practice that is done during spinal breathing and other pranayamas. It involves partially closing the epiglottis (the windpipe door we hold our breath with) while exhaling during pranayama, making a fine hissing sound deep in the throat. This creates additional air pressure in the lungs and pranic pressure throughout the nervous system. It also creates a fine vibration deep in the throat that assists in purifying and opening the neuro-biology in the chest, throat and head.

Upanishads – Commentaries on the Vedas, written in dialog form, forming the basis for vedanta's non-dual philosophy. There are 108 Upanishads.

Vajroli Mudra – A practice enabling a man or woman to draw ejaculative or pre-ejaculative sexual emissions up the urethra and into the bladder. It is performed using uddiyana/nauli and mulabandha/asvini, sometimes combined with conscious control of the ejaculation process. The vajroli effect can also be accomplished by physically blocking ejaculations with the finger pressing on the urethra behind the pelvic bone. In ongoing yoga practice, vajroli has the greatest significance as it evolves naturally to become an automatic biological function in connection with an awakened kundalini. In this case, vajroli is preorgasmic, and provides a constant drawing up of sexual essences into the bladder, GI (gastrointestinal) tract, spinal nerve and other components of the spiritual biology. As the nervous system evolves to become constantly ecstatic, vajroli becomes a constant natural function. The rise of natural vajroli is an important part of the fulfillment of the role of brahmacharya – the preservation and cultivation of sexual energy.

Veda – Means, "knowledge." The Vedas are the most ancient scriptures of India, preserved through oral and written tradition for 5000 years. There are four Vedas: Rig, Sama, Yajur and Atharva.

Vedanta – Means, "the end of the Veda." The monistic (non-dual) branch of Indian philosophy discussed mainly in the *Upanishads*, the *Bhagavad Gita* and the *Brahma Sutra*.

Vigyan Bhairav Tantra – An ancient tantric scripture that identifies many of the methods of yoga practice, including the essential principle involved in tantric sex – the preservation and cultivation of sexual energy.

Vishuddhi – Means, "purity." The fifth chakra, located at the throat. This is a gateway for pranic energy to rise into the head. It is also a key center for speech and communications. With daily yoga practices, purification and opening occur naturally in the throat. The internal and external expressions of energy open up simultaneously.

Yama – Means, "restraint." The first limb of the eight limbs of yoga from the *Yoga Sutras* of Patanjali. The yamas are aspects of conduct that support the process of human spiritual transformation. They are ahimsa (non-violence), satya (truthfulness), asteya (non-stealing), brahmacharya (preservation and cultivation of sexual energy) and aparigraha (non-covetousness).

Yoga – Means, "to join, or union." The vast field of knowledge and practices concerned with promoting the evolutionary process of human spiritual transformation. The methods of yoga are many and diverse. Yet, all are connected by virtue of their common denominator, the human nervous system. All of yoga is derived from the innate ability for divine unfoldment contained within every person.

Yoga Nidra – Means, "yogic sleep." It is the state of remaining conscious during deep sleep. It can be cultivated by specific techniques. It also arises naturally as one advances in daily yoga practices. In that case it is called "turiya" (the fourth state), or the witness.

Yoga Sutras – Means, "stitches of union." The most famous scripture on yoga, written by Patanjali about 500 years ago. The *Yoga Sutras* contain the main elements of yoga practice (the eight-limbed path, plus samyama), and detailed descriptions of the experiences that are encountered on the road to enlightenment, and at the destination. The *Yoga Sutras* are a measuring rod by which all spiritual paths can be measured for completeness.

Yogi – A male practitioner of yoga.

Yogini – A female practitioner of yoga.

Yoni – Means, "womb or origin." It is the female sexual organ, both literally and energetically as the Shakti power in the yogic merging of Shiva and Shakti energies throughout the nervous system.

Yoni Mudra – A yoga practice that purifies and opens the ajna (third eye), and stimulates kundalini/Shakti energy to rise from the pelvic region, up the sushumna (spinal nerve) to the ajna, and permeate the entire nervous system.

Yuga – An age, or era, determined through astronomical calculations of the earth's position over time in relation the sun, planets and constellations. The concept of a yuga is from jyotish (Indian astrology). The concept of ages also exists in Western astrology. Yugas depict rising and falling human spiritual sensitivities over long periods of time, in a repeating cycle that goes round and round over thousands (or millions) of years. Astrologers utilizing various mathematical approaches do not agree on the length of the overall cycle, on the length of the yugas/ages, or on what yuga/age we are in right now. It is a subject of debate. Suffice to say, history records that spiritual sensitivities and knowledge have been slowly on the rise over at least the past 100 years, so perhaps those who say we are entering (or have entered) an age of enlightenment are right. There is still much darkness in the world, but the light of yoga and rising human enlightenment are becoming stronger every day.

Reader Feedback

Thousands of pages of email correspondence have been generated since the Advanced Yoga Practices online lessons began. Readers have often shared their thoughts on the lessons, the practices, and their experiences. The following excerpts are offered to help give a flavor of what these lessons are about. Thank you to all who have shared!

If you would like to submit questions or feedback on the lessons and your experiences in yoga, you are invited to write to the author at the web site provided in the front of the book.

1. "I just had a quick read through some of your posts and I'm blown away at the quality and authenticity contained in what I've read so far. I'm looking forward to studying your inspiring wisdom more closely and working with some of your suggestions. Your words speak intelligently of the Truth and the path that leads there." – SD

2. "I started only few days back, seems to enjoy so far as I have tried other methods also, this seems simple and I understand better." – PM

3. "I want to first thank you for your teaching! I am finding with your lessons that I am actually feeling the process of yoga, the beauty of all." – JF

4. "The reason for my message is to say that for the first time I found a very positive, plain and very well explained approach to yoga practice. Thanks, then, for your precious help; I strongly hope it will be helpful to clean the air from all the commercial fog that is becoming everyday thicker around an important human heritage like yoga. I started my experience 35 years ago. I've been very happy to find in your words the same love for yoga I experience every day." – LB

5. "At any rate, I am very much enjoying your lessons and point of view here. You have a talent for explaining things clearly and without strident religious undertones. What a relief." – BG

6. "I just wanted to let you know I've really enjoyed reading the postings and am glad you're sharing all this information. This is a lot of work for you, and your effort is appreciated. I've practiced hatha yoga for 5 years now, and much that I'm seeing here goes with it beautifully. Plus you're addressing some things that my teacher doesn't, for which I'm grateful – I'm getting some information here exactly when I needed it (funny how things work that way, huh?). I imagine I'll be back along with questions one day, but for now just wanted to drop you a note and tell you how much I'm enjoying this. I too wish everyone on earth could be here!" – NW

7. "I was brought up as a Catholic, but over the years I began to feel that all the different religions were just like clubs, with their own rules and regulations, and that when it all came down to it, it is just God and me ... I am so pleased that you have started this group, I only wish that all this knowledge had been available when I was young (I'm a 'senior citizen' now). I hope that

people today can know how lucky they are to have someone like yourself, who is willing to give so much of their time to pass on the knowledge that has taken so many years to achieve." – BB

8. "I find your article on bhakti (devotion – lesson #67) extremely reader-friendly." – KW

9. "A few words to express my appreciation for the information and effort you have provided. So many of the Tantra sites and groups are thin covers for sex clubs which distort and misappropriate many of the concepts you so generously assist in explaining. For me the joys of Tantric Sex are merely some of the symptoms of Tantric practices, not the practice itself. I feel many miss this point and deny themselves the opportunities of fulfillment the ancient knowledge provides." – LL

10. "I have been reading all your writings in the group and was fascinated by your writing style and knowledge." – NP

11. "I firstly would like to thank you for the lessons which I feel are very beneficial and the program you are putting out seems to be a good one as it covers everything. I am following another yogi's teachings which I'm happy with, but forgot his kundalini meditation which I'm meant to do weekly, so your priceless teachings are well and truly filling the gap that had been left in my spiritual program." – TS

12. "Thank you for the knowledge you are sharing, and for the way you do it." – HN

13. "You say, "the guru is in you." Yes, I agree, but you are greatly helping and improving my inner guru! Thanks again!" – LB

14. "Thank you for your immediate and informative reply! I felt very positive about attempting meditation, and I'll be sure to check out that lesson you recommend. You seem like a beautiful person through your words. Your words have kindness all over them. Thank you for giving me a lift in my day." – SY

15. "Thanks ever so much for your lessons. I'm finding them to be life-enhancing on various levels. The techniques themselves are becoming more and more enjoyable, thus far, even though I am only able practice them once a day. I am finding that they are assisting the other practices that I feel are right for me." – BS

16. "I can't begin to express how much I am enjoying the practices, and I have held at siddhasana for now because I feel so much bliss and at times incredible energy surges as if my whole body pulsates! My whole outlook is bliss. I see God the universal being at times everywhere. Today, driving, I felt so good, I felt as if I should scream out the window and tell everyone I love them and to join the practices. I had to dance when I got home ...." – MF

17. "I really like the simplicity and effectiveness of your instructions. I'm not even sure how I got referred to your group but I'd like to thank whoever did it." – CH

18. "First thank you so much for this group. Your efforts are so appreciated. I'm sure maintaining the group and answering all the questions is time consuming. We, the children of God, needed you, and you came. I have meditated for the past 10 years. I would say that I was never really good at it. So now, fast forward. I joined your group. I really liked the fact that the thoughts that come in meditation are ok. Just keep going and go back to the mantra. I felt like maybe I was doing it right before and that my expectation was off. I've committed to doing the practice twice a day. I wanted to keep the "time line" in mind so that I didn't rush through this. So I added the Advanced Practices slowly. I haven't really had any rush of kundalini energy like some of the people, but I decided to keep practicing. This morning I tried the Yoni Mudra for the 1st time since joining your group. As soon as I started, I saw a bunch of crazy lights. I just watched and kept doing it. Then came circles with a star in the middle. There was a bright circle with a dark circle inside. In the middle was the star. The star would fade in and out. I didn't want it to go away." – QG

19. "First of all, I would like to thank you very sincerely for all the time and effort you put into helping people like me on the path of spiritual development and enlightenment. I find your lessons extremely valuable and you have all my gratitude for it." – DR

20. "Thanks for all that you've done. It's amazing the difference one person can make for so many." – MC

21. "As the saying goes, 'When the student is ready, the teacher appears.' Certainly, this was very timely. I've got a ways to catch up it seems, but I'm enjoying your knowledge." – TK

22. "Wonderful job you are doing! Appreciate your patience and your time!" – PR

23. "I thought that your answer to the question about too much sex was compassionate and practical." – RH

24. "I would like to thank you very much for the lessons you are presenting here. They are wonderful, and I have searched for years to find a method of meditation that I can do. You make this do-able. Thank you." – AN

25. "Hi, and thanks for letting me join this wonderful group. I find the lessons here very useful as I have sort of started over with my yoga practice and right now I am taking things very slowly but still listening more to my body then necessarily following the order of your lessons." – DL

26. "First of all, thank you so much for your very clear and simple instructions. I am someone who has been on a cross-country track up the mountain for quite some time (I will be 70 next year) and have investigated various methods and exercises, picking the ones that seem to suit me best. Your methods are similar in many respects to ones I have been practicing." – RS

27. "What a wonderful group, and your thoughts flow like a river of knowledge!" – KK

28. "I am absolutely fascinated and impressed, and many congratulations to you for creating this group which promotes nothing other than its topic. I think what you have to say is valuable and would like to ask if I might be permitted to include your lessons/discussions one at a time in a local eclectic news letter that goes out monthly." – ZN

29. "Thank you for your encouragement. I will continue my journey with you." – JM

30. "Thanks so much for being! This student was definitely ready, and very happy that you appeared!" – LS

31. "I am immensely enjoying your postings. It is informative and very helpful on my journey. Thank you for your efforts!" – MS

32. "The teachings contained in this newsgroup are wonderful. I would like to thank you for disseminating this information to aspiring yogis." – VT

33. "Thanks for the reply to my earlier query. I also am into yoga practices and have been following your advice very keenly. I have truly benefited from your lessons. I would like to thank you for the same. I firmly believe Yoga is the only path which can lead man past this life of suffering." – SK

34. "I have been experiencing symptoms of spontaneous kechari mudra for some time now but had no idea there even was such a thing. This article (#108 on kechari) was wonderful." – YS

35. "I take this opportunity to convey my deep regards to you. Your knowledge is indeed very special. It will be a great help for a discerning seeker." – VQ

36. "I would just like to say that this list/resource is absolutely incredible. I haven't had chance to read every message yet, but so far I have found them extremely insightful. There seems to be an overwhelming amount of information available on the Internet regarding yoga, but nothing as complete as this." – NC

37. "I wish I could explain in words or even make you feel how I feel about being here. With that said, thank you so much for inviting me here. Words cannot describe what being on this board with these additional kriya techniques and information to help me progress mean to me. I am forever grateful and in your debt." – LB

38. "I have been wondering about bhakti for a few years, trying to understand it. What you said opened a door for me. It feels I have been slightly off track and out of touch with that basic desire toward my ideal, and my ability to maintain it, for quite some time. Hence my speech,

emotions, motivation, and spiritual practice have all suffered somewhat. Thanks for your inspiration." – HF

39. "I am practising Patanjali yoga for a long time. It's part of my life and enjoy it very much. I went through some of the posts and find them very interesting and helpful. I wish the group years and years of successful life." – VG

40. "I have gone through some of the lessons and they are indeed very beautiful. The membership speaks of itself for the usefulness and integration." – MA

41. "Thank you for inviting me to your wonderful group! I've read some of the material and it looks like it could be very helpful to anyone who would pause, be still ..." – DJ

42. "I want to say again how impressed I am by the dedication you give to guiding and enlightening people like me. Your advice is invaluable and I am deeply thankful. I also read with great interest your last posting on Kechari. It's a first class description of what appears to be a key factor in reaching ecstatic bliss and of what needs to be done in order to attain it. In my case, since the experience of 'spontaneous kechari' is a very recent one, I am going to stick with it for a while and then move up gradually to Stage 2, using your method." – DR

43. "Thank you for reminding me of my divinity." – BA

44. "I am appreciative and grateful for your advice in the group and giving us the tools to progress. I am currently keeping my practice fairly simple, but it's great to read about the more advanced practices. I will delve into the advanced practices when I feel the time is right." – NA

45. "Thank you for sharing your gift of knowledge and for your sincere guidance. This is a wonderful group. Thank you. Om Shanti, Shanti." – MV

46. "Too much coincidence here – all along you've been answering questions I have, many that my yoga teacher of 6 years can't or won't address. A friend pointed me to your message board in early January 2004 and I was thrilled to read what you had to say. But right now I'm astounded. Just last week I started using an Om Shree mantra, and tonight I find your message suggesting almost the same thing (2nd mantra enhancement). We are SO on the same wavelength, and I truly appreciate the work you're doing here!" – DE

47. "Hello and thank you for your group. You have developed wonderful practices, which I feel I will continue for a long time." – LS

48. "I wanted to take the time to thank-you for your extremely inspired writings. I have been meditating for years and I have been searching for the teachings that you so graciously give to us. I guess it's like the saying, "when the student is ready the guru appears". Your teachings speak so much truth to me. I have been doing spinal breathing for the past 9 months and can feel the energy moving up and down the spine. My wife joined your discussion group just after

Christmas 2003. I cannot tell you how wonderful it is to have her on the same path. She also joined the tantric part of the discussion and together we travel down our spiritual path." – LO

49. "I am feeling great results with the spinal breathing so far!" – CH

50. "Thank you so much for your quick response to some questions I asked. I have been trying to learn awhile now on my own and I am so happy to have found this group as it is the answer to my prayers." – SV

51. "Thank you for this wonderful group. You are a God send. I read #69 (on kundalini symptoms and remedies), which is also extremely informative and very helpful. Thank you ever so much for all your knowledgeable insight. Know that you are doing a good thing here. All good things to you!" – BB

52. "I am enjoying your posts and find them very useful. I started meditating many years ago and have done several methods looking for one that worked and actually made life better. Your mantra meditation is very fine." – DC

53. "I have only gotten halfway through the posts but I am tired and will be retiring to my room to meditate before I go to sleep and wanted to write to you. I am very glad that you have created this group, and it seems to be another cosmic synchronicity that I am now a member." – KM

54. "It's good to have everything so well organized. Thank you." – WB

55. "Thanks you so much! Now I am really happy that there is someone whom I can ask my questions." – AK

56. "Thank you very much for that illuminating discourse on siddhasana and padmasana; my experience with these two asanas are fully in-tune with what you have described." – YM

57. "I would add a phrase often said by my own teacher – or rather one of my teachers – 'Without action, all is for not.' I have to say, I really like the look of this group. These posts are excellent and very pleasing to see ..." – ACK

58. "I have begun meditation practices this week and I have been voraciously absorbing your lessons. I have quickly caught up to message #39 – Pranayama. Thank you for providing this valuable knowledge, I look forward to developing my meditation practices with your guidance." – MN

59. "I've just started reading your lessons and I find them very supportive of the yoga practices I'm already enjoying. I can feel the energy and constructive vibrations coming from what you are sharing. No sooner did we ask for assistance, than we were introduced to your group. We truly appreciate the sharing of your path towards achieving that ultimate union with what we call Cosmic Consciousness. Understanding that no matter how much we may have already learned

and achieved, there is always room for more, a next step, in a manner of speaking. Once again, thank you for sharing." – EL

60. "First of all I'd like to say 'thank you' for this wonderful forum and the priceless wisdom you give so generously to everyone interested. I love everything about your teachings: Your writing style, clear, concise, without any fluffy new age slang, always making sense on a practical day-to-day basis but also depicting blissfully the heights human conscious can ascend to. And the contents: Priceless Wisdom. This resonates with the deepest parts of my being, showing me the way back to the most precious gift that exists in heaven or earth: 'Myself.' After practising since February 2004 "merely" meditation using the powerful mantra "Ayam" (*I AM*) I start feeling like being in love more and more of the time. I don't mean this in a metaphorical sense, it's exactly the feeling of being in love, this indescribable happiness from a cellular level upwards ... I'm running around in town, constantly with a big smile on my face, this happy feeling inside which is accompanied by an almost physical feeling of radiance from the inside out." – AY

61. "I am very happy, and I wish for great success for everything in your path. You definitely came across many traditions. Continue your service with God's Bliss!" – AK

62. "Even though I'm not familiar with your terminology, I grasp your explanations, and they are indeed profound. I understand now with a deeper appreciation why it is vital to transform or, as you say it, purify the central nervous system. Your spinal exercise, has helped me to be more focused in my intentions." – EL

63. "I heartily thank you for service you are devoting to all yoga enthusiasts by emailing the lessons regarding yoga discipline." – GK

64. "Thank you so much for providing all the info and encouragement. It is much-valued!" – MK

65. "That response (lesson #132) was just incredibly awesome! I've never heard sin put that way. It was beautiful and very encouraging. I always knew that guilt/sin was not an intention of God. We do it to ourselves and each other. Religions teach "the giving to get" idea, i.e., if I go to church every Sunday, I will get into heaven. I'm beginning to understand the importance of meditation. Why can't there be more teachers like you in the world? What a wonderful world it could be. You're just so gentle. Thank you for being here." – DW

66. "Thank you so much for sharing these valuable techniques. I'm very grateful for this seva. I am a yoga teacher of several styles, classical hatha, ashtanga, and raja yoga. All are the same meaning, different focus. I also teach prenatal and work with autistic children. The last two groups of students I feel would benefit immensely from these practices ... (very toned down, of course)" – BM

67. "Please accept my thanks for lively and helpful answers to the questions posed by sadhakas and it is very helpful for me in my sadhana." – CR

68. "Once again I want to thank you for the time and effort that you put into this discussion group. Your responses to others questions certainly put things in perspective and provide assurance. You must understand that I (and probably most) cannot just talk about these things in general. There are not many that would even attempt to understand this 'non-conventional' path." – LO

69. "This (chin pump) is just wonderful. I tried a couple of times the best to my understanding and it is indeed very powerful. Thank you for sharing such precious teachings." – MT

70. "I've read more of your notes and especially was grateful for your #69 on kundalini. So mine must have gone to the crown too soon. It is such a relief to be able to write this to someone who I do not know, who seems to Know. I can not tell anyone for fear of ego-attachment to their reaction. With you, I do not have this because you do not know me, or anyone related to me. Thank you." – ES

71. "I have been reading your mail for a short time and think it's great. I have been meditating, doing yoga, and such, for many years. I have done a lot of work with mantra, and had wonderful experiences. I like what you say so much, and have all the bits and pieces already, I would like to put it together the way you suggest. The Guru is within me ... and you." – DV

72. "Excellent article (on bhakti #67). Congratulations. To reach so many people with such wise words is wonderful. Every red light I stop at will now remind me of this. Hopefully this will be the case for many others as well. I have this vision of seeing a queue at a red light and everyone there topping up their meditation – well you never know." – LB

73. "Dude ... I love the yoga links section you added. Thanks for keeping control of what is placed there. It will be an excellent resource. Your time spent on this group is sooo appreciated. I just got lucky finding you." – DW

74. "Yours is a Great group ... It vibrates to the resonance of my own soul. I thank you from the bottom of my heart for helping me to clarify understand and remember the truth within. I'm sure you shall hear more from me as I progress in enlightenment and I desire to share some of my experiences." – JM

75. "Thank you for your views on sex. As I've mentioned before, the teachings I practice deal with attainment differently, yet in the end all paths towards the truth will be of great assistance if one will but apprehend their purport. I have read and now I review your posts daily, they are an inspirational reminder of the goal – my goal – towards conscious awakening." – EL

76. "I am very thankful for the response regarding spinal breathing." – GU

77. "I am a 21 year old male. I am a member of your yahoo group about Yoga and Tantra. I am deeply touched by your wisdom and insight reflected in the messages that you post on this group. I was surprised and happy to receive such a long and proper reply from you. Thank you

very much for replying to my mail. It was so nice of you to do that. You are a highly spiritually developed master and yet so humble. Hats off to you. God Bless you." – SP

78. "Have been practising 3-5 minutes of Bastrika after mediation for the last 2 days – wow! Could not sleep last night I was so charged after the practice. Will continue as is with the practices for a while with no further changes to see how stable I am in this routine ... Thank you for the reminder on Kerchari. After sending the e-mail I remembered the article (lesson #108) and have since re-read it. I have been at Stage 1, almost Stage 2, now for a couple of weeks and maintaining Kechari during the whole of my pranayama practice time." – BR

79. "Boy ... you come packed with a lot of information, don't you? You are like a concentrated pill of knowledge." – AS

80. "I want to thank you for your suggestion of spinal breathing! It is wonderful! I have regained the bliss I once had. Now, when I even think of it, the souls of my feet tingle and so does the base of my spine and third eye! I feel an inward laughter that is like a giddiness that spreads throughout my entire system and I want to squeal or giggle or dance about. I've been in this state when I was practicing kundalini yoga for hrs. every day, but I'm not putting as much into it this time and it's here ..." – ES

81. "Thanks for your immediate response to my problem. I will follow as said and I will mail you the change within me. thank you once again ..." – RA

82. "Thanks for your excellent way of giving the yoga lessons and clarifying the doubts of the participants in the group." – MV

83. "Thanks for all the time you put into this group – it's a real gold mine!" – IR

84. "I think that it is time for me to thank you for the time and energy and dedication to the work and wisdom you have made available through this medium. Words cannot do justice to express how thankful I am for the daily lectures and food for the soul. This last presentation on Samyama (#150) was so good. I am really lost for word to say thanks. These presentations are so helpful to me for my personal progress. Before these lectures I felt that I needed something more to keep me going on a daily basis – and I was offered to be part of this group. Thank you from the bottom of my heart. We are so blessed to have you, a gem, in our midst." – SS

85. "In working with the sutras (in samyama) I found my chest feel as if it was expanding, as well as my head. It was quite extraordinary. Is this normal? You spoke of the different ways of the energy manifesting and I was just wondering if this too is one of those manifestations? With love and unity." – MF

86. "I thank you very much for a great service you are doing. It is good work and please keep it up." – KR

87. "Thank you so very much for starting the group and all the advice that you have given. You've literally saved my life! I had a spontaneous awakening about 9 years ago and it has driven me crazy ... many times to such a deep depression that I contemplated suicide." – AM

88. "Your explanation of samyama is excellent." – VG

89. "I have recently joined advanced yoga practises. I am very grateful to you for imparting knowledge which I consider priceless." – RK

90. "I am passing on your article (on bhakti) to our web site. Will give you the URL as soon as they put it up. God bless. Incidentally, the piece on Kechari Mudra was superb. Thank you for being." – KW

91. "Your messages have helped my practises very much. Thanks for the guidance. My meditation has improved greatly after I joined this group ..." – AK

92. "Inspired by my practices following your lessons, my wife too has started meditating." – HR

93. "I have recently become a member of your Advanced Yoga Meditation group. I have been greatly inspired by its contents. So far I have been practicing simple meditation, on very low doses. Now I am willing to embark on a journey towards a higher level of spiritual living." – TO

94. "I would like to express my gratitude for the attention that you have given me, and more so for the grace with which you express these yoga teachings. You are doing great good, and helping many." – BR

95. "With a mind which is a little bit more silent now (with meditation), I still can perceive all the emotions the artist expresses in the music as well as my reactions, but besides all that I can listen on a more "analytical level". I'm hearing single notes instead of big clusters of emotional reactions. I also experienced an internal "visualization" of the parallel tunes – and, most surprising I discovered another tune in the tracks I had listened to so often before. The silence between the notes emerged like a very important new instrument I didn't perceive at all before. All those pieces had become more "airy", somehow "thinner" with lots of empty silent spaces in them ... very surprising and very interesting ... Mmmh ... I wonder how the world will look like if this musical experience kind of generalizes, more detachment more huge empty silent spaces everywhere around and maybe more creative joy in a universe which is much easier to move around and handle? Expecting change (and saying thank you for your continuous support)" – AY

96. "Thank you very much for giving the time to write such thorough replies. I greatly appreciate your willingness and dedication." – TO

97. "Many, many thanks for your kind clarifications, guidance and encouragement for daily Sadhana. Really, I am extremely grateful for your prompt, proper, and inner guidance for the advancement of this soul and I feel extremely indebted for the same. In the meanwhile I anxiously await for your further lesson on Spinal Bastrika." – RA

98. "I was really touched with the simple explanation you have offered on how individual meditation can help the entire humanity." – VS

99. "I've started reading your posts and I'm on my way to go through the whole board ... I like it!" – MJ

100. "I am practising meditation regularly. I experience inner silence. I would like to know more about inner silence, energy (that we actually are), and space and the relationship between them." – SK

101. "I'm still a greenhorn in all that yoga stuff – but I am aware of the tremendous irresistible power behind it. I'm very, very happy that I'm being fed it in small units I can easily digest. Probably I'll take up Pranayama this week or next. And I want to go all the way." – AY

102. "Today is my 10th day of meditation and in the evening as I was taking my walk I felt a different emotion. It wasn't joy or ecstasy or an impulse of pleasure. It was something deeper ... sublime ... deep ... like the memories of our childhood. Then for some time there was a lingering pain which gradually went away. Then the mind started to flow again with tremendous clarity and sharpness. I never had an experience like this and was extremely excited, and wanted to share this with someone." – NN

103. "I've practiced asanas for some 30 years and read a fair amount of yoga literature, but I've learned more about *progressing* in yoga since discovering this group 4 months ago than in the previous 30 years. You are being exceptionally generous with your time and providing an invaluable gift to all of us aspiring yogis." – SL

104. "The suggestions provided by you are really good. Please continue doing the same. It relieves a lot of mental stress just by the reading." – SD

105. "I am reading through your messages on your yahoo group and finding them very clear, informative and balanced. This is a very valuable inspiration for people taking up and maintaining their meditation practice. So thank you for the hard work you have put into this resource. I have forwarded the URL on your Yahoo group to over 1,800 people on my distribution list and I'm sure many of them will gain help from it."– DB

106. "I am very thankful to you for your valuable advice on pranayama and yoga." – DS

107. "Loved your lesson on paying it forward (#166)." – BR

108. "I shall tell my yoga students to check out the lessons if they want to deepen their meditation practice. Thank you for sharing these lessons in such an accessible and informed manner!" – BM

109. "I recently joined this magnificent group. It is a wonderful group for me because I have started doing yoga from 3 months before, and recently (15 days) I am also doing meditation so the importance for me for the group is endless." – SKC

110. "I have been practising meditation for nearly a month now. It gives me tremendous energy and peace." – NN

111. "I tend to agree with your opinion on not spoon feeding (yoga lessons) and allowing others to tune in on levels they are ready for themselves. I think your explanation on that has helped me even over the past few days on allowing others pick up information on various levels even if I would have previously assumed they were not ready for it ... so, thanks." – DB

112. "I have been reading about Kundalini for a few years, and have been interested from the start. The best and most moving account I read was by Gopi Krishna. Kundalini arousal in his case was probably not the norm, since it was quite traumatic and violent. I am very pleased at finding your group, where I can continue my studies. The number of postings you have personally done will alone keep me busy for a long time. Meditation will come soon." – PR

113. "The spinal breathing makes me feel so ecstatic that I want to do all the time (all things in moderation!). The lessons that you have been posting are so outstanding that I am tempted to ask – who are the teachers who have helped you and guided you? I know you have stated that this list not about you and you wish to remain anonymous, but I am intensely curious..." – YM

114. "Once again I find myself with a steady stream of tears after reading your lesson. Because of your group, for the first time I have access to grounded and tried perspectives on practices that my body has been intuitively seeking for the past few years. Seeing the Samyama practice laid out in front of me yielded the first objective look at the subjective experience I was having, and enjoying the most. The power of a practice grounded in objective knowledge and subjective experience is so powerful. It's also great to have one of the most pleasurable states I've encountered so far, the lightness of air, as well as the others too, devised, rather than stumbled upon. It's such an amazing level of vibration; the spaciousness, and the freedom to expand into the infinite with feeling of pure ecstasy. I know not to get caught up with experiences, you and others profess this enough, but the pleasure would certainly indicate movement in the right direction. Thank you so much for Being." – KL

115. "I have been member of this group for quite a long time and enjoy reading the postings immensely." – SU

116. "I am getting so much out of this group, your wisdom, and the practise. You have a gift for description and simplicity. I am college degreed professional who has lived such a stressful life

even though I have been practising yoga for over 10 years and now am a certified yoga teacher. I have tried meditation and breathing for some time, but to no avail until now. I am really starting to feel such an awakening and I love the way you explain everything, so simple, yet logical, yet so safe. I have been so ready for your teachings. I was starting to practice spinal breath on my own naturally and did not know why! " – RY

117.   "As much I am into being spiritual and doing yoga, etc., I always ask myself, 'why are we doing this, and where did this come from?' I have never been able to turn that voice off – even in meditation I have all the brain research about it and the effects. And, now, I am comfortable in it. That's your special gift and talent I see, appealing to those who will never have a guru, or follow a cult. I understand the *pay it forward* concept and want to share this with others. Part of me wonders if people are ready and the other part now thinks, why not? Just because it took me many years does not mean it has to take others the same." – TC

118.   "I do feel great doing the spinal breathing and yoni mudra ... They have really helped my practice! I feel like a new person." – CH

119.   "I am reading the previous posts and feeling the desire to return to yoga practice, and most especially meditation." – JS

120.   "I just wanted to tell you how glad I am you started this group. I will be the first person to admit how skeptical I was of Yoga. But after my very first meditation session, I have to admit that I have NEVER felt so relaxed. It was very strange, yet comfortable. The time flew by, my meditation lasted about 26 minutes and it seemed like 5 minutes. A few things did happen that I did not see mentioned in the lessons. I felt "tingly" and numb. I even had small visions if you want call them that, of light "dancing" and forming into small balls of light. Anyway, I just wanted to tell you how "At Peace" I feel with myself after my first lesson. I have a very stressful life and a lot of things that need to be 'flushed' out, and I will be continuing your lessons as long as it takes. I am smiling right now, something I have not done in I do not remember how long. Thank You! You have made me a believer." – JF

121.   "I have been practicing spinal breathing for several months now and have found it has added a valuable dimension to my asana practice." – LS

122.   "Thank you for permitting me membership in your yahoo group. I have been searching ... for something, and I think this may at the least be another step in the right direction. I just completed my first attempt at meditating using *I AM* and found it to be a very good experience. I feel refreshed, clearer, and certainly calmer. It was a good experience, and I am committing myself to this practice, and to continuing to explore your postings. Thank you for taking the time and effort to make your knowledge and this information available to us." – JM

123.   "I have been reading the articles present in this group from about a month or so ... Its really wonderful that I see people are experimenting and experiencing the Yoga practices and finding fruits for their practices." – RKB

124. "I continue to be amazed with your valuable contribution to society through this medium. Your explanations are so simple and so easily understood. You write with such ease and clarity – yet so profound! You amaze me with your knowledge and spirit of sharing your wisdom." – SS

125. "I admire your noble cause and effort because I have found that knowledge and information is surely kept hidden or released in fragments that sometimes it can be very discouraging. I also accept that we at our levels of awareness cannot question everything, but there should be some integration." – AV

126. "As a new member to the group, I first want to thank you for taking time to share this valuable information with those who are interested. I have not read through all the postings, but the postings I have read thus far, make perfect sense to me and 'feel' almost familiar to me in some strange way, yet much of it is completely new to me." – NW

127. "Thanks for your work in sharing your knowledge and experience. Your writings reflected just what I believe about life. The process of unfoldment is built-in and natural. We don't have to superimpose an intellectual system on it for validity. I do think it is obvious from the questions you get ... that yogites have scary experiences in their practice. The purification stuff is perfect to defuse the fear and the advice about going slow at a comfy pace ... that you don't have to act like the sale will end before you get there ... is wonderful. You as teacher here are truly a guide. Excellent." – BC

128. "As I Buddhist monk, a friend sent me some of your site dialogues, thinking that I would appreciate the sensibility. I must say I found much of your discussion group to be refreshing, direct, and simply profound. Is there any way I can find out more about the teachings, other books or web sites? With much appreciation." – RV

129. "The nectar you had referred to in one of the lessons is increasing day by day. Its flow is maximum when I am hungry and goes away when I have my food. I am enjoying it but am not fixated on it thanks to your lesson that scenery is only to be enjoyed but the focus should be the practice." – HR

130. "I greatly appreciate your attempt to assist me managing my way through the infinite capes of techniques, traditions, questions and wanderings." – TO

131. "Thanks a lot for the prompt reply. I really wonder how you find time to reply to each and every query made by people. I hope to become like you one day. I will definitely take it one step at a time. Thanks a lot again for the reply and for maintaining this wonderful group." – MH

132.   "Getting to know a wonderful yogi who loves to share the divine joy of wisdom! Do you have your web site yet? Love to know more about you as you do bring to words what I learnt in silence, and it is apt. All the blossom of divine inspiring joy!" – ND

133.   "Thanks for your opinions. I know I don't have enough meditation practice, but I didn't realize this was unbalancing my path. You have just pointed to where my practice is weak. I will focus more on deep meditation." – PD

134.   "Someone knowing my interest and the URL for Advanced Yoga Practices passed it on to me. I read one lesson, then another and then all of it. Having read Ramakrishna, Yogi Ramacharaka, Arthur Avalon, Rajneesh and anything in between, the subject was not new to me. What was new was a step by step method written in plain English with authority to help the seekers. I wish I had this kind of info when I started some 15 years back. I, having no real directions, mostly followed variations of Raja Yoga with concentrations on one or the other object. Thank you for the wisdom provided in your writings." – AD

135.   "I just read message #20 – from the atheist. I could not have said it better myself. I appreciate the way you make these concepts accessible to my Western-pragmatic-yet-mystic mind." – YB

136.   "Thank you so much for your lessons and the knowledge you are sharing with everyone ... I wrote to you sometime ago about my spontaneous awakening, and for the first time have been able to bring some 'order' to my life by concentrating on the spinal breathing and focusing on finding the peaceful place within." – AM

137.   "Thanks again for your lessons. A point of interest is that several times I have been on the verge of asking a question only to be answered by one of your Q&As before I had a chance to ask the question." – MC

138.   "Once one has experienced some levels of knowing and truth, when he hears the Truth, even through the filters of words, he instantly recognizes them. Such has been my experience with your presentations for the past few months. Thank you." – JM

139.   "My wife's sight has improved from using lenses of 2.75 to 2.5 since she has started meditation. She had to change her lenses. I can't stop from thinking that this incident and her practices are related. Does meditation help in correcting physical problems apart from cleansing the nervous system? Curious to know!" – HR

140.   "You most probably don't need confirmation on the information that you're sharing but I thought I'll let you know my personal experience as a confirmation anyway..." – AM

141.   "Since there are no accidents in the Universe I must thank you for the article on the crown chakra (#199). I choose smooth easeful transition into enlightened states of consciousness. Thank you for the reminder." – JM